O – oxygen
W – weight
E – electricity (Joules)
T – tracheal tube (ETT)
F – fluid bolus
L – lorazepam
A – adrenaline
G – glucose

Weight (kg) over 1 year = (age years + 4) × 2

ETT size (mm) over 1 year = (age years ÷ 4) + 4

ETT length cm = (Age ÷ 2) + 12 for an oral tube

ETT length cm = (Age ÷ 2) + 15 for nasal tube

4 Hs	4 Ts
Hypoxia	Tension pneumothorax
Hypovolaemia	Tamponade (cardiac)
Hypokalaemia/hyperkalaemia/hypocalcaemia	Toxins
Hypothermia	Thromboembolic

CHILDREN IN INTENSIVE CARE

For Mikey, Izzy, and Andy with love, JD

For Shelley, Sara, Shane, and Ian – inspiring mentors –
and Sean, Jenna, and Anthony who keep me smiling.
With love and thanks, MM

For Elsevier

Senior Content Strategist: Alison Taylor

Content Development Specialist: Veronika Watkins and Katie Golsby

Project Manager: Beula Christopher

Publishing Service Manager: Deepthi Unni

Designer: Amy Buxton

Illustration Manager: Amy Heyden

Third Edition

CHILDREN IN INTENSIVE CARE
A Survival Guide

Joanna H Davies BSC (HONS) MSC RGN RSCN ENB 415

Paediatric Retrieval Nurse Practitioner, Paediatric Intensive Care and South Thames Retrieval Service, Evelina London Children's Hospital, Guy's and St Thomas' NHS Foundation Trust, London

Marilyn McDougall MBCHB (UCT SA) DCH(SA) FCPAED (SA) MRCPCH

Paediatric Intensive Care and South Thames Retrieval Service Consultant, Honorary Clinical Senior Lecturer (Postgraduate teaching, Kings College London), Evelina London Children's Hospital, Guy's and St Thomas' NHS Foundation Trust, London

Foreword by

Sara Hanna MSC MRCPCH MB BCHIR (CANTAB)

Medical Director and Consultant in Paediatric Intensive Care, Evelina London Children's Hospital, Guy's and St Thomas' NHS Foundation Trust, London

ELSEVIER

Edinburgh   London   New York   Oxford   Philadelphia   St Louis   Sydney   Toronto 2019

ELSEVIER

First edition 2001
Second edition 2007
Third edition 2019
ISBN 978-0-7020-6744-0

Note

Knowledge and best practice in this field are constantly changing. As new research and experience broaden our understanding, changes in research methods, professional practices, or medical treatment may become necessary.

Practitioners and researchers must always rely on their own experience and knowledge in evaluating and using any information, methods, compounds, or experiments described herein. In using such information or methods they should be mindful of their own safety and the safety of others, including parties for whom they have a professional responsibility.

With respect to any drug or pharmaceutical products identified, readers are advised to check the most current information provided (i) on procedures featured or (ii) by the manufacturer of each product to be administered, to verify the recommended dose or formula, the method and duration of administration, and contraindications. It is the responsibility of practitioners, relying on their own experience and knowledge of their patients, to make diagnoses, to determine dosages and the best treatment for each individual patient, and to take all appropriate safety precautions.

To the fullest extent of the law, neither the Publisher nor the authors, contributors, or editors, assume any liability for any injury and/or damage to persons or property as a matter of products liability, negligence or otherwise, or from any use or operation of any methods, products, instructions, or ideas contained in the material herein.

Printed in China

Last digit is the print number: 9 8 7 6 5

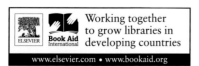

Working together
to grow libraries in
developing countries

www.elsevier.com • www.bookaid.org

The
Publisher's
policy is to use
**paper manufactured
from sustainable forests**

Fig. 1.2 Paediatric cardiac arrest algorithm. *CPR*, Cardiopulmonary resuscitation; *PEA*, pulseless electrical activity; *VF*, ventricular fibrillation; *VT*, ventricular tachycardia. (From Advanced Life Support Group, 2016. Advanced Paediatric Life Support. A Practical Approach to Emergencies, sixth ed. BMJ Books, Wiley and Sons, Chichester.)

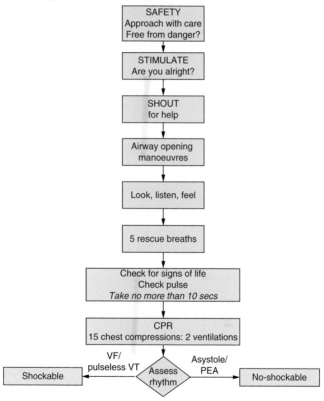

- Perform continuous CPR – establishing ventilation initially via bag/valve/mask with high flow oxygen
- If bag/mask ventilating – use 15 chest compressions to 2 ventilations for all ages, but intubate as soon as possible
- If patient intubated, use continuous chest compressions to a depth of at least one-third of the anteroposterior diameter of the chest
- Compression rate 100–120/min – ensure a cardiac monitor is attached and the rhythm assessed

Fig. 1.1 Paediatric basic life support – health care professionals with a duty to respond. *CPR*, Cardiopulmonary resuscitation. (From Advanced Life Support Group, 2016. Advanced Paediatric Life Support. A Practical Approach to Emergencies, sixth ed. BMJ Books, Wiley and Sons, Chichester.)

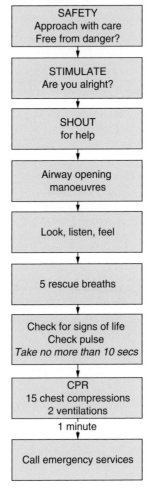

Table 1.1 Normal vital signs – normal values of heart rate, blood pressure, and respiratory rate				
Age of baby/ child	Heart rate (beats/min)	Blood pressure (mm Hg)		Respiratory rate (breaths/min)
		Systolic	Diastolic	
Newborn (3 kg)	100–180	50–70	25–45	30–60
Infant	100–160	85–105	55–65	30–60
Toddler	80–110	95–105	55–65	24–40
Preschool	70–110	95–110	55–65	22–34
School age	65–110	95–110	55–70	18–30
Adolescent	60–90	110–130	65–80	12–16

Source: Adapted from Hazinski, M.F. (Ed.), 1992. Nursing Care of the Critically Ill Child, second ed. Mosby Year Book, St. Louis, MO.

It is also helpful to note the patient's level of consciousness, position, pupil reaction, muscle tone, and urine output.

A quick guide for normal systolic blood pressure in a child 1 year or above

Median systolic blood pressure in children over 1 year of age: 80 mm Hg + (2 × age in years)

THE INITIAL APPROACH TO BASIC LIFE SUPPORT AND LIFE SUPPORT ALGORITHMS (ALSG 2016)

S: Safety – approach with care, free from danger?
S: Stimulate – are you alright?
S: Shout – for help.

Figs 1.1 and 1.2 represent algorithms that are recommended for basic life support and cardiac arrest. Fig. 1.3 is an algorithm for the management of asystole/pulseless electrical activity (PEA). Figs 1.4 and 1.5 represent electrocardiography (ECG) strips of asystole and PEA.

Nonshockable rhythm – asystole/pulseless electrical activity (See Fig. 1.3 for management) (ALSG 2016)

This is the most common arrest rhythm in children as prolonged hypoxia and acidosis lead to bradycardia and then asystole. Asystole appears as an almost flat line on ECG sometimes with occasional P waves (see Fig. 1.4), whereas PEA on an ECG will show recognisable complexes but without a palpable pulse and adequate cardiac output (see Fig. 1.5). PEA will lead to asystole without action. Check that the chest electrodes are still in place and that the ECG is still connected before commencing cardiopulmonary resuscitation (CPR).

ALL ABOUT RESUSCITATION

Recognition and prompt treatment of cardiorespiratory deterioration in children is a vital aspect of paediatric nursing in any environment, but it is particularly pertinent to paediatric intensive care. The airway–breathing–circulation (ABC) method of assessment can be used and children should be frequently reassessed as their condition may rapidly alter. Paediatric cardiorespiratory arrest most frequently occurs as a result of hypoxia, so oxygen delivery rather than defibrillation is often the critical step in life support (Advanced Life Support Group [ALSG] 2016).

CARDIOPULMONARY ASSESSMENT

A: Airway
B: Breathing
C: Circulation

Airway

- Assess patency,
- Assess ability to maintain independently with positioning and suction, or
- Assess need for adjuncts (e.g., rigid airway or endotracheal tube).

Breathing

Assess rate of breathing, depth, chest movement, air entry, the work of breathing, the use of accessory muscles, recession, nasal flaring, grunting, wheeze, stridor, and colour of patient.

Circulation

- Assess heart rate, blood pressure, central and peripheral pulses, skin perfusion, colour, mottling, capillary refill time, and temperature – central and peripheral.

Table 1.1 lists normal ranges of heart rate, blood pressure, and respiratory rates for each age group.

Pulse volume is related to pulse pressure, that is, the difference between the systolic and diastolic pressure. When there is decreased cardiac output, the pulse pressure narrows and pulses become weak.

ACKNOWLEDGEMENTS

Jayanthi Alamelu – Consultant Paediatric Haematologist, Evelina London Children's Hospital

Tom Breen – Consultant Paediatric Anaesthetist, St George's Hospital, London

Ruth Chalmers – Principal Allergy Dietician, Evelina London Children's Hospital

Steve Colthurst – Senior Respiratory Physiotherapist, PICU, Evelina London Children's Hospital

Matt Edwards – Doctor, Kent, Surrey and Sussex Air Ambulance

Juliet Gray – Associate Professor and Consultant Paediatric Oncologist, Southampton General Hospital

Joanna Gribben – Principal Metabolic Dietician, Evelina London Children's Hospital

Sophie Hallowes – Senior Paediatric Dietician, Evelina London Children's Hospital

Sarah Hardwick – Retrieval Nurse Practitioner PICU, Evelina London Children's Hospital

Julia Hopkins – Senior Specialist Paediatric Dietician, Evelina London Children's Hospital

Dawn Knight – Retrieval Nurse Practitioner PICU, Evelina London Children's Hospital

Mary-Anne Leung – Senior Specialist Dietician, Evelina London Children's Hospital

Fiona Lynch – Nurse Consultant, PICU, Evelina London Children's Hospital

Ellie Melkuhn – Specialist Respiratory Physiotherapist, PICU, Evelina London Children's Hospital

Emma Morton – Retrieval Nurse Practitioner and Ward sister PICU, Evelina London Children's Hospital

Jo Perkins – Consultant Paediatric Anaesthetist, Evelina London Children's Hospital

Shelley Riphagen – Consultant Paediatric Intensivist, Evelina London Children's Hospital

Will Thornhill – Paediatric Pharmacist, Evelina London Children's Hospital

We would like to thank all our friends and colleagues in PICU at The Evelina London Children's Hospital who have supported, inspired, and guided us.

PREFACE

Much has changed in paediatric intensive care in the last decade which has inspired new sections and extensive updates in this third edition. The two new chapters are Oncology Emergencies and Pain and Sedation, which provide a broader perspective for those caring for children in intensive care. The cardiac chapter has been comprehensively expanded with new surgical approaches, and inclusion of practical tips on pacing, care of chest drains, and basic echocardiograph terminology. The expanded Handy Hints chapter now provides guidance on sepsis, the collapsed neonate, care of children after spinal surgery; and the drug chapter includes reversal agents, new drug profiles, and an updated compatibilities chart.

It is always tempting to keep writing, but the premise of this book was a pocket-sized guide not a huge text book. It is supposed to be useful at the bedside as a quick reference which also stimulates a thirst for extra knowledge as experience is increased.

This edition provides a new perspective with the additional expertise of a Senior Paediatric Intensive Care Consultant. The combined doctor/nurse approach provides valuable insights and nuggets of practical bedside knowledge that have been acquired through decades of caring for children in intensive care. As always, we have asked experts and referenced national and international evidence, but drugs, dosages, and therapies change rapidly. We carefully tried to avoid any errors but no book is perfect so please do cross-reference local advice, guidelines, and up-to-date evidence.

We have been guided and supported by colleagues from the wider Paediatric Intensive Care community, listened to feedback, and tried to address any areas where we felt more information was needed. We are very grateful for any feedback.

Joanna H. Davies
Marilyn McDougall

FOREWORD

More than 20,000 children are admitted to paediatric intensive care (PICU) in the United Kingdom each year with survival rate in excess of 96% (PICANET report 2016). Centralisation of services, advances in technology and surgical expertise have contributed to the improved survival. However, the speciality remains a clinical one where the clinician is faced with a set of symptoms, signs and investigations in need of distillation. There is also often a degree of time pressure in making a diagnosis and plan which can add to the pressure experienced by the less experienced doctor or nurse. Despite the technological advances, children do not present with a label. We still need to be able to apply the knowledge gained from textbooks and the scientific literature with experience to 'see the wood for the trees' to provide timely and appropriate management of a critically ill child. This handbook, which fits comfortably into a pocket, provides useful tips to negotiate some of the practical challenges, jargon and technology of the intensive care unit. The handbook is not designed to replace traditional textbooks or university courses but rather to supplement those with 'nuggets' gained from years of collective experience of the multidisciplinary teams working in The Evelina London.

The third update of the handbook has maintained the successful formula of previous editions combining concise information with useful drawings, tables and graphs. The latest version has expanded cardiac, respiratory and neurology sections focusing on common and important conditions which are the leading causes of admission to intensive care. There are also two new chapters and an expanded chapter on 'syndromes' which explains some of the more common genetic conditions highlighting the characteristics of children with these conditions that may impact on their requirement for and clinical course on PICU. Key tips are included in the safeguarding, nutrition and pain and sedation chapters to remind us, lest we forget, that the child we are looking after is not a collection of comorbidities but a whole person within their family whose overall wellbeing is our primary concern. There are also some practical insights to help reduce the anxiety of managing the death of a child in PICU and transportation of critically ill children.

The authors intended this book to become a regularly used pocketbook that can ease the stress of working in PICU. This little book not only provides helpful tips but also captures the essence of caring for children that can only be gained from years of experience. It is hoped that this book will be a useful starting point for those who intend to pursue the ultimately rewarding, ever-challenging career provided by PICU.

CONTENTS

Fig. 1.6 Protocol for management of ventricular fibrillation/pulseless ventricular tachycardia. *CPR*, Cardiopulmonary resuscitation; *DC*, direct cardioverison; *IO*, intraosseous; *IV*, intravenous; *ROSC*, return of spontaneous circulation. (From Advanced Life Support Group, 2016. Advanced Paediatric Life Support. A Practical Approach to Emergencies, sixth ed. BMJ Books, Wiley and Sons, Chichester.)

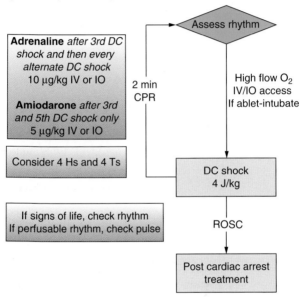

- Continue CPR for 2 minutes; the chest compression rate for all ages is 100–120/min. In all children, a ratio of 15 compressions to 2 ventilations should be used
- Pause briefly to check monitor and if still VF/pulseless VT, give a **third shock** at 4 J/kg, resume CPR, then give adrenaline 10 μg/kg (0.1 mL/kg of 1:10 000) and amiodarone 5 mg/kg IV or IO
- After 2 minutes of CPR, pause briefly to check monitor and if still VF/pulseless VT, give an immediate **fourth shock** at 4 J/kg
- Continue with a further 2 minutes of CPR, pause briefly to check the monitor and if still in a shockable rhythm, give an immediate **fifth shock** at 4 J/kg; resume CPR then give a second dose of adrenaline 10 μg/kg and a second dose of amiodarone 5 mg/kg IV or IO. Continue giving shocks every 2 minutes, minimising pauses in CPR – but briefly check the monitor after each 2 minutes of CPR to assess rhythm; if rhythm changes on ECG then continue to treat according to the changed rhythm protocol
- Give adrenaline 10 μg/kg after every alternate shock until ROSC

Fig. 1.7 Electrocardiography strip showing ventricular fibrillation.

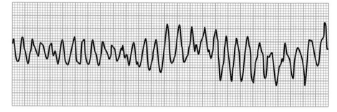

Fig. 1.8 Electrocardiography strip showing pulseless ventricular tachycardia.

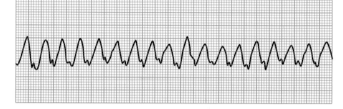

EARLY TREATMENT OF VENTRICULAR TACHYCARDIA (WITH PULSE) ALGORITHM (ALSG 2016)

- Early consultation with paediatric cardiologist (Fig. 1.9)
- May suggest use of amiodarone (5 mg/kg over 20 minutes or 30 minutes in neonates) or procainamide (15 mg/kg over 30–60 minutes) – both can cause hypotension, which should be treated with volume expansion
- If the child is cardiovascularly unstable, then synchronised cardioversion starting at 2 J/kg is the recommended treatment
- Where VT has been caused by drug toxicity, sedation and anaesthesia, DC shock may be the safest approach; use synchronised shocks initially as these are less likely to produce VF but, if they are ineffectual, subsequent attempts will have to be asynchronous if the child is in shock
- Look at ECG for signs of torsades de pointes (polymorphic VT with QRS complexes that change in amplitude and polarity and appear to rotate around an isoelectric line). The treatment for this is emergency defibrillation, followed by magnesium sulphate by rapid IV infusion (25–50 mg/kg [maximum 2 g] over several minutes)
- Check serum potassium, calcium, and magnesium levels.

Resuscitation drug doses – cardiac arrest

- Adrenaline 10 µg/kg (0.1 mL/kg of 1:10 000) via IV or IO route (maximum dose is 10 mL of 1:10 000) every 4 minutes if required in an arrest situation

Fig. 1.3 Protocol for management of asystole/pulseless electrical activity. *CPR,* Cardiopulmonary resuscitation; *IO,* intraosseous; *IV,* intravenous; *ROSC,* return of spontaneous circulation. (From Advanced Life Support Group, 2016. Advanced Paediatric Life Support. A Practical Approach to Emergencies, sixth ed. BMJ Books, Wiley and Sons, Chichester.)

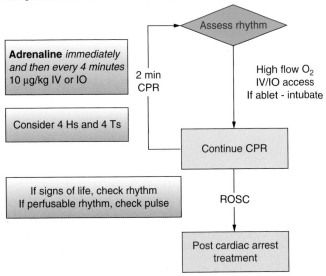

Fig. 1.4 Electrocardiography strip showing asystole.

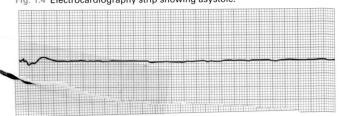

- Give adrenaline (epinephrine) 10 μg/kg (0.1 mL/kg of 1:10 000 adrenaline) every 4 minutes (maximum single dose is 10 mL of 1:10 000 [1 mg])
- Consider and correct reversible causes **(4 Hs and 4 Ts).**
  Causes of PEA include 4 Hs and 4 Ts:
- Hypoxia
- Hypovolaemia

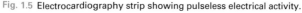
Fig. 1.5 Electrocardiography strip showing pulseless electrical activity.

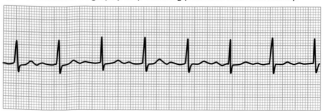

- Hypothermia
- Hyperkalaemia/hypokalaemia, hypocalcaemia
- Tamponade
- Tension pneumothorax
- Thromboembolism
- Toxicity – that is, drug overdose (commonly tricyclic antidepressants)

The underlying cause of PEA must be sought, but PEA should be treated and managed like asystole until the specific cause has been identified and treated.

- Every 2 minutes, briefly pause chest compressions and check the monitor to assess rhythm. If there is no pulse and no signs of life, continue resuscitation until deemed futile by the resuscitation team (usually if there is no return of spontaneous circulation [ROSC] following at least 20 minutes of CPR – but there is no single predictor for when to stop resuscitation, and expert help should be sought in patients with a history of poisoning or a primary hypothermic insult where prolonged resuscitation may occasionally be successful). If there is an ROSC, continue postresuscitation care.

Shockable rhythm (ventricular fibrillation/pulseless ventricular tachycardia)

Fig. 1.6 provides protocol for management (ALSG 2016).

- Assess rhythm (Figs 1.7 and 1.8 for ECGs showing ventricular fibrillation [VF] and pulseless ventricular tachycardia [VT], respectively), give high flow oxygen, simultaneously gain intravenous/intraosseous (IV/IO) access and intubate, proceed to defibrillation without delay if VF or pulseless VT
- Give **shock** of 4 J/kg then immediately resume CPR starting with chest compressions without reassessing rhythm or feeling for a pulse
- Continue CPR for 2 minutes
- Pause briefly to check monitor and if still VF/pulseless VT, give **second shock** at 4 J/kg
- Resume CPR immediately after second shock. Consider and correct reversible causes (4 Hs and 4 Ts)

Fig. 1.9 Algorithm for the management of ventricular tachycardia with pulse. *VF*, Ventricular fibrillation. (From Advanced Life Support Group, 2016. Advanced Paediatric Life Support. A Practical Approach to Emergencies, sixth ed. BMJ Books, Wiley and Sons, Chichester.)

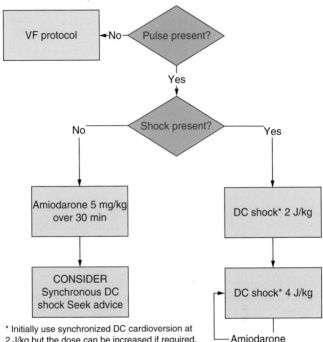

* Initially use synchronized DC cardioversion at 2 J/kg but the dose can be increased if required.

Adrenaline will increase aortic diastolic pressure, increase coronary and cerebral perfusion pressure, and enhance the contractions of the heart through α-adrenergic-mediated vasoconstriction. Subsequent doses of adrenaline will be the same and should be given every 4 minutes. The use of a higher dose of adrenaline via the IV or IO route is not recommended in children as this may worsen the outcome (Enright et al 2012).

Adrenaline can be given via the tracheal tube route at 10 times the IV dose (100 μg/kg) but its effects are not convincing and therefore is it not recommended (ALSG 2016).

- Sodium bicarbonate 8.4% 1 mL/kg

This may be indicated if profound acidosis persists during an arrest situation, but beware as this will increase intracellular carbon dioxide levels so the patient should be receiving assisted ventilation. Sodium bicarbonate is recommended in the treatment of hyperkalaemia and tricyclic antidepressant overdose.

Sodium bicarbonate inactivates adrenaline and dopamine so the IV line should be flushed well after use. Bicarbonate cannot be given via the endotracheal route. Bicarbonate cannot be given via the same IV line as calcium as precipitation will occur.

- **Atropine** 10–20 µg/kg (minimum dose 100 µg to prevent paradoxical bradycardia and maximum dose of 600 µg) is no longer recommended except in a patient who has developed bradycardia from vagal stimulation
- **Calcium gluconate 10%** (0.5 mL/kg maximum 20 mL) is no longer recommended in the treatment of PEA and asystole. However, it is indicated in documented hypocalcaemias, in hyperkalaemia, and in the treatment of hypermagnesaemia and calcium channel overdose.

Emergency antiarrhythmic drugs

- Amiodarone 5 mg/kg diluted to 4 mL/kg with 5% dextrose given over 30 min, IV or IO for shock-resistant VF and pulseless VT. Use central vein if access available or a large peripheral vein (ALSG 2016). Amiodarone is INCOMPATIBLE with normal saline, so do not use this for dilution.
- Adenosine initially:

  Neonate 150 µg/kg, increasing dose if required by 50–100 µg/kg until tachycardia terminated or maximum dose of 300 µg/kg reached (ALSG 2016).

  1 month–1 year 150 µg/kg increasing dose if required by 50–100 µg/kg every 1–2 minutes until tachycardia terminated or up to a maximum single dose of 500 µg/kg (maximum dose 12 mg) (ALSG 2016).

  1–12 years 100 µg/kg increasing dose if required by 50–100 µg/kg every 1–2 minutes until tachycardia terminated or up to a maximum single dose of 500 µg/kg (maximum dose 12 mg) (ALSG 2016).

  12–18 years Initially 3 mg, followed by 6 mg after 1–2 minutes and if still required 12 mg after a further 1–2 minutes (ALSG 2016).

- Adenosine should be given as a fast IV bolus through a large peripheral or central vein and followed immediately by a rapid saline flush for the treatment of supraventricular tachycardia (SVT) resistant to vagal manoeuvres in patients who are not in shock (ALSG 2016). If the patient is in shock, then synchronised cardioversion should be considered.
- Magnesium 25–50 mg/kg (to maximum of 2 g) IV infusion over several minutes. It is indicated in documented hypomagnesemia or torsade de pointes (ALSG 2016).
- Procainamide loading dose is 15 mg/kg IV given slowly over 30–60 minutes with ECG and BP monitoring. Stop the infusion if QRS widens or hypotension occurs (ALSG 2016).
- Lidocaine (lignocaine) 1% 1 mg/kg (maximum dose 100 mg) may be considered in VF or VT but is only recommended when amiodarone is unavailable.

In emergencies, it is often difficult but essential to establish IV access in infants and children; IO access is a very effective alternative.

INTRAOSSEOUS ACCESS

IO access uses the vascular network in long bones to transport fluids or drugs from the medullary cavity into the circulation.

Sites for IO infusions include the proximal tibia, the medial malleolus, and the distal femur; in postpuberty the humerus has been used.

Advantages of intraosseous access

- Quick, safe, and easy to insert
- Medication can be given in the same dose as the IV route.
- Absorption time has been found to be as effective as IV injections in maintaining drug levels.

Contraindications

Not recommended for use:
- on recently fractured bones
- on the same bone as a previous IO insertion attempt
- in osteogenesis imperfecta

Guidelines on the insertion of an intraosseous needle in the proximal tibia

- Use universal precautions.
- Immobilise limb and paint with antiseptic – use a towel to support the leg.
- Use local anaesthetic down to the periosteum if required, that is, if the patient is conscious.
- Use landmarks to assess the correct placement and select the correct sized needle according to weight, anatomy, and tissue depth
- Palpate tibial tuberosity and grasp the medial aspect of the tibia with the thumb – the optimal site of insertion is halfway between these points and 1–2 cm distal (Spivey 1987).
- The needle is inserted perpendicular to the bone at a 15- to 30-degree angle toward the foot; that is, away from the epiphyseal plate.
- Apply downward pressure in a boring motion until a 'pop' is heard and resistance suddenly decreases, indicating that the needle has entered the medullary cavity, or if using the EZ-IO drill, insert the needle into the skin until you reach hard bone; hold at 90 degrees to the skin, then use the drill to enter the bone until there is a loss of resistance (indicating that it has entered the cortex).
- The needle should stand up without support.
- Penetration from the skin through the cortex is around 1 cm in an infant or child.
- Remove inner stylet; bone marrow content (like blood) should be aspirated to confirm needle placement. If using the EZ-IO, attach the stabilisation device before attaching the primed connection tubing.

- A transparent dressing may be placed around the entry site.
- Medication must be administered under pressure and then flushed well. Complications include needle clotting, extravasation and, rarely, infection. If fluid is seen to be entering surrounding tissues, stop the infusion immediately, remove the needle, and apply pressure to the site. An intraosseous needle can remain in place until other intravascular access is obtained.

 NB In a conscious patient, pain associated with IO infusion under pressure is severe (Fowler 2007).

Sinus tachycardia or supraventricular tachycardia (ALSG 2016)

- Sinus tachycardia is typically characterised by a heart rate of less than 200 bpm in infants and children, whereas infants with SVT usually have a heart rate greater than 220 bpm.
- P waves may be difficult to identify in both sinus tachycardia and SVT once the ventricular rate exceeds 200 bpm. If P waves are identifiable, they are usually upright in leads I and AVF in sinus tachycardia while they are negative in leads II, III, and AVF in SVT.
- In sinus tachycardia, the heart rate varies from beat to beat and is often responsive to stimulation, but there is no beat-to-beat variability in SVT.
- Termination of SVT is abrupt, whereas the heart rate gradually slows in sinus tachycardia in response to treatment.
- A history consistent with shock (e.g., gastroenteritis or septicaemia) is usually present with sinus tachycardia.

Vagal manoeuvres

These include:
- Application of a rubber glove filled with iced water over the patient's face – or wrapping the infant in towel and immersing its face in iced water for 5 seconds
- One-sided carotid sinus massage
- Valsalva manoeuvre, for example, blowing hard through a straw
- **Do not use ocular pressure in infants or children** as it may cause damage
- If SVT persists, Fig. 1.10 provides an algorithm for the management of SVT.

USE OF THE DEFIBRILLATOR

The defibrillator can be used both for defibrillation and for synchronised cardioversion. All oxygen should be removed from the area before using the defibrillator.

Fig. 1.10 Algorithm for the management of supraventricular tachycardia. (From Advanced Life Support Group, 2016. Advanced Paediatric Life Support. A Practical Approach to Emergencies, sixth ed. BMJ Books, Wiley and Sons, Chichester.)

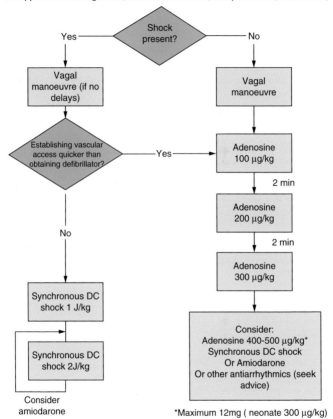

Defibrillation

- Is the definitive treatment for VF or pulseless VT
- Is the passage of an electrical current through the heart
- Is an asynchronous depolarisation of a critical mass of myocardial cells to allow spontaneous reorganised myocardial depolarisation to resume.

 When using a manual defibrillator, the shock energy for defibrillation in children is 4 J/kg for all shocks (ALSG 2016).

Automated external defibrillators

- A standard automated external defibrillator (AED) can be used for all children over 8 years.
- Purpose-made pads or programmes that attenuate the energy output of AED are recommended for children between 1 and 8 years.
- If no such system or manually adjusted machine is available, an unmodified machine may be used for children over 1 year.
- There is insufficient evidence to support a recommendation for or against the use of AEDs in children less than 1 year old. ALSG 2016.

Synchronised cardioversion

- Is the treatment of choice in patients who have tachyarrhythmias (e.g., SVT, VT with palpable pulses, atrial fibrillation, and atrial flutter) who are haemodynamically unstable (ALSG 2016)
- Results in depolarisation of the myocardium but provides depolarisation that is timed with the patient's own intrinsic electrical activity (on the R wave of the QRS complex).

Select synchronised function on defibrillator prior to each shock delivered.

Initial dose: 1 J/kg

A subsequent dose can be increased if required (ALSG 2016).

The discharge buttons on the paddles must be pressed and held for several QRS complexes when cardioverting.

Choice of pads or paddle

- Infant paddles or pads: 4.5 cm, should be used for infants up to 1 year of age or up to 10 kg in weight
- Adult paddles or pads: 8–13 cm, should be used in patients older than 1 year of age and more than 10 kg in weight

Defibrillation pads

Defibrillation pads are recommended for use rather than electrode gel or KY jelly.

Electrode paddles should be placed so that the heart is in between them. Anterior to posterior electrode and pad position is superior but difficult. Normally, one pad is placed on the upper right chest below the clavicle and the other to the left of the left nipple in the anterior axillary line. Fig. 1.11 shows correct anterolateral pad placement for defibrillation in children; Fig. 1.12 shows correct anteroposterior pad placement for infants.

SHOCK

Shock is defined as inadequate delivery of oxygen and metabolic substrates to meet the metabolic demands of the tissues, which results in

Fig. 1.11 Correct pad placement for defibrillation – anterolateral in children. (From Advanced Life Support Group, 2016. Advanced Paediatric Life Support. A Practical Approach to Emergencies, sixth ed. BMJ Books, Wiley and Sons, Chichester.)

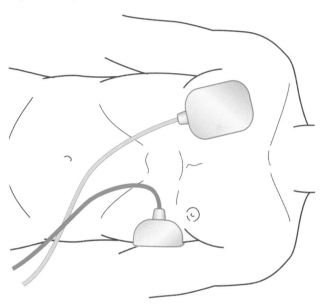

inadequate organ and tissue perfusion. This, in turn, can lead to anaerobic metabolism, lactic acidosis, multisystem organ failure, and death.

Usually, shock is associated with low cardiac output, but in early septic shock there may be a high-output state with bounding pulses. At this stage, there is low systemic vascular resistance and increased blood flow to the skin, but there may be a mismatch in distribution of blood flow to the tissues. This can result in tissue hypoxia and eventually a lactic acidosis.

In shock with a low cardiac output there is an increased sympathetic drive raising the systemic vascular resistance, maintaining the blood pressure and hence perfusion. This diverts blood flow away from nonessential areas (e.g., skin and gut) to increase flow to essential areas (e.g., brain and heart). Clinically, a patient in this state will appear pale, feel cool to the touch, and have poor peripheral perfusion (American Heart Association 1997).

Shock may be:

- hypovolaemic
- cardiogenic

Fig. 1.12 Correct pad placement for defibrillation anteroposterior in infants. (A) Pad on the back of the patient. (B) Pad placed on the front of the patient's chest. (From Advanced Life Support Group, 2016. Advanced Paediatric Life Support. A Practical Approach to Emergencies, sixth ed. BMJ Books, Wiley and Sons, Chichester.)

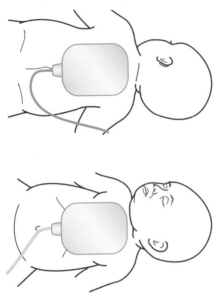

- septic
- neurogenic
- anaphylactic

A child in shock will require cardiovascular support with fluid resuscitation and/or inotropic support.

It is useful to classify shock as either compensated or decompensated. Table 1.2 lists the classification of haemorrhagic shock.

Compensated shock

(↓ cardiac output, normal blood pressure and ↑ systemic vascular resistance index)

The child will have a tachycardia and signs of poor peripheral perfusion (e.g., increased capillary refill time) but will have normal blood pressure at this stage. The child may have a normal level of consciousness but some signs of inadequate tissue perfusion may become apparent (e.g., increasing lactic acidosis).

Table 1.2 Classification of haemorrhagic shock: the effect on five systems

Degree of shock	I: Very mild – haemorrhage, <15% blood volume loss	II: Mild – haemorrhage, 15–25% blood volume loss	III: Moderate – haemorrhage, 26–39% blood volume loss	IV: Severe – haemorrhage, >40% blood volume loss
Cardiovascular	Heart rate normal or mildly raised, normal pulses, normal blood pressure	Tachycardia, peripheral pulses may be diminished, normal blood pressure	Significant tachycardia, thready peripheral pulses, hypotension	Severe tachycardia, thready central pulses, significant hypotension
Respiratory	Normal pH, rate normal	Normal pH, tachypnoea	Metabolic acidosis, moderate tachypnoea	Significant acidosis, severe tachypnoea
Central nervous system	Slightly anxious	Irritable, confused, combative	Irritable or lethargic, diminished pain response	Lethargic, coma
Skin	Warm, pink, capillary refill time brisk (<2 s)	Cool extremities, mottling, delayed capillary refill time (>2 s)	Cool extremities, mottling or pallor, prolonged capillary refill time	Cool extremities, pallor or cyanosis
Kidneys	Normal urine output	Oliguria, increased specific gravity	Oliguria, increased urea	Anuria

Source: Modified from American College of Surgeons, 1989. Advanced Trauma Life Support Course. American College of Surgeons, Chicago, IL and as cited in Hazinski, M.F. (Ed.), 1992. Nursing Care of the Critically Ill Child, second ed. Mosby Year Book, St. Louis, MO and Fleisher, G.R., Ludwig, S., 1988. Textbook of Pediatric Emergency Medicine, second ed. Williams & Wilkins, Baltimore, MD. © Lippincott Williams & Wilkins, reproduced with permission.

Decompensated shock

(↓ cardiac output, ↓ blood pressure as ↑ systemic vascular resistance index is no longer able to compensate)

The child will now be hypotensive with weak or absent central pulses and will have an increasing metabolic acidosis, increased capillary refill, a decreased urine output, and an altered level of consciousness, which is reflective of poor end-organ perfusion. This child will need immediate resuscitation as cardiopulmonary arrest will occur if no treatment is given.

Management of shock

- 100% oxygen
- Assess airway and breathing, using adjuncts as necessary
- Establish vascular access – intravenous or intraosseous if necessary
- Use volume expanders and inotropic drugs as required
- Monitor closely

USEFUL MNEMONICS

Quick assessment tool for measuring responsiveness is AVPU:

A: awake
V: voice
P: pain
U: unresponsive

(American Heart Association 1997)

Assessment tool: **ABCDEFG**

A: airway
B: breathing
C: circulation
D: don't
E: ever
F: forget
G: glucose – particularly in the fitting child

Common postresuscitation airway complications: **DOPE**

D: displacement of endotracheal tube
O: obstruction of endotracheal tube
P: pneumothorax
E: equipment failure

Drugs that can be given via endotracheal tube: **LEAN**

L: lidocaine (lignocaine)
E: epinephrine (adrenaline)
A: atropine
N: naloxone

NEWBORN RESUSCITATION

Paediatric intensive care nurses are not often required to resuscitate newborn infants but do need to know the principles if required to do so. Fig. 1.13 provides the algorithm for newborn life support (Resuscitation Council (UK) 2015). Additional guidance from the Resuscitation Council (2015):

- Delay cord clamping for at least 1 minute if the term or preterm baby is not compromised (Wyllie et al 2015).

Fig. 1.13 Algorithm: newborn life support. *ECG*, Electrocardiography. (Reproduced with the kind permission of the Resuscitation Council (UK))

Newborn Life Support

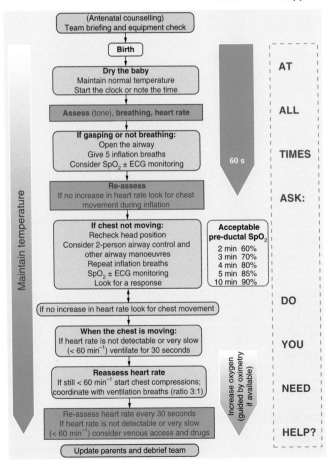

(Antenatal counselling)
Team briefing and equipment check

Birth

Dry the baby
Maintain normal temperature
Start the clock or note the time

Assess (tone), breathing, heart rate

If gasping or not breathing:
Open the airway
Give 5 inflation breaths
Consider SpO$_2$ ± ECG monitoring

Re-assess
If no increase in heart rate look for chest movement during inflation

If chest not moving:
Recheck head position
Consider 2-person airway control and other airway manoeuvres
Repeat inflation breaths
SpO$_2$ ± ECG monitoring
Look for a response

Acceptable pre-ductal SpO$_2$
2 min 60%
3 min 70%
4 min 80%
5 min 85%
10 min 90%

If no increase in heart rate look for chest movement

When the chest is moving:
If heart rate is not detectable or very slow (< 60 min^{-1}) ventilate for 30 seconds

Reassess heart rate
If still < 60 min^{-1} start chest compressions; coordinate with ventilation breaths (ratio 3:1)

Re-assess heart rate every 30 seconds
If heart rate is not detectable or very slow (< 60 min^{-1}) consider venous access and drugs

Update parents and debrief team

60 s

AT

ALL

TIMES

ASK:

DO

YOU

NEED

HELP?

Maintain temperature

Increase oxygen (guided by oximetry if available)

MANAGEMENT OF A BLOCKED TRACHEOSTOMY

Infants and children with established tracheostomies will have a well-formed stoma track and it should be straightforward to change a blocked tracheostomy tube if you are unable to suction down the tube to clear it. If the tracheostomy is recent, the stoma site will appear small when the blocked tracheostomy tube is removed and it may be difficult to pass a new trachy tube through the stoma, as occasionally a blind-end false track may be created. Remember to position the child, and using a rolled towel under their shoulders may help to expose the tracheostomy site.

When caring for an infant or child with a tracheostomy, it is important to know whether the child has a patent or partially patent upper airway so that if the tracheostomy becomes blocked and you are unable to replace the tracheostomy tube, you may be able to give rescue breaths via the mouth with a bag or valve mask, but if the upper airway is not patent, these rescue breaths must be delivered via the stoma. This information should be easily visible at the child's bed space (Fig. 1.14 provides an example of daily checklist/plan that should be immediately available at the bed space in case of emergency. Fig. 1.15 lists the equipment required for an emergency tracheostomy change. Fig. 1.16 outlines the steps required to manage a blocked tracheostomy tube.).

NEEDLE THORACOCENTESIS

This may be a life-saving procedure with a tension pneumothorax and should precede chest drain placement.

Information taken from Advanced Paediatric Life Support (ALSG 2016):

Absolute minimum equipment required: alcohol swabs, large over-the-needle intravenous cannula (16 gauge or commercially available product), 20-mL syringe

Procedure:
- Identify the second intercostal space in the midclavicular line on the side of the pneumothorax.
- Swab the chest wall with surgical preparation solution or an alcohol swab.
- Attach the syringe to the cannula. Fluid in the cannula will assist in the identification of air bubbles.
- Insert the cannula vertically into the chest wall, just above the rib below, aspirating all the time (Fig. 1.17).
- If air is aspirated remove the needle leaving the plastic cannula in place.
- Tape the cannula in place and proceed to chest drain insertion as soon as possible.

MANAGEMENT OF ANAPHYLAXIS

Anaphylaxis is a severe, life-threatening allergic reaction that all nursing and medical staff should know how to treat. A child may present to hospital with an anaphylactic reaction to food products, bee stings, drugs, etc.

Fig. 1.14 Tracheostomy care: daily checklist and plan.

Patient Name
Patient Number
Date of Birth
(or affix patient label)

PICU Tracheostomy Care: Daily Checklist and Plan

Complete on admission and display clearly at bedspace for duration of ICU stay

Date of trachy:	_____	
Size / type of trachy tube (ie Neo or Paed)	_____	
Depth of suction to trachy tip (cm)	_____	
Suction catheter Size (Fr)	_____	
Stay Sutures in-situ	Yes ☐ No ☐	
Date 1st planned trachy change	_____	
X-ray seen post-tracheostomy	Yes ☐ No ☐	
Face mask bagging /orotracheal intubation contraindicated? (occlusive laryeal/subglottic obstruction such as silicone stent/ granulations)	Yes ☐ No ☐	*NB: Must ventilate through trachy stoma!*
Wired tracheal stent presnt (eg.Palmaz)	Yes ☐ No ☐	Risk of granulomas on deep suctioning
Grade of laryngoscopy (circle)	I II III IV	

Daily equipment check list

The following must be at the bedside and visible at all times:

☐ Tracheostomy tubes of same size and type and one size smaller available

☐ Tracheostomy dilators clearly labelled

☐ Trachy Tapes appropriate for patient size

☐ Scissors

Admitting nurse name:	Signature:	Date:
Admitting doctors name:	Signature:	Date:

Fig. 1.15 Emergency equipment required for tracheostomy tube change. (From Advanced Life Support Group, 2016. Advanced Paediatric Life Support. A Practical Approach to Emergencies, sixth ed. BMJ Books, Wiley and Sons, Chichester.)

- Usual size tracheostomy tube with tapes attached
- Half size smaller tracheostomy tube with tapes attached
- Suction catheter of appropriate size
- Resuscitation trolley: self-inflating bag and face masks, oxygen sources, simple airway adjuncts such as oropharyngeal airways, nasopharyngeal airways and laryngeal mask airways
- Scissors
- Spare tape
- Gauze swab
- Gloves

In hospital, however, anaphylaxis may be caused by latex, blood products, colloids, radiocontrast media, or drugs (Ryder & Waldmann 2003). A spectrum of reactions may occur from minor clinical changes to acute cardiovascular collapse and death. A child may present with several of the signs and these may include:

- hypotension
- bradycardia
- tachycardia
- dysrhythmias
- cardiac arrest
- bronchospasm
- laryngeal obstruction
- periorbital oedema
- generalised oedema
- rash
- urticarial
- nausea, vomiting
- diarrhoea
- hoarseness, dry cough
- sneezing
- shortness of breath
- metallic taste in mouth
- chest tightness
- flushing
- feeling faint
- aura of doom (Sampson 2003)

Management includes ABC approach – Fig. 1.18 for emergency treatment of anaphylaxis.

Dose of intramuscular adrenaline for acute anaphylaxis

All ages 10 μg/kg (0.1 mL/kg of 1:10 000 infants and young children OR 0.01 mL/kg of 1:1000 in older children) (ALSG 2016).

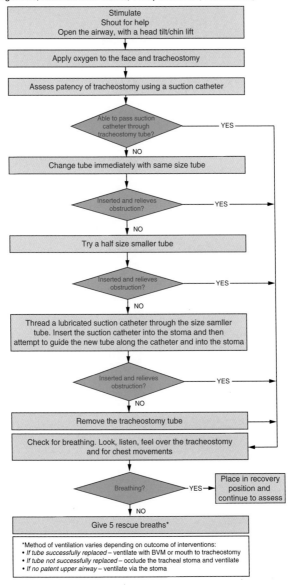

Fig. 1.16 Management of a blocked tracheostomy. (From Advanced Life Support Group, 2016. Advanced Paediatric Life Support. A Practical Approach to Emergencies, sixth ed. BMJ Books, Wiley and Sons, Chichester.)

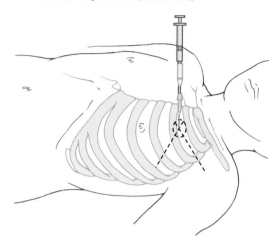

Fig. 1.17 Needle thoracocentesis. (From Advanced Life Support Group, 2016. Advanced Paediatric Life Support. A Practical Approach to Emergencies, sixth ed. BMJ Books, Wiley and Sons, Chichester.)

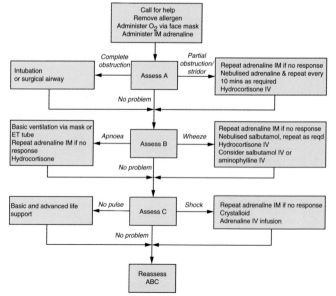

Fig. 1.18 Emergency treatment of anaphylaxis. *ABC*, Airway–breathing–circulation; *ET*, endotracheal tube; *IM*, intramuscular; *IV*, intravenous. (From Advanced Life Support Group, 2016. Advanced Paediatric Life Support. A Practical Approach to Emergencies, sixth ed. BMJ Books, Wiley and Sons, Chichester.)

Fig. 1.19 Algorithm for the management of hyperkalaemia. *IV*, Intravenous. (From Advanced Life Support Group, 2016. Advanced Paediatric Life Support. A Practical Approach to Emergencies, sixth ed. BMJ Books, Wiley and Sons, Chichester.)

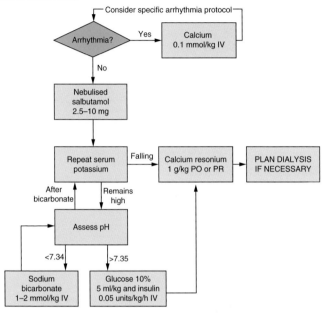

Management of hyperkalaemia

Hyperkalaemia (serum K + >5.5 mmol/L) is a dangerous condition that may cause arrhythmias or death. It is most commonly caused by renal failure, but may also be caused by potassium overload, loss of potassium from cells due to acidosis or cell lysis, hypoaldosteronism, and hypoadrenalism. If potassium is very high, more than one treatment can be used simultaneously. Fig. 1.19 provides an algorithm for the management of hyperkalaemia (ALSG 2016).

A summary for the management of hyperkalaemia can be found in Table 1.3 (ALSG 2016).

Table 1.3	Summary of emergency management of hyperkalaemia in children
Basics	Definition: K^+ significantly above upper end of normal for age and/or rising ABC
	Monitoring: continuous ECG (first signs are tented T waves then loss of P waves), SaO_2, blood pressure, urine output, weight
	Recheck urea and electrolytes urgently – hours may have elapsed since last sample. Sample may have haemolysed
	Consider the cause: high K^+ intake, high production or low output
Stop K^+ intake	Stop any potassium in diet and in any fluids being infused
	Stop drugs that can cause hyperkalaemia, for example, angiotensin-converting enzyme inhibitor (ACE inhibitor), angiotensin II blockers and β-blockers
Stabilise myocardium	10% calcium gluconate
	0.5–1 mL/kg IV over 5 min, maximum 20 mL; give undiluted
	Give if ECG changes or K^+ significantly above upper end of normal for age or rising
	Effect occurs within minutes. Duration of action approx. 1 h, repeat within 5–10 min as necessary
Shift K^+ into cells	Nebulised salbutamol
	<2 years: 2.5 mg or ≥2 years: 5 mg; repeat 2-hourly as necessary
	Onset of action: within 30 min, maximum effect at 60–90 min
Seek specialist advice	
The following strategies can be used depending on clinical situation:	
Shift K^+ into cells	*Sodium bicarbonate 1–2 mmol/kg IV over 30 min*
Dialysis	*(1 mmol = 1 mL of 8.4% $NaHCO_3$, dilute 1:5 in 5% dextrose)*
	Glucose (± insulin):
	by rectum: 250 mg/kg (maximum 15 g) 6-hourly, repeat if expelled within 30 min
	by mouth: 250 mg/kg (maximum 15 g) 6-hourly
	Limited role for oral route as it is unpalatable. Takes 4 h for full effect
	In specialist environment

ABC, Airway, breathing, circulation; *ECG*, electrocardiography; *IV*, intravenous.
From Advanced Life Support Group, 2016. Advanced Paediatric Life Support. A Practical Approach to Emergencies, sixth ed. BMJ Books, Wiley and Sons, Chichester.

REFERENCES

Advanced Life Support Group (ALSG), 2016. Advanced Paediatric Life Support: A Practical Approach to Emergencies, sixth ed. BMJ Books, Wiley and Sons, Chichester.

American Heart Association, 1997. Pediatric Advanced Life Support, third ed. American Heart Association, Dallas, TX.

Enright, K., Turner, C., Roberts, P., et al., 2012. Primary cardiac arrest following sport in children presenting to an emergency department: chest compressions and early defibrillation can save lives, but is intravenous epinephrine always appropriate? Pediatr. Emerg. Care 28, 336–339.

Fleisher, G.R., Ludwig, S., 1988. Textbook of Pediatric Emergency Medicine, second ed. Williams & Wilkins, Baltimore, MD.

Fowler, R., Gallangher, J.V., Isaacs, S.M., et al., 2007. The role of intraosseous vascular accessin the out-of-hospital environment (resource document to NAEMSP position statement). Prehosp. Emerg. Care 11 (1), 63–66.

Resuscitation Council (UK), 2015. Resuscitation guidelines 2015. Resuscitation Council (UK), London.

Ryder, S.A., Waldmann, C., 2003. Anaphylaxis. Care. Crit. Ill 19, 174–176.

Sampson, H.A., 2003. Anaphylaxis and emergency treatment. Pediatrics 111, 1601–1608.

Spivey, W.H., 1987. Intraosseous infusions. J. Pediatr. 111, 639–643.

Wyllie, J., Bruinenberg, J., Roehr, C.C., et al., 2015. European Resuscitation Council Guidelines for Resuscitation 2015: Section 7. Resuscitation and support of transition of babies at birth. Resuscitation 95, 242–262.

USEFUL WEBSITE

www.resus.org.uk – also, a free app is available from the Resuscitation Council (UK) iResus, which allows access to the latest algorithms for resuscitation.

AIRWAY AND BREATHING

2

Respiratory failure is the most common reason for admission to a paediatric intensive care unit (PICU), so recognition of respiratory distress and a good understanding of respiratory failure is a fundamental part of working in PICU. In addition, the paediatric airway anatomy differs from that of an adult patient, which makes infants and young children particularly vulnerable to upper and lower airway obstruction. Respiratory failure, as opposed to cardiac failure, is often the primary reason for cardiopulmonary arrest in children. Early recognition and treatment may prevent an arrest. Simple interventions may help alleviate respiratory distress (Table 2.1). Normal respiratory rates are shown in Box 2.1.

Table 2.1 Practical tips to help manage the airway in neonates and infants	
Anatomic challenge	**Solutions**
The occiput is large, so the neck may be flexed in the supine position. This may lead to airway obstruction.	Placing the head and neck in a more neutral position may help relieve obstruction and improve the view for intubation.
Neonates are predominantly nasal breathers, prone to blockage with secretions.	Simple nasal suction can help alleviate respiratory distress.
Infants have a relatively large tongue.	Optimising head position and use of oral pharyngeal airways may help.
The epiglottis is floppier and is more difficult to displace on laryngoscopy in neonates and infants. Watch out for loose teeth in older children.	Choose an appropriate type and size of laryngoscope.
The anterior commissure of the glottis is directed caudally and the infant trachea is angled posteriorly, which may hamper the easy passage of the endotracheal tube.	Rotation of the endotracheal tube may help to guide it into the subglottis.

Continued

Anatomic challenge	Solutions

Anatomic challenge	Solutions
Larynx is high and anterior in infants, which may make it more difficult to visualise the laryngeal inlet.	Keep the head in a neutral position rather than the traditional 'sniffing the morning air position.'
Narrowest part of airway is subglottic at level of the cricoid so any condition which effects subglottis (e.g., postextubation oedema) will be poorly tolerated in comparison to an adult.	At extubation – always be prepared for complications related to postextubation oedema.
Immature cartilage in the upper larynx and the trachea may collapse during the respiratory cycle causing airway obstruction (laryngo- and tracheobronchomalacia).	PEEP may be required to overcome dynamic compression.
Respiratory mechanics are less efficient in the paediatric population.*	Be aware that children will desaturate more rapidly than adults particularly at induction of anaesthesia and be prepared to intervene.
Abdominal distension for any reason will also impede diaphragmatic excursion.	Placement of an NG tube and aspiration of any air or fluid can improve respiratory distress and aid airway management.

*The chest wall is more compliant, which will cause it to retract in respiratory distress reducing functional residual capacity and limiting tidal volume. The intercostal muscles are not fully developed in children until school age, so they have reduced ability to lift ribs. The diaphragm muscles insert horizontally rather than obliquely, which affects ability to lift chest outwards.
NG, Nasogastric tube; *PEEP*, positive end-expiratory pressure.

Box 2.1   Normal respiratory rates for infants and children

<1 year: 30–40 breaths/min
2–5 years: 20–30 breaths/min
5–12 years: 15–20 breaths/min
>12 years: 12–16 breaths/min
At rest, tachypnoea indicates that increased ventilation is needed because of either lung or airway disease or metabolic acidosis.

UPPER RESPIRATORY TRACT

Common conditions that affect the upper respiratory tract include viral respiratory tract infections, croup, and subglottic stenosis. Any respiratory condition that leads to an increase in respiratory secretions can cause significant airway obstruction in infants and young children.

The airway of infants and children is much smaller than that of adults. Poiseuille's law states:

$$\text{resistance} = 1/\text{radius}^4,$$

that is, the resistance to airflow is inversely proportional to the fourth power of the radius. In other words, a small amount of mucus in the airway, oedema, or subglottic stenosis will significantly increase resistance to airflow and will increase the work of breathing.

A child with upper airway obstruction will be most comfortable sitting up and leaning forward, may be anxious, restless, tachypnoeic, tachycardic, have an inspiratory stridor, drool, have nasal flaring, and be using the accessory muscles to breathe.

Precautions and action in upper airway obstruction

- Avoid unnecessary stress for the child, let her/him sit with parents/carers
- Avoid blood gases and x-ray if this will cause distress
- Give oxygen to maintain oxygen saturations prior to intubation
- Give adrenaline (epinephrine) nebulisers (1:1000)
- Give budesonide nebulisers (1 mg total dose)
- Intravenous antibiotics if required
- Advanced airway intervention is a clinical decision

If child requires intubation:

- Call ENT team prior to start
- Use most experienced anaesthetist/operator
- Gas induction in theatre
- Have a wide range of endotracheal (ET) tubes ready, especially smaller sizes
- Have a bougie, introducer, and laryngeal mask to hand
- Anticipate potential need for a surgical airway
- Use HELPKIDS mnemonic for intubation (Breen & Edwards 2016, unpublished)

 Avoid muscle relaxants until you have confirmed that it is possible to ventilate the patient with a mask and bag technique.

Causes of airway obstruction (stridor)

Consider the age of the child presenting with stridor (Table 2.2) and the differences between epiglottitis and stridor (Table 2.3).

Table 2.2 Common causes of stridor	
Age	**Most common causes of stridor**
Neonate	Laryngomalacia, vascular ring, subglottic stenosis, laryngeal web
Toddler	Croup, foreign body aspiration, anaphylaxis
Older child	Mediastinal mass, recurrent croup, acquired subglottic stenosis, anaphylaxis

Table 2.3 Differentiating between epiglottitis and croup		
	Epiglottitis	**Croup (laryngotracheobronchitis)**
Age	2–7 years	1–3 years
History	Hours	1–2 days
Appearance	Toxic, unwell, sits up, mouth open	Anxious, lethargic
Fever	+ + + (>38, 5°C)	+
Voice	Hoarse, weak	Hoarse
Cough	+	+ + (usually barking)
Drooling	+ + +	Unusual
Respirations	Laboured, stridor	Increased, stridor
Hypoxia	Common	Uncommon

Also consider speed of onset as some diagnoses may be more likely:

- If minutes – foreign body aspiration, anaphylaxis
- If hours – epiglottitis, tracheitis
- If days – croup, mediastinal mass
- If weeks – subglottic stenosis, laryngomalacia, vascular ring

Croup (laryngotracheobronchitis)

Croup is the most common acute upper airway obstruction in children; it can be caused by a number of respiratory viruses, most commonly parainfluenza. It usually affects children between 6 months and 5 years of age. The most effective treatment is steroid therapy either nebulised, oral or intravenous, depending on the clinical state of the patient. Steroid therapy takes up to 6 hours to reach a peak effect. In the acute setting an adrenaline nebuliser may alleviate the symptoms. However, children who do not respond to nebulised adrenaline and steroids are likely to require intubation.

If intubation is required to maintain a secure airway:

- Secureness of tube is vital – tapes may need to be changed daily because of secretions and movement of child

- Use of arm splints effective in preventing self-extubation
- Regular suction – if child is active, likely to cough up secretions frequently
- Child is likely to be on a course of steroids from admission to PICU – wait to hear leak around tube prior to extubation, can take 3–5 days
- Wean ventilation and allow child to self-ventilate via a Swedish nose filter on the end of the ET tube if adequate tube size.
- Encourage the family and visitors to play with the patient and become involved in daily care routine to minimise the patient's distress and boredom.

Epiglottitis

Epiglottitis is most often caused by *Haemophilus influenzae,* and the incidence of epiglottitis has fallen dramatically since Hib vaccine has been introduced. It is now a rare cause of upper airway obstruction. If a diagnosis of epiglottitis is made, the child will require immediate assessment by a senior anaesthetist or someone who can perform advanced airway procedures, probable intubation under gas induction of anaesthesia, and intravenous antibiotics. These patients are often pyrexial with systemic signs of infection; early administration of antibiotics intravenous such as coamoxyclavulanic acid or cefuroxime is an important part of their care.

Foreign-body aspiration

History: Usually sudden-onset cough and stridor; however, the act of inhalation may not have been witnessed.

Examination: Often child appears well and active, has stridor and may have wheeze; there may be differential air entry or signs of pneumonia in case of delayed presentation. Chest x-ray may show differential hyperinflation.

Bacterial tracheitis

Often presents with symptoms similar to croup, but this is a much more serious illness and the child will develop pyrexia and become more unwell. When this child is intubated, pus may be observed in the airway. Intravenous antibiotics will be required.

LOWER RESPIRATORY TRACT

Common conditions that affect the lower respiratory tract include bronchiolitis, asthma, pneumonia, and foreign-body aspiration, all of which may progress to acute respiratory distress syndrome (ARDS). Bronchospasm, increased mucous production, oedema, and inflammation of airway mucosa can lead to diffuse air trapping, decreased air movement, decreased compliance, and increased work of breathing. A child with lower respiratory tract disease may have an expiratory wheeze, have a prolonged expiratory time, be tachypnoeic or cyanotic, use accessory muscles, cough, and have hyperinflated lungs.

Signs of respiratory distress and inadequate ventilation in children

Tachypnea, cricoid tug, sternal, intercostal or subcostal recession, shoulder rolling, nasal flaring, weak cry, stridor or wheeze, head bobbing, lethargy, decreased responsiveness, irritability, decreased level of consciousness, hypoxaemia, hypercarbia
   Late signs: bradycardia, decreased air movement, apnoea or gasping, poor systemic perfusion

Bronchiolitis

This is a viral respiratory condition most commonly caused by respiratory syncytial virus but also by many other viruses, including rhinovirus, influenza, parainfluenza, human metapneumovirus, and adenovirus. It mainly affects infants younger than 1 year, but certain groups of babies are at higher risk and these include premature babies and neonates, those with congenital heart disease, neuromuscular conditions, or interstitial lung disease or babies with immunodeficiency. Mortality is less than 1% and high-risk group is at highest risk.

The bronchioles become acutely inflamed and oedematous, and there is necrosis of epithelial cells which line the small airways, as well as increased mucous production.

CLINICAL PRESENTATION

Bronchiolitis is a seasonal, common lower respiratory tract infection with symptoms of fever, rhinitis, cough, intercostal and subcostal recession, tachypnea, fine inspiratory crackles and/or expiratory wheeze, apnoea, cyanosis, poor feeding.

Whilst the majority of neonates and infants with bronchiolitis can be cared for at home, a small percentage will require hospital care and, of those, approximately 2% will require mechanical ventilation.

Criteria for severe disease include:
- Tachypnea (RR ≥70/minute) (Wang et al 1995)
- Saturations <92% despite oxygen therapy
- Apnoea (Damore et al 2008)
- Severe respiratory distress (Mansbach et al 2012)
- Decreased level of consciousness

(Principles of Management in High Dependency: STRS Guideline 2016, www.evelinalondon.nhs.uk/resorces/our-services/hospital/south-thames-retrieval-service/severe-bronchiolitis.pdf)
- Maintain oxygen saturations ≥92% unless congenital heart disease
- Apnoea monitoring
- Minimal handling

- Suction nasal secretions
- Noninvasive respiratory support by humidified high-flow nasal cannula (HFNC) at 2 L/kg/minute or continuous positive airway pressure (CPAP) 5–6 cm H_2O. Reassess frequently.
- Small-volume nasogastric (NG) feeds if possible
- Reduce enteric fluid intake to 50 mL/kg/day (risk of fluid overload/ hyponatraemia/seizures)
- If IV fluid required, give isotonic (e.g., 0.9% saline plus 5% dextrose)
- There is no role for nebulised salbutamol, ipratropium bromide, adrenaline, 3% saline, or steroids (Chavasse et al 2009; Zorc & Hall 2010; Hartling et al 2011; Fernandes et al 2013)
- Antibiotics are not routinely recommended in bronchiolitis because it is a viral infection. However, in PICU there may be secondary bacterial infection in 30%–40% cases, in which case IV coamoxiclav is often chosen as first line cover with CNS cover of cefotaxime and aciclovir, if concerns.

(Intubation and Ventilation in Bronchiolitis, STRS Guideline 2016, www.evelinalondon.nhs.uk/resorces/our-services/hospital/south-thames-retrieval-service/severe-bronchiolitis.pdf)

- Optimise preoxygenation
- Decompress stomach by NG tube aspiration
- Consider volume bolus (10 mL/kg) prior to anaesthesia
- Anticipate noncompliant chest once anaesthetised and muscle relaxed. Mask ventilate with slow respiratory rate (20–30) to achieve good chest movement
- Ensure end-tidal CO_2 monitoring available
- Initial ventilation: inspired time (IT) 0.8 second, RR 20–30, positive end-expiratory pressure (PEEP) 5 cm H_2O, enough peak inspiratory pressure (PIP) to move chest (ideally <30 cm H_2O)
- Secure ETT and do chest x-ray to ensure optimal position (T2)
- Review chest and ventilator settings regularly
- Target oxygen saturations ≥92% unless congenital heart disease
- Target end-tidal CO_2 5–10 kPa
- Sedate with morphine and muscle relax as required
- Suction of ETT may be helpful
- Arterial line not usually required for management

Ventilation may cause lung injury in children; therefore lung protective ventilation is essential to prevent harm, and these measures include (Turner & Arnold 2007):

- Low tidal volume pressure limited approach (target 5–8 mL/kg)
- Permissive hypercapnia (tolerating high CO_2 if pH >7.2)
- Controlling oxygen exposure (tolerate saturations >88%)

PNEUMONIA

Bacterial pneumonia should be considered the likely diagnosis in febrile children (temperature > 38.5°C) with increased respiratory rate and subcostal recession. Viruses account for 30%–60% of community-acquired infections, especially in children younger than 1 year. Streptococcus pneumonia is the most common cause of bacterial pneumonia. Group A streptococcus and staphylococcus are more likely to be complicated with an effusion or require PICU admission. Children younger than 5 years, with immunodeficiency, congenital heart conditions, and sickle cell are particularly vulnerable to respiratory tract infections. Local antibiotic guidance and the clinical condition of the child should guide antibiotic administration.

Patients with saturations less than 92% in air should receive supplemental oxygen. Auscultation usually identifies crackles and bronchial breathing; however, if reduced breath sounds and dullness to percussion, a potential effusion or empyema should be investigated. Frontal x-ray can be used to confirm the diagnosis and areas of consolidation and identify any complications (e.g., effusion or lobar collapse). Microbiologic tests such as blood culture, nasal secretions, and bronchoalveolar lavage should be used for viral detection (via PCR) and bacterial culture.

If children remain hypoxic despite supplemental oxygen, early consideration of invasive ventilation is pragmatic.

To ensure safe induction of anaesthesia:
1. Adequate preoxygenation is key.
2. Fluids and inotropes to ensure blood pressure are maintained at safe levels throughout the procedure.

Care of intubated patients on PICU:
1. Regular suctioning may be necessary due to large volumes of secretions.
2. Adequate ventilation to provide reasonable tidal volumes (6–8 mL/kg) without excessively high peak pressure (PIP limit 28–30 cm H_2O).
3. Respiratory rate should be set at a level that is appropriate for a self-ventilating patient of that age. This can be adjusted to maximise ventilation and CO_2 clearance.
4. Early enteral feeding is appropriate.
5. Daily chest x-rays to exclude empyema or effusion.
6. Enough sedation to keep the patient comfortable and allow ventilation and regular physiotherapy.
7. Pneumonia may progress to ARDS, patients should be carefully monitored with attention to changes in FiO_2.

PAEDIATRIC ACUTE RESPIRATORY DISTRESS SYNDROME

ARDS is the end point of a cascade of events: a primary insult (e.g., direct lung such as pneumonia or an indirect problem such as systemic infection) triggers a process of inflammation in the host which leads to hypoxic respiratory failure. Table 2.4 includes a list of causes of paediatric ARDS. Fortunately, the incidence is rare in PICU (2% of all admissions), but the mortality remains high (35%).

A new paediatric definition was agreed in 2015 by a consensus group of international PICU experts (new definition Table 2.5).

Table 2.4 Causes of paediatric acute respiratory distress syndrome

Causes	Condition	Incidence
Direct	Viral pneumonia/bronchiolitis	16%
	Bacterial pneumonia	15%
	Near drowning	9%
	Aspiration	
	Burns	
Indirect	Septic shock	34%
	Nonpulmonary trauma	

From Dahlem, P., van Aalderen, W.M., Bos, A.P., 2007. Pediatric acute lung injury. Paediatr. Respir. Rev. 8 (4), 348-362.

The key features of ARDS include:
1. Hypoxia despite oxygen and respiratory support defined by a low P_aO_2/FiO_2 ratio or high oxygenation index (OI)
2. Bilateral x-ray changes
3. Onset of respiratory failure within 7 days of clinical insult

Children with ARDS require careful attention to management to improve their survival and avoid aggravating the lung injury. The consensus panel recommended some key points regarding management of patients with ARDS:
1. Cuffed ET tubes are recommended to minimise the leak in conventional ventilation.
2. Tidal volumes should be patient-specific according to lung severity. In controlled ventilation, use 6–8 mL/kg for moderate disease and 3–6 mL/kg for patients with severe disease and very poor lung compliance.
3. PEEP level should be increased to 10–15 cm H_2O titrated to the improvement in oxygenation without compromising blood pressure and cardiac output (CO).
4. Inspiratory pressures should be limited to 28 cm H_2O.
5. Although there is no consensus regarding absolute target saturation levels, if PEEP has been optimised, it may be necessary to target saturations of 88%–92%. Monitoring of oxygen index and central venous saturation is highly recommended in this setting.
6. Permissive hypercapnia maintaining a pH 7.15–7.30 is recommended.
7. High-frequency ventilation should be considered as an alternative for patients who remain hypoxic with high inspiratory pressures on conventional ventilation.
8. There is insufficient evidence to recommend nitric oxide (NO), exogenous surfactant, prone positioning, or corticosteroid therapy in this group of patients. Local guidelines and policies should guide these specific treatment options.

Table 2.5 Definition of acute respiratory distress syndrome

	Noninvasive mechanical ventilation	Invasive mechanical ventilation		
Age	Exclude patients with perinatal-related lung disease			
Timing	Within 7 days of known clinical insult			
Origin of Oedema	Respiratory failure not fully explained by cardiac failure or fluid overload			
Chest Imaging	Chest imaging findings of new infiltrate(s) consistent with acute pulmonary parenchymal disease			
Oxygenation	PARDS (No severity stratification)	Mild	Moderate	Severe
	Full-face-mask bilevel ventilation or CPAP	$4 \leq OI < 8$	$8 \leq OI < 16$	$OI \geq 16$
	≥ 5 cm H_2O[b]	$5 \leq OSI < 7.5$[a]	$7.5 \leq OSI < 12.3$[a]	$OSI \geq 12.3$[a]
	PF ratio ≤ 300			
	SF ratio ≤ 264[a]			
Special Populations				
Cyanotic Heart Disease	Standard criteria above for age, timing, origin of oedema, and chest imaging with an acute deterioration in oxygenation not explained by underlying cardiac disease.[c]			
Chronic Lung Disease	Standard criteria above for age, timing, and origin of oedema with chest imaging consistent with new infiltrate and acute deterioration in oxygenation from baseline which meet oxygenation criteria above.[c]			
Left Ventricular Dysfunction	Standard criteria for age, timing, and origin of oedema with chest imaging changes consistent with new infiltrate and acute deterioration in oxygenation which meet criteria above not explained by left ventricular dysfunction.			

[a]Paediatric acute respiratory distress syndrome (PARDS) definition. Use PaO_2- based metric when available. Use PaO_2- based metric when available. (if PaO_2 not available, wean FiO_2 to maintain $SpO_2 \leq 97\%$ to calculate oxygen saturation index (OSI):[FiO_2 x mean airway pressure x 100]/SpO_2:(SF) ratio.

[b]ARDS severity groups stratified by oxygenation index (OI);[FiO_2 x mean airway pressure x 100]/PaO_2 or OSI should not be applied to children with chronic lung disease who normally receive mechanical ventilation or children with cyanotic heart disease.

[c]ARDS severity groups stratified by OI or OSI should not be applied to children with chronic lung disease who normally receive invasive mechanical ventilation or children with cyanotic congenital heart disease.

From Khemani, R.G., Smith, L.S., Zimmerman, J.J., Erickson, S., for the Pediatric Acute Lung Injury Consensus Conference Group. 2015. Pediatric acute respiratory distress syndrome: definition, incidence, and epidemiology: proceedings from the pediatric acute lung injury consensus conference. Pediatr. Crit. Care Med. 16 (5 Suppl 1), 23–40.

9. Sedation should be targeted to achieve tolerance of ventilation and minimal oxygen requirements by adhering to local policies and guidelines.
10. Neuromuscular blockade may be necessary if sedation alone is not adequate to allow effective ventilation.
11. Enteral nutrition if tolerated if preferential to the parenteral route.
12. Blood transfusion should be considered if the haemoglobin levels are <70 g/L.
13. Monitoring of ventilator parameters, capnography, and flow-time and pressure-time curves to ensure optimal ventilator patient synchrony.
14. A peripheral arterial catheter should be considered in patients with ARDS to allow careful monitoring of haemodynamic status and facilitate regular blood gas analysis.
15. Extracorporeal membrane oxygenation (ECMO) should be considered in children with severe ARDS where the cause of respiratory failure is likely to be reversible. This decision should be based on a structured evaluation of the case history and clinical status.

Management of severe asthma

Asthmatics have:
- Airway inflammation with wall thickening and increased vascular permeability
- Mucous hypersecretion
- Bronchial smooth muscle contraction (wheeze)

This leads to air trapping and atelectasis. Increased intrathoracic pressure induced by air trapping can reduce CO (tamponade effect).

It is essential to assess the severity of symptoms correctly (Table 2.6) before a child can be effectively treated.

The principles of therapy include:
- Eliminate symptoms and improve lung function
- Correct hypoxia
- Reverse inflammation with steroids
- Relieve smooth muscle constriction with bronchodilators
- If required, supportive ventilation

MANAGEMENT OF ASTHMA

- Assess airway, breathing, and circulation
- High-flow oxygen mask with reservoir if oxygen saturations (S_pO_2) <92%.
- Nebulised salbutamol 2.5–5 mg with oxygen as driving gas (repeat if necessary)
- Nebulised ipratropium bromide 0.25 mg (<2 years 0.125 mg)
- Oral prednisolone 1 mg/kg or IV hydrocortisone 4 mg/kg

Table 2.6 Assessing severity of asthma

Management of acute asthma in children in emergency department

Age 2–5 years				Age >5 years			

Assess and record asthma severity

Age 2–5 years			Age >5 years		
Moderate asthma • SpO₂ ≥ 92% • No clinical features of severe asthma **NB: If a patient has signs and symptoms across categories, always treat according to their most severe features**	**Acute severe asthma** • SpO₂ < 92% • Too breathless to talk or eat • Heart rate > 140/min • Respiratory rate > 40/min • Use of accessory neck muscles	**Life-threatening asthma** SpO₂ < 92% plus any of: • Silent chest • Poor respiratory effort • Agitation • Confusion • Cyanosis	**Moderate asthma** • SpO₂ ≥ 92% • PEF ≥ 50% best or predicted • No clinical features of severe asthma **NB: If a patient has signs and symptoms across categories, always treat according to their most severe features**	**Acute severe asthma** • SpO₂ < 92% • PEF 33–50% best or predicted • Heart rate > 125/min • Respiratory rate > 30/min • Use of accessory neck	**Life-threatening asthma** SpO₂ < 92% plus any of: • PEF < 33% best or predicted • Silent chest • Poor respiratory effort • Altered consciousness • Cyanosis

First line treatments

Oxygen via face mask/nasal prongs to achieve SpO₂ 94–98%

Age 2–5 years			Age >5 years		
• β₂ agonist 2–10 puffs via spacer ± facemask (given one puff at a time inhaled separately using tidal breathing) • Give one puff of β₂ agonist every 30–60 s up to 10 puffs according to response • Consider oral prednisolone 20 mg	• β₂ agonist 2–10 puffs via spacer ± facemask or nebulised salbutamol 2.5 mg • Oral prednisolone 20 mg or IV hydrocortisone 4 mg/kg if vomiting **If poor response** add 0.25 mg nebulised ipratropium bromide to every nebulised β₂ agonist • Repeat β₂ agonist and ipratropium up to every 20 min for 2 h according to response	• Nebulised β₂ agonist: salbutamol 2.5 mg ± nebulised ipratropium bromide 0.25 mg nebulised • Repeat bronchodilators every 20–30 min • Oral prednisolone 20 mg or IV hydrocortisone 4 mg/kg if vomiting **Discuss with senior clinician, PICU team or paediatrician**	• β₂ agonist 10 puffs via spacer or nebulised salbutamol 5 mg • Oral prednisolone 30–40 mg or IV hydrocortisone 4 mg/kg if vomiting	• β₂ agonist 10 puffs via spacer and mouthpiece (given one puff at a time inhaled separately during tidal breathing) • Give one puff of β₂ agonist every 30–60 s up to 10 puffs according to response • Oral prednisolone 30–40 mg	• Nebulised β₂ agonist: salbutamol 5 mg plus ipratropium bromide 0.25 mg nebulised • Repeat bronchodilators every 20–30 min • Oral prednisolone 30–40 mg or IV hydrocortisone 4 mg/kg if vomiting **Discuss with senior clinician, PICU team or paediatrician**

Reassess within 1 h (Age 2–5 years) / Reassess within 1 h (Age >5 years)

Second line treatments

Age 2–5 years	Age >5 years
• Consider second line treatments – see Annex 7 • Admit all cases if features of severe attack persist after initial treatment • Arrange transfer to PICU/HDU if poor response to treatment as per local guidelines	• Consider second line treatments – see Annex 7 • Admit all cases if features of severe attack persist after initial treatment • Arrange transfer to PICU/HDU if poor response to treatment as per local guidelines

Discharge plan

Age 2–5 years	Age >5 years
• Continue β₂ agonist 4 hourly as necessary • Consider prednisolone 20 mg daily for 3–5 days until symptoms have settled • Advise to contact GP if not controlled on above treatment • Provide a written asthma action plan • Review regular treatment • Check inhaler technique • Arrange GP follow up within 48 h • Arrange hospital asthma clinic follow up in 4–6 weeks if second or subsequent attack in past 12 months.	• Continue β₂ agonist 4 hourly as necessary • Consider prednisolone 30–40 mg daily for 3–5 days until symptoms have settled • Seek medical advice if not controlled on above treatment • Provide a written asthma action plan • Review regular treatment • Check inhaler technique • Arrange GP follow up within 48 h • Arrange hospital asthma clinic follow up in 4–6 weeks if second or subsequent attack in past 12 months.

HDU, high dependency unit; *PICU*, Paediatric intensive care; *PEF*, peak expiratory flow.

Reproduced from BTS/SIGN British Guideline on the management of asthma by kind permission of the British Thoracic Society. From BTS/SIGN 2016.

- If worsening respiratory distress or no improvement in severe or life-threatening categories, progress to:
  - IV salbutamol infusion 06.–2mcg/kg/min (consider bolus IV salbutamol 15 µg/kg of 200 µg/mL solution over 10 minutes if older than 2 years; maximum IV bolus dose is 250 µg) – monitor ECG and serum potassium for detection of hypokalaemia
  - Consider IV magnesium sulphate 40 mg/kg (maximum 2 g) of 50% solution over 20 minutes. One dose only (Ciarallo et al 2000)

 Magnesium sulphate is contraindicated in renal failure. Excessive or repeated doses of magnesium sulphate may induce moderate hypotension and muscle weakness.

- Consider IV aminophylline 1 mg/kg/h after bolus of 5 mg/kg over 20 minutes (unless receiving oral theophyllines)
- IV antibiotics if focal areas on chest x-ray
- Contact senior anaesthetist, PICU, and the retrieval service for advice about possible transfer

 Monitor serum potassium if salbutamol is used and give potassium supplements if serum potassium is low.

CRITERIA FOR INTUBATION (Phipps & Garrard 2003; ALSG 2016)

- Increasing exhaustion, respiratory muscle fatigue
- Decreased chest movement with breathing
- Quiet chest, absent audible wheeze
- Pulsus paradoxus (systolic pressure change >20 mm Hg with dip in pulse wave amplitude during inspiration)
- Lethargy, agitation, confusion, coma
- Severe mucous plugging and lobar collapse
- Hypoxaemia – decreasing saturations and/or increasing oxygen requirement or rising $P\text{co}_2$

 Intubation

Avoid atracurium for intubation because it causes histamine release, which may aggravate bronchospasm. (Vecuronium or rocuronium can be used, e.g., with ketamine for intubation.)
- Volume bolus at intubation may be necessary because hyperinflation compresses the heart and may lead to hypotension. It would also be sensible to prepare and/or start inotropes if hypotension is refractory to fluid boluses.

STRATEGIES FOR VENTILATION

- Suggested initial settings – tidal volume 6–8 mL/kg or PIP to generate chest movement, low rate (e.g., 12–16 breaths/min, inspiratory time 1.0, I:E (inspiratory:expiratory) ratio 1:3 or 1:4, PEEP 5, $F_i\text{o}_2$ 0.6)

- Humidification essential, plus regular ET suction
- Permissive hypercapnia, permissive hypoxia to avoid barotrauma (saturations >88%, pH >7.2)
- May require high levels of sedation while ventilated
- Switch to pressure support ventilation (PSV) mode as soon as possible

PEAK PAUSE PRESSURES

Airflow obstruction in asthma can be quantified by a peak inspiratory pause manoeuvre: closing the inspiratory valve at the end of inspiration (i.e., holding the pause knob on the Servo ventilator). This results in a full breath being delivered into the lungs. In 'normal' lungs, there will be a very small drop in the PIP after an inspiratory pause because there is no change in flow (i.e., no obstruction in the airways). In asthma, pressure will be dissipated by overcoming the resistance in the major airways due to obstruction to airflow by bronchospasm or mucous plugs. As a result, a fall in pressure will occur on inflation of the lungs, reaching a plateau only when airflow resistance is overcome. This fall in pressure (from peak to plateau pressures) is proportional to airway resistance.

AutoPEEP can be measured by an expiratory hold manoeuvre (closing the expiratory valve on expiration). This will be positive if airflow is still occurring at the end of expiration (i.e., the alveoli are still emptying). The higher the expiratory pause pressure (autoPEEP), the higher the flow limitation during expiration. It has been suggested that low-level externally applied PEEP (<7.5 cm H_2O) or matched to the level of autoPEEP may overcome the obstruction to flow without increasing alveolar pressure.

CRISIS MANAGEMENT

- Hand-ventilate 100% oxygen, no PEEP for 1 minute, giving only very low rate
  - Exclude tension pneumothorax and drain if necessary
  - Consider intratracheal DNase to treat mucous plugs with physiotherapy/bronchoscopy (Patel 2000)
- Ketamine infusion (bronchial smooth muscle dilator)
- Isoflurane/heliox administration via ventilator
- ECMO

 Anticipate arrhythmias, barotraumas, and hypotension due to overdistension – treat with volume.

Pertussis

Pertussis (whooping cough) is a highly contagious respiratory infection caused by the bacteria *Bordetella pertussis* that is characterised by coryzal symptoms, paroxysmal cough with typical inspiratory 'whoop,' sometimes followed by vomiting. All suspected cases should be nursed in isolation. Whilst admission to PIC is rare, clinicians should consider pertussis as a differential diagnosis of babies with respiratory illness. Unvaccinated infants younger than 12 months of age have highest risk for severe and life-threatening complications, such as apnoea, pneumonia, seizures, encephalopathy, pulmonary hypertension, renal failure, or death. Babies may require intubation and ventilation. Notify Public Health of all suspected cases and consider chemoprophylaxis of contacts.

A predictor of more severe *B. pertussis* disease in young babies is an elevated and rapidly rising white cell count ($>50 \times 10^9$/L), which may require double volume exchange transfusion for leucodepletion (Murray et al 2013). Target white cell count less than 20 after exchange transfusion. If the infant remains in cardiorespiratory failure, a referral should be made to an ECMO centre.

Suspected pertussis is treated with antibiotics:
- Neonates (<1 month) – clarithromycin
- Older than 1 month – azithromycin or clarithromycin
- Pregnant women – erythromycin (NICE 2015)

Oxygenation

Oxygen delivery (D_{O_2}) is the amount of oxygen delivered to the tissues per minute. The following formulae demonstrate the relationships between *haemoglobin, D_{O_2}, and CO*.

D_{O_2}	=	Arterial oxygen content × CO
CO	=	Heart rate × stroke volume
Arterial oxygen content (mLO$_2$/100 mL)	=	Hb (g/dL) × 1.34 (mLO$_2$/gHb) × oxyhaemoglobin saturation + (0.003 × P_aO_2)

Haemoglobin that is 100% saturated contains 1.34 mL of bound oxygen. Normal arterial oxygen content is 18–20 mL of O_2 per 100 mL blood. Children may be able to cope with mild hypoxia for a short time by increasing their CO but, when they become unable to compensate, cardiorespiratory failure will ensue.

Oxyhaemoglobin dissociation curve

The oxyhaemoglobin dissociation curve (Fig. 2.1) shows the nonlinear relationship between haemoglobin saturation and the partial pressure of oxygen (P_aO_2). Each molecule of haemoglobin is made up of a protein (globin) and a combination of ferrous iron and protophyrin (haem), of which there are four. Each haem group has a different affinity to oxygen. Looking at the oxyhaemoglobin dissociation curve, the first haem group binds moderately easily with oxygen and there is a gentle curve. The second and third haems have the greatest affinity for oxygen and there is a steep slope as the haemoglobin saturation rises with a relatively small change in the P_aO_2. The fourth haem has the greatest difficulty binding to oxygen and so the curve flattens out, relatively less oxygen being taken up per unit change in P_aO_2 as the haemoglobin is reaching near-total saturation (i.e., 97%–100%). This occurs when P_aO_2 reaches approximately 13.3 kPa; there is therefore no additional benefit in keeping a patient's P_aO_2 any higher than this.

Fig. 2.1 Oxyhaemoglobin dissociation curve, showing the relationship between haemoglobin saturation and pH.

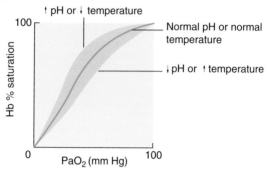

If the curve is shifted to the right, then haemoglobin binds less oxygen and is less well saturated at any P_aO_2. Factors that shift the curve to the right include acidosis, hypercapnia, and hyperthermia.

If the curve is shifted to the left, haemoglobin binds more oxygen at any P_aO_2. Factors that shift the curve to the left include alkalosis, hypocapnia, and hypothermia.

How do we assess oxygenation?

This can be assessed clinically by looking at the child's tongue or oral mucosa. It is more accurately measured using pulse oximetry or blood gas analysis. In a critically ill child, it is important to elicit:

- Oxygen saturation (S_aO_2)
- Arterial oxygen content. The arterial oxygen content can be used in calculations to assess the severity of respiratory failure

P_aO_2/F_iO_2 ratio

This ratio is used to estimate the severity of the hypoxia in relation to the amount of inspired oxygen delivered to the patient. The ratio is greater than 450 in healthy patients.

ARDS is present if P_aO_2/F_iO_2 (%) ratio is <200.

Oxygenation index

The OI is a tool used to assess the degree of hypoxia related to the amount of mechanical support and the inspired oxygen tension. It can be calculated as follows:

$$OI = \frac{\text{Mean airways pressure} \times (\text{fraction of inspired oxygen} \times 100)}{P_aO_2 \times 7.5 \text{ mm Hg}}$$

It is sometimes calculated when patients are nearing maximal conventional ventilator settings and clinicians are considering adjunct therapy (e.g., high-frequency oscillation ventilation [HFOV] or ECMO). It is useful to observe trends in OI and response to interventions.

In the adult population with ARDS, HFOV may be considered when OI is 22–46, but OI greater than this figure in patients who were not on HFOV led to 100% mortality (Fort et al 1997). ECMO may be considered in the neonatal population when OI is ≥40, indicating failure of conventional ventilator strategies.

Pulse oximetry

This is a noninvasive, reliable and easy-to-use method of calculating a patient's S_aO_2. The pulse oximeter consists of a photodetector that is wrapped around a pulsatile tissue bed where skin is thin (i.e., on a finger, toe, ear, lip or indeed penis in males), and two light-emitting diodes that transmit red and infrared light. Oxygenated and deoxygenated haemoglobin absorb these two lights differently, and the haemoglobin saturation (percentage of total haemoglobin oxygenated) is inversely related to the amount of red light absorbed.

Inaccurate readings may occur as a result of
- poor peripheral perfusion
  - hypotension or low CO state
  - vasoconstriction
  - hypothermia
- oedema
- environmental
  - nail polish
  - high ambient light levels
  - motion artefact
- abnormal haemoglobins (e.g., methaemoglobin, carboxyhaemoglobin foetal and sickling red cells)

The federal U.S. Food and Drug Administration requires documented accuracy within 3% in the range 70%–100% for pulse oximeters. However, these are generally based on studies involving healthy adult volunteers. A recent study in paediatrics (Ross et al 2013) comparing pulse oximetry with arterial gases shows that S_pO_2 typically overestimates throughout the range 70%–97%. The bias was greatest in the range 81%–85%. This could have significant clinical implications, particularly in children with congenital heart disease who are persistently desaturated or in neonates for whom hyperoxia may be hazardous.

Mixed venous oxygen saturations (S_vO_2)

Mixed venous oxygen saturation reflects the percentage of oxygen that is bound to haemoglobin in blood returning to the right side of the heart; that is, the amount of oxygen that is 'left over' after the tissues have extracted what they need to function. A normal mixed venous saturation is 60%–80%. A mixed venous saturation measurement can help to determine if CO and Do_2 are sufficient to meet a patient's needs.

If the amount of oxygen required by tissues falls to below the level required, the body will try to compensate by:

- increasing CO
- increasing tissue oxygen extraction
- increasing anaerobic metabolism

A low mixed venous S_aO_2 measurement may indicate the need to increase patient ventilation of increase cardiac supportive medication.

Blood gas analysis
PARTIAL PRESSURES P_AO_2 AND P_ACO_2

Partial pressure is the contribution each gas in a mixture makes to the total mixture. When a gas is dissolved in a liquid, the partial pressure is the same as the gas in contact with that liquid. This allows us to measure the P_aO_2 and carbon dioxide in blood.

CO-OXIMETRY

A co-oximeter is a device that measures the oxygen carrying state of haemoglobin, including oxygen-carrying haemoglobin, as well as car-boxy-haemoglobin and methhaemoglobin.

METHAEMOGLOBINAEMIA

Methaemoglobin is abnormal haemoglobin in which the iron molecule is oxidised to the ferric state (Fe^{3+}) rather than the normal ferrous state (Fe^{2+}), and this means that the molecule is incapable of binding to oxygen and can lead to cyanosis (Curry 1982; Goldfrank et al 1985). Methaemoglobinaemia may be congenital or acquired. Acquired methaemoglobinaemia is the most common form, where exposure to certain drugs or chemicals increases the rate of oxidation so that it exceeds the rate of reduction by methaemoglobin reductase systems and methaemoglobinaemia may occur.

Methaemoglobinaemia can also occur as a result of NO therapy, as NO binds to haemoglobin to produce methaemoglobin. During NO therapy, blood should be routinely tested to measure levels of methaemoglobin.

Normal methaemoglobin level is <1%. Methaemoglobinaemia should be suspected (Pow 1997) if:

- Cyanosis fails to respond to oxygen therapy (Goldfrank et al 1985)
- Po_2 is normal or elevated in the presence of decreased measured S_aO_2 (Goldfrank et al 1985)
- Blood is brown in colour and remains dark on aeration (Mansouri 1985)

Carboxyhaemoglobin

Carbon monoxide is a toxic, odourless gas produced by car exhausts and fires, among other causes. Carbon monoxide has a greater affinity for haemoglobin than oxygen and when bound to haemoglobin forms carboxyhaemoglobin. This impairs oxygen transport, produces decreased D_{O_2} and tissue hypoxia, and can result in metabolic acidosis if carbon monoxide levels are high. Levels of carboxyhaemoglobin >60% are often fatal (Hazinski 1992).

ACID–BASE BALANCE AND INTERPRETATION OF BLOOD GASES

pH is a term used to describe the acidity or alkalinity of a solution. The pH scale is based on the concentration of hydrogen ions, expressed in moles per litre, which is the negative logarithm of the hydrogen concentration.

- The pH of a normal arterial blood sample lies between 7.35 and 7.45.
  - pH <7.35 is acidaemia (more H+ ions than OH− ions)
  - pH >7.45 is alkalaemia (more OH− ions than H+ ions)

Routinely we use the terms *acidosis* and *alkalosis* to describe these situations. This actually refers to the processes which lead to the changes in pH.

Three major mechanisms homeostatically control blood pH:

- Buffers which offer a temporary solution to the production of acids
  - Intracellular: proteins, phosphates, and haemoglobin
  - Extracellular: proteins and bicarbonate
- Respiration
- Renal excretion

See Table 2.7 for normal arterial blood gas values in infants and children.

Buffers

The most important buffer is the carbonic acid–bicarbonate buffer system in which carbonic acid (H_2CO_3) is the weak acid and sodium bicarbonate ($NaHCO_3$) is the weak base. In solution dissociation occurs:

H_2CO_3	$\rightleftharpoons$	H^+	$+$	HCO_3^-
Carbonic acid		hydrogen		bicarbonate

$NaHCO_3$	$\rightleftharpoons$	Na^+	$+$	HCO_3^-
Sodium bicarbonate		sodium		bicarbonate

Table 2.7 Normal arterial blood gas values for neonates and children		
	Normal infant/child values	**Normal neonatal values**
pH	7.35–7.45	7.3–7.4
P_{CO_2} (kPa)	4.5–6.0 (35–45 mm Hg)	4.6–6.0 (35–45 mm Hg)
P_{O_2} (kPa)	10–13 (75–100 mm Hg)	7.3–12 (55–90 mm Hg)
Bicarbonate (mmol/L)	22–26	18–25
Base (mmol/L)	−2 to +2	−4 to + 4

If the blood becomes very acidic, sodium bicarbonate disassociates to buffer the acid, thus increasing concentration of carbonic acid and decreasing sodium bicarbonate, but the net result is an increase in pH (as carbonic acid is weak). If there is a strong base in the blood (i.e., the blood is alkaline), the concentration of sodium bicarbonate increases and carbonic acid is used up as the buffer.

Respiration

CO_2 is a waste product of metabolism. In the body, it behaves as an acid. Any increase in P_aCO_2 will increase production of H+ ions.

$$CO_2 + H_2O \leftrightarrow H_2CO_3 \leftrightarrow H^+ + HCO_3^-$$

If metabolic production is constant, what affects the amount of CO_2 in the blood is its removal by respiration. Any decrease in alveolar ventilation will cause a rise in P_aCO_2, a rise in H+ concentration, and what we describe as respiratory acidosis. Any increased alveolar ventilation eliminates CO_2 and less H_2CO_3 and H^+ are formed, increasing pH. This is described as respiratory alkalosis.

Renal secretion

Kidney tubular secretion helps control the pH of blood. If the pH of blood is acidic, there is increased secretion of H^+, which displaces another cation, usually Na^+, which then diffuses from the urine into the tubule cell where it combines with bicarbonate to form sodium bicarbonate, which then gets absorbed into the blood stream. Thus H^+ is lost from the body and the pH becomes less acidic (Tortora & Anagnostakos 1984).

Interpretation of blood gas analyses

The primary problem in an acid–base disorder is defined by its initiating process, which may be metabolic (changes in HCO_3) or respiratory (changes in P_aCO_2). A compensatory response describes the secondary physiologic response to the primary disturbance. Box 2.2 lists common causes of acidosis and alkalosis.

To interpret blood gas values (Resuscitation Council [UK] 2004):

- Assess oxygenation – is the child hypoxic?
- Assess pH
- Assess respiratory component
  - P_aCO_2 >6 kPa: respiratory acidosis (or renal compensation for a respiratory alkalosis)
  - P_aCO_2 <4.7 kPa: respiratory alkalosis (or respiratory compensation for a metabolic acidosis)
- Assess metabolic component
  - HCO_3 <22 mmol/L: metabolic acidosis (or renal compensation for a respiratory alkalosis)

Box 2.2 Common causes of acidosis and alkalosis

Respiratory acidosis
Any cause of hypoventilation:
- Obstructive airways disease (e.g., asthma)
- CNS depression (e.g., head injury, encephalitis)
- Neuromuscular disease (e.g., myasthenia gravis, Guillain–Barré syndrome)
- Artificial ventilation

Respiratory alkalosis
Any cause of hyperventilation:
- Psychogenic (e.g., hysteria, pain)
- Central (e.g., raised intracranial pressure, meningitis)
- Pulmonary (e.g., hypoxia, pulmonary embolus or oedema, pneumonia)
- Metabolic (e.g., fever, acute liver failure)
- Drugs (e.g., acute salicylate poisoning)
- Artificial ventilation

Metabolic acidosis
Normal anion gap:
- Intestinal losses (e.g., diarrhoea)
- Renal losses (e.g., renal tubular acidosis)
  - Excessive chloride administration or accumulation (Cl/Na >0.8)
Increased anion gap:
- Overproduction of organic acid (e.g., diabetic ketoacidosis, lactic acidosis)
- Decreased ability to conserve HCO_3 (e.g., chronic renal failure)
- Advanced salicylate, methanol, or ethylene glycol poisoning
- Inborn errors of metabolism (e.g., maple syrup urine disease)

Metabolic alkalosis
- Excess acid loss (e.g., persistent vomiting as in pyloric stenosis, low chloride relative to Na [Cl/Na ratio < 0.72])
- Diuretic therapy
- Excess intake of alkali

- HCO_3 >26 mmol/L: metabolic alkalosis (or renal compensation for a respiratory acidosis)
- Determine primary disturbance and whether there is any metabolic or respiratory compensation

Metabolic disturbances are compensated acutely by changes in ventilation and chronically by appropriate renal responses. Respiratory disturbances are compensated by renal tubular secretion of hydrogen.

In chronic conditions where $P\text{CO}_2$ is increased, there is renal compensation and retention of bicarbonate, with pH returning to near normal levels. Table 2.8 shows effects of acid-base disorders on pH, $P_a\text{CO}_2$, and HCO_3.

Anion gap

It may be useful to calculate the anion gap if the cause of a metabolic acidosis is not known. The anion gap is calculated as the difference

Table 2.8 Changes in pH, P_aco_2, and HCO_3 in acid-base disorders			
Acid-base disorder	**pH**	**P_aco_2**	**HCO_3**
Respiratory acidosis	↓	↑	N
Metabolic acidosis	↓	N	↓
Respiratory alkalosis	↑	↓	N
Metabolic alkalosis	↑	N	↑
Respiratory acidosis with renal compensation	↓*	↑	↑
Metabolic acidosis with respiratory compensation	↓*	↓	↓
Respiratory alkalosis with renal compensation	↑*	↓	↓
Metabolic alkalosis with respiratory compensation	↑*	↑	↑
Mixed metabolic and respiratory acidosis	↓	↑	↓
Mixed metabolic and respiratory alkalosis	↑	↓	↑

*If compensation is virtually complete, the pH may be in the normal range – overcompensation does not occur. *N*, normal.
Source: Resuscitation Council (UK), 2004. Acid–Base Balance: Interpreting Arterial Blood Gases. Advanced Life Support Manual, Appendix. Resuscitation Council (UK), London, p. 142.

between the sum of plasma sodium and potassium and the sum of plasma bicarbonate and chloride concentration:

Anion gap = (sodium + potassium) − (total bicarbonate + chloride).

The normal anion gap ranges from 5 to 12 mmol/L. A patient who has a metabolic acidosis with a normal anion gap will have lost base (e.g., with diarrhoea). A patient with a metabolic acidosis who has an increased anion gap will have gained acid (e.g., in ketoacidosis) (Hinds & Watson 1996).

 NB The anion gap will be underestimated with hypoalbuminaemia.

Stewart model (STRS 2016)

(www.evclinalondon.nhs.uk/resources/our-services/hospital/south-thames-retrieval-service/Acid-base-interpretation-2017.pdf)

In some circumstances it may not be possible to explain all the acid-base disturbances by changes in bicarbonate and base excess alone, especially in sick children when there are electrolyte and blood component problems as well. The Stewart strong ion pH methodology explains pH changes for three major buffer systems: (1) bicarbonate (2) electrolytes (NA, K, Cl, lactate, Ca and Mg), and (3) weak acids and phosphate.

In practice, in addition to looking at the standard acid-base measures, it is also useful to consider the role of sodium and chloride in a patient with metabolic acidosis. This can be simplified by calculating the base excess due to chloride and sodium.

Formula to base excess due to sodium and chloride = Na − Cl − 32

For example, if the base excess $= -10$ mEq/L and Na $=140$ and Cl $=113$, then $140 - 113 - 32 = -5$ mEq/L

Therefore the chloride is contributing to 5 mEq/L of the acid levels.

Another easy way to check if the chloride is contributing is to consider the **chloride to sodium ratio:**
- Normal chloride to sodium ratio $= 106/140 = 0.75$
- Chloride acidifying if ratio >0.80
- Chloride alkalising if ratio <0.72

High chloride to sodium ratio is usually due to administration of resuscitation with fluids that have a relatively high Cl content (e.g., 0.9% NaCl); this can be reduced by using fluids such as Hartmann, which has a lower concentration of chloride. Low chloride levels may be due to excessive loss of chloride (e.g., vomiting or use of diuretics).

SYSTEMATIC REVIEW OF CHEST X-RAY

This should include:
- Bones and soft tissues
- Mediastinum, including thymus
- Heart and great vessels
- Lungs
- Abdomen

See Fig. 2.2 chest x-ray interpretation and Figs 2.4, 2.5, 2.6 and 2.7 for striking abnormalities on chest x-ray.

Bones and soft tissue

Observe clavicles, ribs, scapulae, and vertebra – follow the edges of each bone to look for fractures or areas of calcification. Look for any enlargement of areas of soft tissue or vertebral abnormalities. Observe if there is any rib crowding, which could indicate atelectasis.

Mediastinum including thymus

The thymus is usually apparent on the chest x-ray until the age of approximately 2 years, although it may still be seen in older children up to 4 years (Schelvan et al 2002). It can typically be seen on both sides of the superior mediastinum, has a smooth lateral border, and blends inferiorly with the cardiac contour (although sometimes there is a little notch at the junction). The edge of the mediastinum should be clear, and a fuzzy edge may suggest consolidation or collapse in the adjacent lung field.

 Thymus is absent in DiGeorge syndrome.

The trachea should be central but deviates slightly to the right around the aortic knuckle. Check the position of the right and left main bronchi (splaying of the left bronchi could indicate left atrial enlargement).

Fig. 2.2 Chest x-ray interpretation. *AP*, Anteroposterior; *ETT*, endotracheal; *NG*, nasogastric tube; *PA*, posterioranterior. (Based on Corne, J., Carroll, M., Brown, I., Delany, D., 2002. Chest X-Ray Made Easy, second ed. Churchill Livingstone, London.)

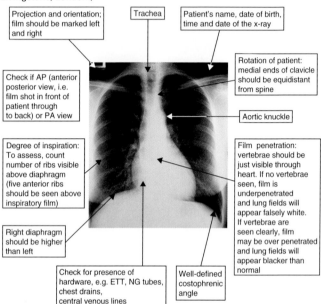

Projection and orientation; film should be marked left and right

Trachea

Patient's name, date of birth, time and date of the x-ray

Rotation of patient: medial ends of clavicle should be equidistant from spine

Check if AP (anterior posterior view, i.e. film shot in front of patient through to back) or PA view

Aortic knuckle

Degree of inspiration: To assess, count number of ribs visible above diaphragm (five anterior ribs should be seen above inspiratory film)

Film penetration: vertebrae should be just visible through heart. If no vertebrae seen, film is underpenetrated and lung fields will appear falsely white. If vertebrae are seen clearly, film may be over penetrated and lung fields will appear blacker than normal

Right diaphragm should be higher than left

Check for presence of hardware, e.g. ETT, NG tubes, chest drains, central venous lines

Well-defined costophrenic angle

Heart and great vessels

Assess the heart size. This should be approximately 50% of the cardio-thoracic ratio, but this is slightly increased in neonates. The heart is usually situated one-third on the right of the spine and two-thirds on the left.

 The thymic shadow may give a false impression of cardiomegaly in infants.

The right heart border on the x-ray is the right atrium of the heart. The left heart border comprises the aorta, the pulmonary arteries, the left atrium, and the right ventricle.

(An enlarged right ventricle in the heart may be observed on x-ray if the apex is uplifted. An enlarged left ventricle moves the apex left laterally towards the chest wall.)

Fig. 2.3 Diagram showing lung lobes and fissures.

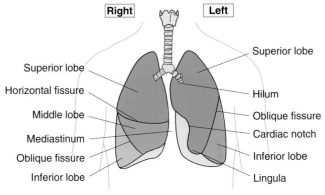

Right	**Left**
	Superior lobe
Superior lobe	
Horizontal fissure	Hilum
Middle lobe	Oblique fissure
Mediastinum	Cardiac notch
Oblique fissure	Inferior lobe
Inferior lobe	Lingula

Observe and note:
- Heart position and orientation
- Aortic arch orientation
- Size of heart
- Any enlarged chambers or vessels
- Perfusion of lung fields
- Congestion of lung fields
- Other findings (e.g., prosthesis – valves, stents, calcification)

SIGNS OF HEART FAILURE ON CHEST X-RAY

- Cardiomegaly
- Upper lobe venous equilibration
- Alveolar oedema – 'fluffy appearance'
- Hepatomegaly
- Fluid in fissures and pleural effusions sometimes present.

 Cardiomegaly may not just indicate cardiac failure. You may also need to consider cardiomyopathy, Ebstein anomaly, and pericardial effusions.

Lungs

Lung fields should appear black in colour, which indicates the presence of air except for the pulmonary vessel markings. The lung fields should be of equal translucency. See Fig. 2.3 for lung anatomy.
- Identify the horizontal fissures.
- Check lung volumes – if asymmetric, consider inhalation of a foreign body, or if hyperinflated, consider bronchiolitis in a baby or asthma in an older child.

- Observe for any focal pathology (e.g., mediastinal mass, consolidation, or collapse).
- Observe for any diffuse abnormality (e.g., pulmonary oedema or fibrosis).
- Observe for pulmonary shadows within lung tissue – look for symmetry (i.e., reticular nodular appearance [interstitial fluid]), look for reduced pulmonary markings that could indicate bullae (ringlike appearance).
- Observe for extrapulmonary shadows (i.e., outside lung tissue, pleural effusion, pneumothorax, empyema [loculated white areas]).

The right diaphragm should be higher than the left diaphragm (<3 cm). The costophrenic angles should be acute, well-defined angles, and if the cardiophrenic angles (adjacent heart border) are fuzzy and indistinct, consider that the adjacent area of lung has collapse/consolidation.

Abdomen

- Check the position of all visible abdominal organs on the x-ray (e.g., for situs solitus).
- Check for the gastric air bubble.
- Look for air under the diaphragm or obviously dilated loops of bowel.

Striking abnormalities on chest x-ray – what to look out for

Fig. 2.4 Consolidation

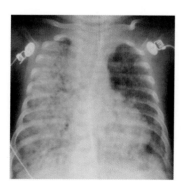

Fig. 2.4 This is a term used to describe lung tissue where air-filled spaces are replaced by products of disease (e.g., water, pus, mucus, or blood). **Radiologic findings:** shadowing with ill-defined markings, air bronchograms, silhouette sign (where the border of a structure is lost by consolidation), no volume loss.

Fig. 2.5 Atelectasis

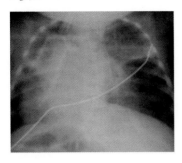

Fig. 2.5 This refers to a loss of aeration in the lung, which leads to collapse. It is not usually an infective process but may be caused by a foreign body, aspiration, tumour or mucous plug. **Radiologic findings:** crowding of ribs, shift of mediastinum usually toward the white lung field, elevation of the hemidiaphragm, compensatory hyperinflation.

Fig. 2.6 Pleural effusion

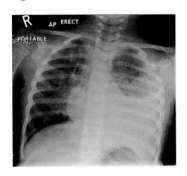

Fig. 2.6 This refers to fluid in the pleural space. **Radiologic findings:** will be different in erect and supine films; the effusion will be white in colour and a visible meniscus may be present. Look for air bronchograms as this finding may lead you to suspect consolidation rather than effusion. An absence of mediastinal shift suggests an effusion but collapse with an effusion can occur with some mediastinal shift.

Fig. 2.7 Pneumothorax

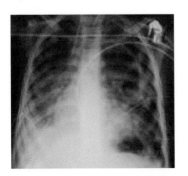

Fig. 2.7 This refers to air within the pleural space. **Radiologic findings:** black area with loss of vascular markings to the pleural edge.

Fig. 2.8 Tension pneumothorax

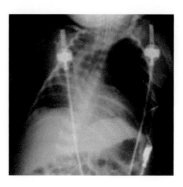

Fig. 2.8 If air enters the pleural space during inspiration and cannot leave during expiration, this will lead to a rapid increase in pressure and a life-threatening tension pneumothorax. **Radiologic findings:** a hyperlucent *(black)* lung field with a complete absence of vascular markings on that side, shift of mediastinum to the opposite side and flattening of the ipsilateral diaphragm.

Life-threatening tension pneumothorax requires immediate intervention – placing a large-bore cannula in the second intercostal space in the midclavicular line on the side of the pneumothorax then following this up with a pleural drain. It does not need an x-ray urgently; it requires intervention first.

LUNG PERFUSION

An x-ray must be normally penetrated to be able to see if lungs are underperfused or overperfused. In a normally penetrated x-ray, vertebrae should be visible through the cardiac silhouette but not through the liver. Underperfused lung fields are blacker to the edge (oligaemic). Overperfused lung fields have increased vessel markings to the peripheries (hyperaemic).

MEANS AND METHODS OF OXYGEN DELIVERY

This can be divided into high- or low–flow methods. See Table 2.9 demonstrating oxygen concentration versus flow rates.

Low flow

Mask (e.g., Venturi) can give wide range of concentrations, from 35% to 60% oxygen with a flow rate of 6–10 L/min. The inspired oxygen can reach only 60% because air mixes with oxygen through the exhalation ports in the side of the mask. A minimum flow of 6 L/min must be used to maintain an increased oxygen concentration to prevent rebreathing of exhaled carbon dioxide.

Nasal cannula: A maximum flow rate of 2 L/min is usually prescribed because higher flow rates will irritate the nasopharynx. However, this could vary up to 4 L/min according to manufacturers' instructions.

Table 2.9 Oxygen concentration versus flow rates	
Oxygen concentration (%)	**Oxygen flow (litres)**
28	4–5
31	6
35	8
40	9
60	10

High flow

- Paediatric HFNC oxygen therapy (e.g. Optiflow and Vapotherm) may be indicated in mild to moderate respiratory failure. This may be secondary to bronchiolitis or pneumonia. It has been used in asthma and post extubation on PICU. It is contraindicated in severe respiratory failure, recurrent apnoeas, upper airway obstruction, basal skull fracture, epistaxis or in the presence of an air leak and must be used with caution in the presence of trauma or surgery to the nasopharynx (Brink et al 2013).

SETTING UP OPTIFLOW

Optiflow is a non-invasive therapy which delivers warmed, humidified high-flow air/oxygen mix via nasal cannula.

- To select Junior mode, you must see the 'warm-up' or 'ready for use' symbol to activate. Hold the mode button for 5 seconds. The butterfly/bird icon indicates you are in Junior mode – which limits the settings to a temperature of 34°C and flow of 2–25 L/min.
- Ensure the Optiflow unit is placed on a flat surface BELOW the level of the patient's head. Install humidifying chamber and tubing
- Select correct size nasal cannula and note maximum flow rates for each cannula:

Neonatal size (weight 2–8 kg) – maximum flow rate 8 L/min
Infant size (weight 3–15 kg) – maximum flow rate 20 L/min
Paediatric size (weight 12–22 kg) – maximum flow rate 25 L/min
Adult small – flow rates 10–50 L/min in adult mode

Ensure that the nasal cannula does not fill the nares, but there should be clear space around to allow for expiratory airflow.

Follow local protocols for initiating Optiflow but flows are often commenced on 1–2 L/min.

- Connect oxygen supply if required to the inlet port on the back of the unit. Oxygen flow settings should be titrated to the child's S_aO_2. According to the manufacturer:
  - An oxygen flow rate of 1 L/min with Optiflow of 10 L/min will provide at least 29% oxygen when using an oxygen source as opposed to a home oxygen concentrator.
  - Oxygen flow rate 4 L/min with Optiflow of 10 L/min provides at least 53% oxygen.

- Oxygen flow rate of 4 L/min with Optiflow of 25 L/min will provide at least 34% oxygen.
- Oxygen flow rate of 10 L/min with Optiflow of 25 L/min will provide at least 54% oxygen.

For Optiflow rates <10 L/min, the oxygen fraction varies significantly with very small changes to oxygen flow rates but the manufacturer does not quantify this.

See Figs 2.9 and 2.10 for setup diagram and interpretation of alarms on unit Also see www.fphcare.co.uk for educational videos for fitting Junior Cannula for Optiflow.

Fig. 2.9 H.E.L.P.K.I.D.S. intubation guideline side A. *BAL*, Bronchiolar lavage; *ETT*, endotracheal; *NG*, nasogastric tube.

Intubation Pathway – H.E.L.P.K.I.D.S. - Side A

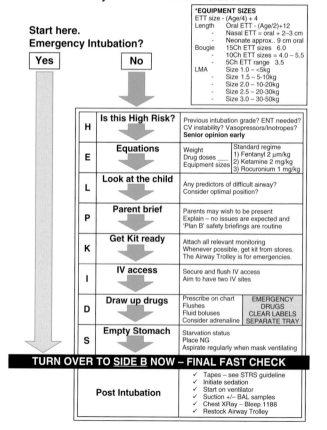

Start here.
Emergency Intubation?

| Yes | | No |

*EQUIPMENT SIZES
ETT size - (Age/4) + 4
Length   Oral ETT - (Age/2)+12
  - Nasal ETT = oral + 2–3 cm
  - Neonate approx.. 9 cm oral
Bougie   15Ch ETT sizes 6.0
  - 10Ch ETT sizes = 4.0 – 5.5
  - 5Ch ETT range 3.5
LMA   Size 1.0 – <5kg
  - Size 1.5 – 5-10kg
  - Size 2.0 – 10-20kg
  - Size 2.5 – 20-30kg
  - Size 3.0 – 30-50kg

H	**Is this High Risk?**	Previous intubation grade? ENT needed? CV instability? Vasopressors/Inotropes? **Senior opinion early**
E	**Equations**	Weight ___ Drug doses ___ Equipment sizes ___ Standard regime 1) Fentanyl 2 µm/kg 2) Ketamine 2 mg/kg 3) Rocuronium 1 mg/kg
L	**Look at the child**	Any predictors of difficult airway? Consider optimal position?
P	**Parent brief**	Parents may wish to be present Explain – no issues are expected and 'Plan B' safety briefings are routine
K	**Get Kit ready**	Attach all relevant monitoring Whenever possible, get kit from stores. The Airway Trolley is for emergencies.
I	**IV access**	Secure and flush IV access Aim to have two IV sites
D	**Draw up drugs**	Prescribe on chart Flushes Fluid boluses Consider adrenaline EMERGENCY DRUGS CLEAR LABELS SEPARATE TRAY
S	**Empty Stomach**	Starvation status Place NG Aspirate regularly when mask ventilating

TURN OVER TO <u>SIDE B</u> NOW – FINAL FAST CHECK

Post Intubation	✓ Tapes – see STRS guideline ✓ Initiate sedation ✓ Start on ventilator ✓ Suction +/– BAL samples ✓ Chest XRay – Bleep 1188 ✓ Restock Airway Trolley

Fig. 2.10 H.E.L.P.K.I.D.S. intubation guideline side B. *ETT*, Endotracheal tube; *PICU*, paediatric intensive care.

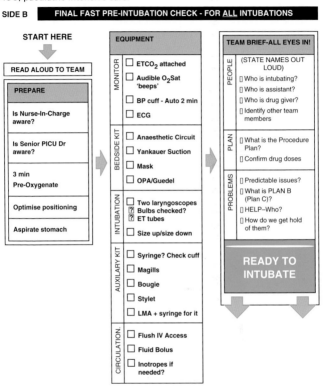

INTUBATION

Intubation of critically ill children may occur in PICU, in theatre, or in other areas, including the ward or the emergency department. Intubation algorithms have been developed to manage anticipated or unanticipated difficult airways (APA DAS 2015). These were primarily designed for the theatre environment and may not always reflect intubation in other areas. There is evidence both in adults and children that the incidence of difficult and failed intubation is higher in intensive care than in theatre environments (Cook et al 2011; Graciano et al 2014). It is therefore very important to plan carefully around time of intubation. Clear communication between all members of the team is vital.

In children younger than 8 years, uncuffed ETT tubes are usually the first choice. However, low-pressure, high-volume cuffed tubes are increasingly being used both in the theatre and PICU environments. A cuff tube may be chosen preferentially if a leak could interfere with ventilation (e.g., ARDS or acute severe asthma). A cuffed tube may be chosen to limit the number of instrumentations of the airway to find the correct size of ETT. If a cuffed tube is used, the cuff should be inflated with 0.2 mL of air initially and then inflated to the minimum to abolish leaks up to 20 cm H_2O. The cuff pressure should be checked using a pressure monitor to ensure that the pressure is not too high. Overinflation or a cuff in the wrong position in the airway may cause airway trauma.

Emergency checklist for intubation – step by step

HELPKIDS is a mnemonic to assist in the safe process of intubation. It is a pathway and emergency checklist providing a safe guide for the intubation of infants and children. It was devised by doctors Matt Edwards and Tom Breen and is used with permission.

> NB Position patient and preoxygenate in 100% oxygen for a few minutes. The exceptions to this will be neonates with congenital heart lesions that lead to potential pulmonary overcirculation. In these patients apply a percentage of oxygen (21%–100%) to achieve saturations in 70–80%.

See Box 2.3 for intubation equipment

Box 2.3   Equipment required for oral intubation
<ul><li>Laryngoscope and appropriate blade:<ul><li>Neonate – small (size 0–1) straight or curved blade</li><li>Young child – small (size 1–2) curved blade</li><li>Older child – large (size 2–3) curved blade</li></ul></li><li>Have alternative blade types and sizes available in case of difficult intubation</li><li>Magill forceps, appropriate size</li><li>Yankauer sucker and suction – to gauge appropriate size: size of ET tube used ×2 = French gauge of catheter required</li><li>Anaesthetic circuit or Ambu bag – appropriate size</li><li>Oxygen supply with oxygen flowing</li><li>Introducer stylet: S, M or L and bougie</li><li>ET tube and end tidal carbon dioxide detector<ul><li>Correct size+</li><li>Spare tube of same size+</li><li>Spare tube one size smaller and one size larger</li><li>Consider using a cuffed tube if high airway pressure required and leak to be avoided</li></ul></li><li>Catheter mount connector attaches from end of ET tube to rebreathe or ventilator circuit</li><li>Nasogastric tube</li><li>Assorted tapes if oral intubation+<ul><li>DuoDERM to protect skin</li></ul></li><li>Drugs prior to intubation according to prescription</li><li>Drugs for resuscitation and fluids in unstable patient.</li></ul>

ET, Endotracheal.

Box 2.4 shows common intubation drugs.

Box 2.5 shows the formula for selecting the correct size ET tube (or see front cover for additional guide).

Capnography

Capnography displays a respiratory waveform representing the profile of expiratory $P\mathrm{CO_2}$ over time with a numerical value for end-tidal CO_2. An infrared sensor is placed between the ET tube and the ventilator tubing, and this analyses the expired CO_2 at the mouth and can be used to monitor trends of alveolar ventilation and CO_2 elimination. The amount of CO_2 expired may not accurately match alveolar CO_2 because of the mixing of alveolar air with dead space. Factors that change the dead space will affect the $P\mathrm{CO_2}$ and end-tidal CO_2 gradient (Laker 2003).

Capnography is useful to determine that the ET tube is correctly placed and the position maintained, particularly on patient transfers. The typical shape of a capnograph waveform (Fig. 2.11) has four distinct phases:

- Phase 1: End inspiration
- Phase 2: Exhalation of dead space in trachea and large airways

---

Box 2.4   Common drug doses used for intubation (check local policy)

Fentanyl 1–2 µg/kg
Ketamine 1–2 mg/kg
Rocuronium 0.6–1 mg/kg
Atracurium 0.3–0.6 mg/kg
Morphine 0.1 mg/kg
Etomidate 0.3 mg/kg
Propofol 1–2.5 mg/kg
Thiopentone 2–5 mg/kg

Box 2.5   Formula for calculating endotracheal tube requirements

ETT diameter <3 kg: 3.0
ETT diameter birth to 1 year: 3.5
ETT diameter >1 years: age/4 + 4
   • Use ½ size smaller if cuffed tube preferred
ETT length (oral) >1 year: age/2 +12
ETT length (nasal) >1 year: age/2 +15

ETT, Endotracheal tube.

Fig. 2.11 Typical capnograph waveform.

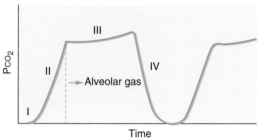

- Phase 3: Alveolar gas
- Phase 4: Early inspiration – fresh gas over sensor (Gravenstein et al 1989)

Interpreting ventilatory function using capnography – examples/ troubleshooting

Oesophageal intubation/tracheal extubation (Fig. 2.12)
This may initially show the presence of CO_2, particularly if the patient has been bag–mask ventilated, but the waveform will diminish then disappear because no CO_2 will be eliminated across the sensor.

Fig. 2.12 Oesophageal intubation/tracheal extubation.

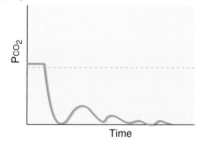

Sawtooth formation = obstructive airways, acute respiratory distress syndrome, asthma (Fig. 2.13)
If the waveform changes from a normal waveform to this, then auscultation will be required to determine whether bronchospasm or secretions are present. Patency of ET tube and ventilator tubing should also be checked (Laker 2003).

Fig. 2.13 Sawtooth formation = obstructive airways.

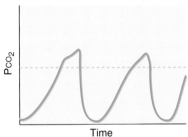

Waveform not returning to baseline (Fig. 2.14)
This indicates rebreathing CO_2. Check expiratory valve not waterlogged or incompetent, which may be preventing expired CO_2 from escaping.

Fig. 2.14 Waveform not returning to baseline.

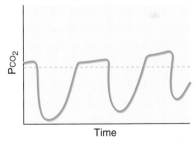

Hypoventilation (Fig. 2.15)
Hypoventilation following bicarbonate injection (i.e., rising CO_2).

Fig. 2.15 Hypoventilation.

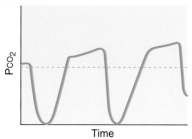

Hyperventilation (Fig. 2.16)
Gradual fall with preservation of waveform, or decreasing CO (i.e., hypovolaemic state).

Fig. 2.16 Hyperventilation.

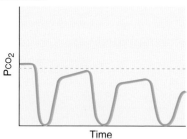

Sudden absence of any waveform (Fig. 2.17)
Check airway disconnection, total obstruction of ET tube or displaced tube, loss of CO.

Fig. 2.17 Sudden absence of any waveform.

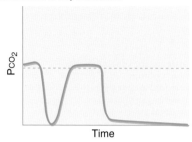

Sudden decrease in waveform amplitude (Fig. 2.18)
Possible kinked or partially occluded ET tube.

Fig. 2.18 Sudden decrease in waveform amplitude.

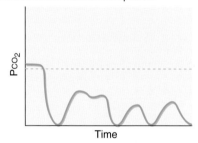

Irregular cleft in waveform (Fig. 2.19)
This could indicate interbreathing (i.e., if paralysis is wearing off or trigger sensitivity in support mode is set too low) (Laker 2003).

Fig. 2.19 Irregular cleft in waveform.

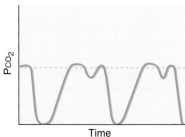

VENTILATION AND DEFINITION OF TERMS

- **Ventilation** is the process of movement of gas between the lungs and the ambient air.
- **Tidal volume** is the volume of gas that is inspired and expired in one normal breath (6 mL/kg).
- **Minute volume** is the quantity of gas expired by the lungs in 1 minute: minute volume = tidal volume × frequency.
- **Functional residual capacity** is the amount of gas that remains in the lungs after normal expiration.
- **The anatomic dead space** (approximately 30% of each tidal volume) fills the conducting airways and no gas exchange takes place there.

INDICATIONS FOR ASSISTED VENTILATION

Apnoea, respiratory distress with either poor oxygenation or increasing P_{CO_2}.

MODES OF VENTILATION

Noninvasive ventilation

Ventilation delivered via nasal mask, nasal pillows, face mask, or mouthpiece is called noninvasive ventilation (NIV). Ventilation may be CPAP or biphasic positive airway pressure (BiPAP).

Although there are comprehensive guidelines from the British Thoracic Society regarding NIV in the adult population, the guidance in children is more limited. However, some of the principles may also be applied to the paediatric population. Guidance has been produced for the use of NIV in children with neuromuscular weakness (British Thoracic Society Respiratory Management of Children with Neuromuscular Weakness Guideline Group 2012). In addition, many paediatric hospitals have developed guidance in this area.

CONTINUOUS POSITIVE AIRWAY PRESSURE

CPAP via nasal prongs or a mask. This is designed to reduce the work of breathing by providing active assistance on both inspiratory and expiratory phases of the respiratory cycle. (This differs from PEEP, which provides positive end-expiratory pressure only.) CPAP restores functional residual capacity and allows normal breathing with normal pressures.

BIPHASIC/BILEVEL POSITIVE AIRWAY PRESSURE

Biphasic positive airway pressure is noninvasive, intermittent, positive-pressure–assisted ventilation that can either be triggered by the patient or fully controlled.

BiPAP can give two levels of respiratory support, CPAP, sometimes known as expiratory positive airway pressure (EPAP), and inspiratory positive airway pressure (IPAP).

CONTINUOUS POSITIVE AIRWAY PRESSURE/EXPIRATORY POSITIVE AIRWAY PRESSURE

- Helps to keep airways open
- Improves alveolar gas exchange
- Improves oxygenation
- Increases lung volume.

INSPIRATORY POSITIVE AIRWAY PRESSURE

- Supports inspiratory effort and decreases work of breathing
- Improves tidal volumes
- Improves CO_2 removal.

INDICATIONS

- Respiratory failure with hypoxia and/or hypercarbia
- To maintain upper airway patency (e.g., in tracheomalacia)
- To prevent intubation and ventilation or planned as step down from mechanical ventilation
- Cardiovascular support
  Selecting the appropriate mask is vital to the success of NIV. Mask types include:
- **Nasal mask** – Use the size gauge to measure for the correct mask. Aim for the smallest fitting mask without sacrificing length from the bridge of the nose. Nasal masks can be used as full-face masks on small children.
- **Full-face masks** – This should fit from the bridge of the nose to just below the bottom lip. Use the foam spacer to attach to the top of the mask to bridge the gap from the forehead to the upright strut of the mask. Alternative designs also include larger full-face masks, which cover all of the forehead, full-head masks, and helmet masks.
  There is now a large range of devices that can be used to deliver both CPAP and bilevel ventilation. Each will have different modes of operation.

SETTING UP BILEVEL POSITIVE AIRWAY PRESSURE

BiPAP is a noninvasive, pressure-controlled ventilation therapy which allows unrestricted spontaneous breathing and is delivered via an orofacial mask. It may be instituted to avoid intubation and ventilation or as a weaning tool following extubation.
  Contraindications include:
- Airway obstruction
- Base of skull fractures
- Undrained pneumothorax
- Bowel obstruction/abdominal distension
- Decreased level of consciousness
- Haemodynamic instability
- Excessive secretions or vomiting
- Severe hypoxia or hypercapnia

- Combative or uncooperative patient
- Recent facial surgery, burns or trauma, or facial shape that does not allow a good seal on facial mask

Setting up BiPAP:
- Position patient appropriately
- Explain to the child and family about NIV
- Apply hydrocolloid dressing (e.g., DuoDERM) to areas in contact with the mask to protect the face in vulnerable areas (e.g., bridge of nose, ears)
- Select nasal or full-face mask – Use full-face mask for pressure support ≥10 cm H_2O. Remove the mask every few hours for pressure area checks. Ensure head strap/bonnet is correctly orientated
- Ensure NG tube in situ for ALL patients
- Hold the mask to the child's face for first few breaths, remove and repeat. Then when child is comfortable, hold the mask on for a few minutes of initiating NIV. Then once child is comfortable and no longer frightened, apply the bonnet or head straps. Check for leaks, but reassure family that the exhalation port must be kept clear (because they may be concerned that this is a leak)
- Stay with child to ensure that he or she is able to tolerate and synchronise with NIV – discuss with medical team if mild sedation may be helpful
- Monitor RR, HR, BP, saturations – sometimes ABG may be used to evaluate
- Observe child closely for signs of fatigue/agitation/increasing work of breathing/sweating and report to medical staff and have a plan B ready in case of NIV failure
  See Table 2.10.

Table 2.10 Suggested starting parameters for noninvasive ventilation	
Mode	**Pressure support/pressure control**
IPAP	5–12 cm H_2O (start low for anxious children and slowly increase)
EPAP	4–5 cm H_2O
Insp time if using pressure control mode	0.4–0.8 s depending on spontaneous rate
Backup rate	5 breaths/min below normal patient rate
F_iO_2	As required to maintain saturations >90%
Trigger	Insp and Exp trigger set to 4 (default setting)
Flow alarms	High alarm 20% max flow recorded at peak pressure
	Low alarm 20% below min recorded at peak pressure

EPAP, Expiratory positive airways pressure; *Exp*, expiratory; *Insp*, inspiratory; *IPAP*, inspiratory positive airways pressure.

Changing NIV Settings –
- If P_{CO_2} ↑, then ↑ IPAP by 2–4 cm H_2O (limit of 25 cm H_2O)
- If P_{O_2} <9 and F_iO_2 >0.5, then ↑ EPAP by 2–3 cm H_2O (limit 10 cm H_2O)

Changes to NIV settings should be made on clinical observation.
Adjust alarm parameters once the flow is established.
Stop if the following occurs:
- Inability to maintain a patent airway
  - Worsening encephalopathy or agitation or inability to clear secretions
  - Worsening oxygenation
- Progressive hypercapnia because patient will need further assessment and possible intubation and ventilation, or
- If the child's condition has improved, then intolerance of BiPAP may indicate that it is no longer required
- Haemodynamic instability

Invasive ventilatory modes via tracheal intubation or tracheotomy

There are many modes of ventilation that can be used in a child requiring ventilatory assistance.

A simple way to look at ventilation is to identify:

1. The control mode

Pressure control ventilation (PCV) is where the inspiratory pressure is chosen, flow is decelerating, and volume is variable. Volume (flow) control ventilation (VCV) is where tidal volume and flow are set and airway pressure is variable. A question may be asked, 'Which is better?' although each control mode has slightly different attributes, for example:

- PCV
  - Alveolar pressure is limited
  - Peak airway pressures will be lower for a given tidal volume
  - For a given peak airway pressure, mean airway pressure (MAP) is higher
  - May be improved distribution of ventilation
- VCV
  - Less variation in tidal volume
  - In vigorous patient inspiratory effort, pleural pressure drops significantly and the transpulmonary pressure may be high with PCV

There is no clear evidence that favours one mode of ventilation over another.

2. The mode of triggering of breaths – this is either the patient or the ventilator (i.e., spontaneous or mandatory)

If it is patient controlled, then the ventilator responds to a change in flow or pressure.

3. The mode of cycling between inspiration and expiration

This depends on the mode of triggering breaths. If breaths are mandatory, then cycling will be time cycled in PCV and volume cycled in VCV. In spontaneous supported breaths (e.g., PSV), they are flow cycled and expiration usually starts at 25%–30% of peak inspiratory flow.

4. Synchrony

This is the agreement between the patient's own (neural) and the ventilator (mechanical) inspiratory and expiratory times and includes the matching of patient effort with delivered tidal volume. This is different between different modes of ventilation. When we compare mandatory modes versus pressure support modes (i.e., synchronised intermittent mandatory ventilation [SIMV] vs. PS/BiPAP), they are identical in a passive patient. In an active patient, patient ventilator interaction in expiration is the same. However, during inspiration, patient effort in SIMV mode is unrecognised, whereas in PS/BiPAP the patient can breathe throughout inspiration.

POSITIVE END-EXPIRATORY PRESSURE

- Increases functional residual capacity(FRC) and maintains lung recruitment
- Improves alveolar ventilation
- Increases arterial oxygen content
- Increases intrathoracic pressure and may impede systemic venous return and thus CO
- High PEEP (i.e., >8) may impede cerebral venous return, which may increase intracranial pressure

OTHER MODES OF VENTILATION

Neurally adjusted ventilator assist

In an ideal world, a ventilator would respond to a signal generated in the respiratory centres of the brain and ensure complete synchrony between patient and ventilator. Neurally adjusted ventilator assist (NAVA) uses diaphragm electrical activity (EAdi) to control the timing and level of assist delivered. It is therefore proportional to the level of activity of the patient's respiratory muscles. An oesophageal array of electrodes mounted on an NG feeding tube detects and quantifies electrical activity in the diaphragm. A signal processing unit enhances the signal to noise ratio, and this is transferred to the ventilator unit to regulate ventilator support. Because the ventilator is triggered directly by EAdi, synchrony between neural and mechanical inspiratory time is guaranteed. EAdi proceeds muscle contraction, as well as pressure flow and volume generation. The signal should not be delayed or dampened by altered respiratory mechanics, PEEP, or air leaks. NAVA relies on intact respiratory centres, phrenic nerves and neuromuscular junctions, and on ventilatory drive not being suppressed by drugs. The amount of support provided by NAVA should correspond to demand.

Positioning of the NAVA catheter is very important to ensure effective operation. There is evidence that it improves patient–ventilator interactions and increases respiratory variability. NAVA reduces the problem of overventilation, including the risks or ineffective or missed inspiratory efforts due to rapid frequency and small tidal volumes in paediatric patients. However, more work is needed to determine optimum time to wean NAVA and to assess patient comfort and dyspnoea on NAVA. NAVA has also been used in conjunction with NIV (Teriz et al 2012).

SETTING UP NEURALLY ADJUSTED VENTILATOR ASSIST

See www.maquet.com for information and online training.
- The respiratory centre in the brain sends an electrical impulse to the diaphragm via the phrenic nerve, exciting the diaphragm.
- This signal is captured by the NAVA probe (transoesophageal placement). See Figs 2.20, 2.21 and 2.22 which show the NAVA probe and placement.
- The Servo-I ventilator is used to provide pressure-supported breaths proportionally to the strength of the electrical signal See Fig. 2.23 for the NAVA screen on the ventilator.

The NAVA level is set by the medical team. It is representative of the amount of ventilatory support that will be given to the patient. The higher the NAVA level, the more support the patient will receive for each microvolt of diaphragmatic electrical activity. This results in the patient receiving an amount of support that is directly proportional to the level of diaphragmatic activity.

Brain wants a bigger breath

↓

Sends more signals to the diaphragm

↓

Diaphragm has a high amount of electrical activity

↓

Higher electrical activity results in higher measurement of Edi

↓

This high Edi is multiplied by the constant NAVA level to assess the amount of pressure required

↓

A higher pressure and hence bigger breath is delivered to the patient

The inspiratory pressure delivered by the ventilator is:
Inspiratory pressure/PIP (cm H_2O above PEEP) = NAVA level × electrical activity of the diaphragm (Edi)
Edi is measured in microvolts. Edi peak demonstrates active contraction of the diaphragm. Edi minimum demonstrates resting state of the diaphragm.
Normal Edi ranges:
Neonates – Edi peak 5–15, Edi minimum 2–4

Fig. 2.20 The Edi catheter: A single-use gastric feeding tube with an array of 10 electrodes. One is a reference electrode, and the remaining 9 are measuring electrodes. The electrodes are made of stainless steel. Interelectrode distance (IED) is the distance between two measuring electrodes. Only 12- and 16-Fr Edi catheters have an evacuation lumen.

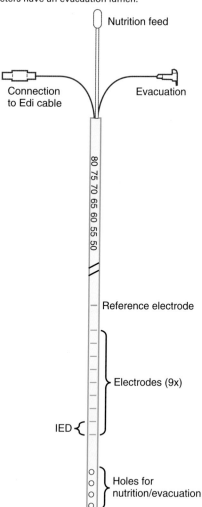

Fig. 2.21 To capture the Edi signal, an Edi catheter is inserted via the oesophagus. The Edi signal is measured 62.5 times a second.

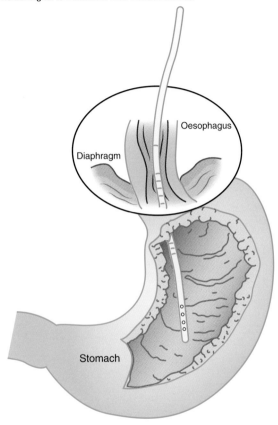

Child – Edi peak 5–10 (>20 indicates patient is working too hard) (Increased Edi amplitude on inspiration indicates a greater inspiratory effort.) NAVA is not affected by leaks.

COMMENCING NEURALLY ADJUSTED VENTILATOR ASSIST

1. Set peak airway pressure alarm to 35 to protect against barotrauma.
2. Start patient on NAVA level of 2, or NAVA level that will ensure that the pressure delivered is the same as, or slightly lower than, the set pressure support level.
   (NAVA level of 1 can indicate patient ready for extubation.)

Fig. 2.22 Edi catheter positioning. (A) Open the 'Neural access' menu. (B) Select 'Edi Catheter positioning.' 1 = Edi deflections, 2 = Blue highlights. The catheter is in the correct position if the middle two wave forms are coloured blue. If the top two are blue, the catheter needs to be pulled back. If the bottom two are blue, the catheter needs to be descended further.

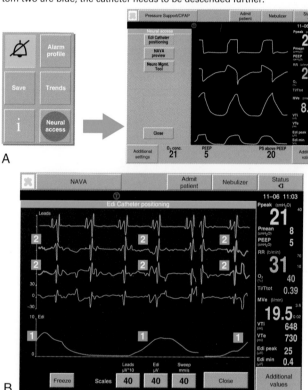

3. Assess the patients' respiratory effort and efficacy and observe Edi measurements.
4. If Edi peak is too high, increase NAVA level to reduce work of breathing. If Edi peak is too low, reduce NAVA level.
5. If Edi minimum is too high, increase PEEP, but if Edi minimum is too low, decrease the PEEP.
6. Pressure limit must be set on the ventilator as the combination of NAVA support and high EADi peaks may lead to excessive peak inspiration pressures. The NAVA mode will not deliver PIP above the

Fig. 2.23 The neurally adjusted ventilator assist (NAVA) screen. Important values to note are: NAVA level *(bottom right)*, F$_i$O$_2$ *(bottom left)*, positive end-expiratory pressure (PEEP) *(bottom centre)*, peak *(top right)* – this value is dependent on the level of Edi; therefore take a rough average of the values, peak alarm value/cut off (small number to the top right of the peak) – setting this value can be used to wean patients, Vti (in the centre of the right-hand side of the screen) Insp tidal volumes, Edi peak (on the right-hand side toward the bottom) – take a rough average.

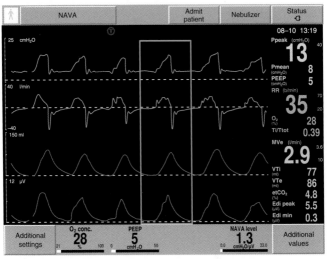

limit; if the ventilator is continuously reaching the set limit with each breath (i.e., PIP too high), it may be necessary to increase the pressure limit if safe to do so, or switch to another mode of ventilation to provide adequate respiratory support without causing lung injury.

WEANING NEURALLY ADJUSTED VENTILATOR ASSIST

1. The patient may be ready to wean NAVA support when the Edi signal and peak pressure reduces, but check this has not occurred as a result of a sedation bolus.
2. NAVA levels should be decreased by 0.1–0.2 cm H$_2$O/microvolt increments.

Record mode, PIP, PEEP, MAP, PS, NAVA level, Edi Max, Edi Min and Trigger.

How can we assess if conventional ventilation is failing, and what other options have we?

Protective lung ventilation is the current standard of care for mechanical ventilation. There is evidence for its use in ARDS, trauma, sepsis, and post high-risk surgery. It aims to maintain plateau pressures <30 cm H_2O and sets tidal volumes of 4–8 mL/kg. It may be combined with an 'open-lung' strategy in ARDS, which uses higher PEEP and recruitment manoeuvres and permissive hypercapnia, where the hypercarbia is tolerated as long as the pH remains >7.2 (Serpa et al 2012). This strategy may need to be modified in children with asthma to prevent dynamic hyperinflation.

HIGH–FREQUENCY VENTILATION

There are four main types, but HFOV will be discussed in more detail because it is most commonly used.

HFOV uses small tidal volumes 0.5–4 mL/kg delivered at high frequencies (3–15 Hz) with an oscillatory pump. It maintains constant lung recruitment and aims to prevent lung injury from overdistention and loss of recruitment. Advantages of HFOV include a decreased risk of ventilator-associated lung injury, dissociation between oxygenation and carbon dioxide clearance, and mobilisation of secretion.

There are a number of proposed mechanisms of gas exchange in HFOV:
- Pendelluft mixing
- Augmented diffusion
- Taylor dispersion
- Coaxial flow patterns
- Cardiogenic mixing

Oxygenation is influenced by MAP (cm H_2O), F_iO_2, and amplitude to some degree. Elimination of CO_2 is influenced by amplitude (ΔP), frequency and, to a much smaller extent, MAP. Oscillatory amplitude (difference between peak and trough pressure) directly determines tidal volumes delivered.

The MAP and ΔP are significantly attenuated as they pass down the ET tube, particularly in the smaller sized ET tubes. Frequencies of 10–15 Hz are most often used in neonates and infants (= 600–900 breaths per minute, with higher frequencies being more lung protective).

Indications for HFOV may include:
- Primary treatment in ARDS or preferentially used in some neonatal units
  - Rescue following failure of conventional ventilation. This can be oxygenation failure despite high F_iO_2 and high PEEP or ventilation failure and inability to clear CO_2 leading to a pH <7.25 with tidal volumes 6 mL/kg and a plateau pressure >30 cm H_2O
- Air leak syndromes (i.e., pneumothorax)

Considerations and contraindications:
- Alternative means or treating respiratory failure available and preferred (e.g., ECMO)
- Severe airflow obstruction
- Intracranial hypertension
- Cardiovascular instability is more common due to high MAP
- Requirement for heavy sedation and paralysis

Recent randomized controlled trails in the adult population have not demonstrated any benefit (Ferguson et al 2013; Young et al 2013), and one trial (OSCILLATE) had a higher mortality in the HFOV group. A recent prospective snapshot of HFOV use in paediatrics over several continents found a trend to use settings that generated higher HFOV frequencies and amplitudes compared with historical data (Rettig et al 2015). Patients who have failed conventional ventilation may be candidates for ECMO, so this should also be considered.

It is important to recognise that the HFOV can be used in many different ways and that a specific strategy should be developed on an individual patient basis when managing specific pathologies. There are several essential factors to be considered when determining the HFO strategy, and these are:

- Air leak
- Pulmonary hypertension
- Impaired cardiac performance

The clinician must also consider the current MAP on conventional ventilation, disease pathology, and inflation of lung fields.

If SensorMedics Oscillator is used, ensure the right ventilator is selected according to patient weight:

Sensormedics HFOV 3100A – neonatal and up to 35 kg
Sensormedics HFOV 3100B – use in patients greater than 35 kg

Ventilator recording for high-frequency oscillation ventilation

Parameters that need to be set and recorded hourly or according to local hospital policy include: F_iO_2, MAP, oscillatory amplitude (ΔP) breath frequency (Hz), IT, and flow.

If using the SLE 2000 ventilator in HFO mode, the amplitude PIP, MAP, positive end-expiratory pressure, IT, rate, patient's own rate, humidifier temperature, and the fraction of inspired oxygen should be recorded hourly or according to local policy. HFO can be superimposed on to a positive-pressure ventilator rate, in which case all the usual ventilator parameters will also need to be recorded.

Nitric oxide may be used in the circuit if required. The patient will still require suction and assessment of secretions (Hazinski 1992).

Consider the need for re-recruitment after suctioning.

Tables 2.11 and 2.12 outline management of oxygenation and ventilation in HFOV.

See www.carefusion.com for further information.

In the literature, four distinct groups of patients have been identified and strategies developed for optimal HFOV (Kohe et al 1988; Clark et al 1994; Clark & Null 1999).

Diffuse lung disease

Caused by ARDS, respiratory distress syndrome (RDS), pulmonary haemorrhage, pneumonia (particularly group B streptococcus).

Table 2.11   Management of oxygenation on HFOV considering P_aO_2 and lung compliance

If P_aO_2 is:	Lung inflation	Primary action	Secondary action
Increased	↑	↓ MAP	↓ F_iO_2
Increased	Normal	↓ F_iO_2	—
Increased	↓	↑ MAP	↓ F_iO_2
Normal	↑	↓ MAP	—
Normal	Normal	—	—
Normal	↓	↑ MAP	—
Decreased	↑	↓ MAP	↑ F_iO_2
Decreased	Normal	↑ F_iO_2	—
Decreased	↓	↑ MAP	↑ F_iO_2

HFOV, High-frequency oscillation; *MAP*, mean airway pressure.
Reproduced with permission from Avila, K., Mazza, L., Morgan-Trujillo, L., 1994. High frequency oscillatory ventilation: a nursing ap-proach to bedside care. Neonat. Netw. 13 (5), 23–30; Adapted from HFO Study Group, 1993. Randomised study of high frequency oscillation ventilation in infants with severe respiratory distress syndrome. J. Pediatr. 122, 609–619.

Table 2.12   Management of high-frequency oscillation and action to take to rectify P_aCO_2

P_aCO_2	Primary action	Secondary action
Increased	↑ oscillation amplitude	↓ frequency
Normal	—	—
Decreased	↓ oscillation amplitude	↑ frequency

Reproduced with permission from Avila, K., Mazza, L., Morgan-Trujillo, L., 1994. High frequency oscillatory ventilation: a nursing ap-proach to bedside care. Neonat. Netw. 13 (5), 23–30; Adapted from HFO Study Group, 1993. Randomised study of high frequency oscillation ventilation in infants with severe respiratory distress syndrome. J. Pediatr. 122, 609–619.

Goal of ventilation is to improve lung inflation, compliance and ventilation/perfusion matching while avoiding barotrauma and cardiac compromise.

HFOV strategy:
- Initially MAP approximately 2–5 cm H_2O above MAP on conventional ventilator to maintain recruitment in the face of pressure attenuation by the ET tube (Ventre & Arnold 2004), then increase MAP in 1 cm H_2O increments until arterial oxygenation improves or there is a rise in central venous pressure with signs of decreased systemic blood flow, or until the chest x-ray shows normal lung inflation, or a sustained inflation manoeuvre to increase lung volume and oxygenation by reexpanding atelectatic alveoli

- Then aggressive weaning to bring the lung on to the deflation limb of the pressure volume curve (i.e., same volume at lower pressure)
- Chest x-ray required to assess degree of lung inflation
- If P_aO_2 continues to rise, wean F_iO_2 until less than 0.6 then wean MAP

Initial settings IT% 0.33, F_iO_2 1.0, MAP as described previously, Hz range 8–15 depending on age and size of patient. If adequate P_aCO_2 cannot be achieved with maximal power output (ΔP), decrease rate to increase tidal volume.

Unilateral or patchy lung involvement

For instance, in meconium aspiration syndrome, focal pneumonia.

Goal of ventilation is to improve oxygenation with low MAP and to avoid lung overinflation.

HFOV strategy:

PATHOLOGY WITH AIR-TRAPPING

- MAP on HFOV should be initiated at similar level as on continuous mandatory ventilation (CMV)
- Amplitude should be set to achieve good chest wall movement
- Use lower range of frequency to allow more time for the delivery of larger tidal volumes distally in an effort to overcome some of the airway obstruction (i.e., 10–15 Hz).

Patients least likely to respond to HFOV are those with evidence of air-trapping and overinflation on CMV. Focal air-trapping may be accentuated by HFOV, and the result may be pneumothorax and airway rupture.

PATHOLOGY WITH DIFFUSE HAZE (ACUTE RESPIRATORY DISTRESS SYNDROME)

- MAP above MAP on CMV
- Frequency in lower range
- Amplitude set to achieve good chest wall movement

Lung hypoplasia

For instance, in congenital diaphragmatic hernia, uniform pulmonary hypoplasia. These infants have small, abnormal lungs.

Goal of ventilation is to improve oxygenation at the lowest possible MAP and minimise ventilator-associated barotrauma.

HFOV strategy

UNIFORM PULMONARY HYPOPLASIA

- MAP set at same level as CMV, then increase gradually to achieve maximum S_aO_2. If MAP is increased by 5–6 cm H_2O without an increase in saturations, recheck chest x-ray for lung and vessel positioning

- Frequency 10–15 Hz
- Amplitude set to achieve **minimal** chest wall movement to minimise lung injury

NONUNIFORM PULMONARY HYPOPLASIA (CONGENITAL DIAPHRAGMATIC HERNIA)

- MAP started ≥CMV dependent on the contralateral lung. The MAP should be initiated in the 10–12 cm H_2O range and increased by 1 cm H_2O increments to optimise the lung volume of the unaffected lung
- Increase MAP slowly while observing cardiac function. When over-inflation occurs, the mediastinum become narrowed or may be shifted away from its optimal position and will compromise cardiac filling and output
- Frequency usually set at 10 Hz
- Amplitude set to achieve adequate chest wall movement

Air leak syndromes

Goal of ventilation is use of the lowest possible ventilator settings, accept low P_aO_2 and high P_aCO_2 (with pH >7.25)
   HFOV strategy

RECURRENT PNEUMOTHORACES

- If the patient has poor inflation, then the goal is to improve inflation by slightly increasing MAP from CMV.

SEVERE AIR LEAK – WITH OR WITHOUT CYSTS IN LUNGS

- MAP ≤ MAP on CMV
- Reduce MAP by 1 cm H_2O increments until the target P_aO_2 is reached or chest x-ray shows normal lung inflation with signs of resolution of the air leak
- Wean MAP in preference to F_iO_2 in these patients
- Put most severely affected lung in dependent position to increase resistance to gas delivery in that lung
- Avoid hand bagging these patients if possible.
   In general, after an appropriate degree of lung inflation has been achieved, a typical sequence for addressing hypercarbia would be:
- increasing ΔP in increments of 3 cm H_2O until the power is maximised
- decrease the frequency in increments of 0.5–1.0 Hz
- partially deflating the ET tube cuff to allow the additional exit of CO_2 (but the decrease in MAP should be corrected by an increase in bias flow) (Mehta et al 2001; Derdak et al 2002; VandeKieft et al 2003; Ventre & Arnold 2004).

USE OF INHALED NITRIC OXIDE

NO is a powerful pulmonary vasodilator that does not cause systemic hypotension. It can be used in patients who have reversible pulmonary hypertension and/or ventilation perfusion mismatch, e.g., neonates with persistent pulmonary hypertension of the neonate; children with congenital heart disease, pulmonary hypertension and right heart failure; primary graft failure post lung transplant or children with ARDS. It may be used as a bridge to another treatment (e.g., HFOV, ECMO). In neonates, it has been shown to increase oxygenation, decrease pulmonary hypertension, and reduce the need to go on ECMO. Several studies suggest transient improvement in oxygenation in ARDS with inhaled nitric oxide (iNO) therapy; however, no study has found clinically meaningful benefits in mortality or duration of ventilation in ARDS. A systematic review of nine trials showed no reduction in mortality in severe ARDS or mild-moderate ARDS (Adhikari et al 2014).

Nitric oxide must be prescribed. The starting dose is usually 5-20 parts per million in the PICU population; however, higher doses may be used in neonatal populations. NO may be started at maximum dose and weaned slowly in response to effect; however, regulation of this is sometimes difficult. Consideration may be given to adding an oral agent (e.g., sildenafil) to children with pulmonary hypertension to aid weaning from inhaled NO.

In addition to normal observations and blood tests, when using NO, blood levels of nitrogen dioxide (NO_2) and methaemoglobin should be tested, and both, ideally, should be <1%. (Methaemoglobin levels should be taken 12–24 hourly.) Other complications include a risk of bleeding and renal failure.

NO cylinders should be checked regularly to ensure that they do not run out. Infants and children can become very dependent on NO, and the rebound effect if the NO supply failed could be fatal.

Analysers must be used to measure NO and NO_2 concentrations.

Scavenger systems can be used (i.e., a charcoal filter can be placed on the exhaust of the ventilator, which gets rid of NO and NO_2 from the circuit).

A circuit should be set up to hand-ventilate the child with NO if s/he is particularly sensitive to it.

Closed-circuit suction should be considered if the child is very sensitive to NO. If normal suction is used, consider giving extra breaths using the manual breath button on the ventilator prior to suction. Record NO concentration hourly on the ITU chart.

Prone positioning

Prone positioning can:
- Optimise ventilation/perfusion ratio (V/Q) mismatch
- Increase FRC
- Reduce atelectasis
- Facilitate secretion drainage

The benefits of proning may result from:
- less lung deformation in the prone position leading to increased ventilation,
- less abdominal distension,
- less compression of the lung by the heart as it sits against the sternum,
- recruitment manoeuvres being more effective, and
- more uniform alveolar ventilation as plateau pressure is more uniformly distributed.

There have been conflicting randomised controlled trials; however, evidence now suggests prone ventilation is of benefit in selected patients with severe ARDS. Cautions and contraindications to prone positioning include increased intracranial and intra-abdominal pressure, abdominal and chest wounds, and patients with C-spine precautions. When proning, it is important to assemble sufficient staff to turn the patient safely, provide padding and support for potential pressure areas, ensure the abdomen is not compressed, and to place the patient supine for a minimum of 6 hours in a 24-hour period to relieve pressure areas. Care must be taken not to dislodge ET tubes or chest drains. Enteral feeding may be affected by proning. As with other interventions, response to treatment must be evaluated and consideration given to other options if unsuccessful (Guerin et al 2013).

BRONCHOALVEOLAR LAVAGE (BAL) (NONBRONCHOSCOPIC) IN A VENTILATED CHILD

(Guideline developed by Steve Colthurst – Physiotherapist and used with permission)

Equipment required: Universal specimen pot labelled with patient details, plus

If weight <10 kg, use 2 mL of 0.9% normal saline (NOT PER KG), in a 5-mL syringe with a size 6 french gauge (FG) NG tube

If weight ≥10 kg, use 5 mL of 0.9% normal saline (NOT PER KG), in a 10-mL syringe with size 8 FG NG tube

Method:
- Monitor patient, including S_aO_2 during procedure
- Clear large airway secretions by preoxygenation then suction as per unit protocol
- Prefill syringe with designated amount of normal saline, draw in approximately 2 mL of air into the syringe before attaching and priming the appropriate sized NG tube (to ensure all the fluid is pushed into the airways, leaving the NG tube before being aspirated back)
- Use clean gloves to disconnect the patient from the ventilator and advance the NG tube down the ET tube until resistance is felt in a wedged position
- Instil the normal saline slowly to limit the amount of reflux up the airway and immediately aspirate the normal saline back up using the syringe

- Withdraw the NG tube and reconnect the patient to the ventilator
- Remove the NG tube from the syringe and place the contents of the syringe into the labelled specimen pot and send for analysis
- In some patients with ARDS, re-recruitment of the lungs may be required before putting back on ventilator
- Further suctioning may be required to remove excess normal saline or secretions left after BAL
- Adjust the ventilator to achieve target S_aO_2

REFERENCES

Adhikari, N.K., Dellinger, R.P., Lundin, S., et al., 2014. Inhaled nitric oxide does not reduce mortality in patients with acute respiratory distress syndrome regardless of severity: systematic review and meta-analysis. Crit. Care Med. 42 (2), 404.

Advanced Life Support Group, 2016. Advanced Paediatric Life Support, sixth ed. Wiley Blackwell.

Association of Paediatric Anaesthetists. Difficult Airway Society, 2015. Paediatric difficult airway guidelines 2015 Paediatric airway group. www.das.uk.com.

Avila, K., Mazza, L., Morgan-Trujillo, L., 1994. High frequency oscillatory ventilation: a nursing approach to bedside care. Neonat. Netw. 13 (5), 23–30.

British Thoracic Society Standards of Care Committee, 2002. Non-invasive ventilation in acute respiratory failure. Thorax. 57, 192–211.

British Thoracic Society respiratory management of children with neuromuscular weakness guideline group, 2012. British Thoracic Society Guidelines for respiratory management of children with neuromuscular weakness. Thorax. 67 (1), i1–40.

British Thoracic Society (BTS) / Scottish Intercollegiate Guidelines Network (SIGN), 2016. British Guideline on the management of asthma. Edinburgh: SIGN. (QRG 153), http://www.sign.ac.uk.

Chavasse, R.J.P.G., Seddon, P., Bara, A., et al., 2009. Short acting beta2-agonists for recurrent wheeze in children under two years of age. Cochrane Database Syst. Rev. (2), CD002873.

Ciarallo, L., Brousseau, D., Reinert, S., 2000. Higher-dose intravenous magnesium therapy for children with moderate to severe asthma. Arch. Pediatr. Adolesc. Med. 154, 979–983.

Clark, R.H., Yoder, B.A., Sell, M.S., 1994. Prospective, randomised comparison of HFO and conventional ventilation in candidates for ECMO. J. Pediatr. 124, 447–454.

Clark, R.H., Null, D.M., 1999. High frequency oscillation ventilation: clinical management strategies. Critical Care Review. SensorMedics Corporation, Yorba Linda, CA.

Cook, T., Woodall, N., Frerk, C., 2011. NAP4 – Major complications of airway management in the U.K.: results of the 4th National Audit Project of the Royal Collage of Anaesthetists and the Difficult Airway Society, Br. J. Anaesth, UK 106, 617–642.

Corne, J., Carroll, M., Brown, I., et al., 2002. *Chest X-ray Made Easy*, second ed. Churchill Livingstone, London.

Curry, S., 1982. Methaemoglobinaemia. Ann. Emerg. Med. 11, 214–221.

Dahlem, P., van Aalderen, W.M., Bos, A.P., 2007. Pediatric acute lung injury. Paediatr. Respir. Rev. 8 (4), 348–362.

Damore, D., Mansbach, J.M., Clark, S., et al., 2008. Prospective multicenter bronchiolitis study: predicting intensive care unit admissions. Acad. Emerg. Med. 15 (10), 887–894.

Derdak, S., Mehta, S., Stewart, T.E., et al., Multicenter Oscillatory Ventilation for Acute Respiratory Distress Syndrome Trial (MOAT) Study Investigators, 2002. High-frequency oscillatory ventilation for acute respiratory distress syndrome in adults: a randomised controlled trial. Am. J. Respir. Crit. Care Med. 166, 801–808.

Ferguson, N.D., Cook, D.J., Guyatt, G.H., et al., The OSCILATE Trial Investigators and the Canadian Clinical trials Group, 2013. High frequency oscillation in early acute respiratory distress syndrome. N. Engl. J. Med. 368 (9), 795.

Fernandes, R.M., Bialy, L.M., Vandermeer, et al., 2013. Glucocorticoids for acute viral bronchiolitis in infants and young children. Cochrane Database Syst. Rev. (6), CD004878.

Fort, P., Farmer, C., Westerman, J., et al., 1997. High-frequency oscillatory ventilation for adult respiratory distress syndrome – a pilot study. Crit. Care. Med. 25, 937–947.

Frerk C, Mitchell V.S, McNarry A.F, et al., 2015. Difficult Airway Society 2015 Guidelines for management of unanticipated difficult intubation in adults. Br. J. Anaesth. 115 (6), 827–848.

Goldfrank, L.R., Price, D., Kirstein, R.H., 1985. *Goldfrank's Toxicological Emergencies*, third ed. Appleton & Lange, Norwalk, CT.

Graciano, A.L., Tamurro, R., Thompson, A.E., et al., 2014. Incidence and associated factors of difficult tracheal intubations in pediatric ICUs: a report from National Emergency Airway Registry for Children. NEAR4KIDS Intensive Care Med. 40 (11), 1659–1669.

Gravenstein, J.S., Paulus, D., Hayes, T.J., 1989. *Capnography in Clinical Practice*. Butterworth Publishers, Stoneham, MA.

Guerin, C., Reignier, J., Richard, J.C., et al., PROSEVA Study Group, 2013. Prone positioning in severe acute respiratory distress syndrome. N. Engl. J. Med. 368 (23), 2159.

Hazinski, M.F. (Ed.), 1992. Nursing Care of the Critically Ill Child, second ed. Mosby Year Book, St Louis, MO.

Hartling, L., Fernandes, R.M., Bialy, L., et al., 2011. Steroids and bronchodilators for acute bronchiolitis in the first two years of life: systematic review and meta-analysis. BMJ 342.

HFO Study Group, 1993. Randomised study of high frequency oscillation ventilation in infants with severe respiratory distress syndrome. J. Pediatr. 122, 609–619.

Hinds, C.J., Watson, D., 1996. second ed. W B Saunders, London.

Khemani, R.G., Smith, L.S., Zimmerman, J.J., et al., for the Pediatric Acute Lung Injury Concensus Conference Group, 2015. Pediatric acute respiratory distress syndrome: definition, incidence, and epidemiology: proceedings from the Pediatric Acute Lung Injury Consensus Conference. Pediatr. Crit. Care Med. 16 (5 Suppl. 1), S23–S40.

Kohe, D., Perlman, M., Kirpalani, H., et al., 1988. High frequency oscillation in the rescue of infants with persistent pulmonary hypertension. Crit. Care Med. 16, 510–516.

Laker, S., 2003. Part 2: Capnography in respiratory monitoring. In: Flight Nursing News, Autumn. Royal College of Nursing, London.

Mansbach, J.M., Piedra, P.A., Stevenson, M.D., et al., 2012. Prospective multi-center study of children with bronchiolitis requiring mechanical ventilation. Pediatrics 130 (3).

Mansouri, A., 1985. Review: methaemoglobinaemia. Am. J. Med. Sci. 289, 200–208.

Medivent Ltd, 2002. RTX Operator's Manual. Medivent Ltd, Lucan, Co, Dublin.

Mehta, S., Lapinsky, S.E., Hallett, D.C., et al., 2001. Prospective trial of high frequency oscillation in adults with acute respiratory distress syndrome. Crit. Care Med. 29, 1360–1369.

Miller, M.J., Martin, R.J., Carlo, W.A., et al., 1985. Oral breathing in newborn infants. J. Pediatr. 107, 465.

Miller, M.J., Carlo, W.A., Strohl, K.P., et al., 1986. Effect of maturation on oral breathing in sleeping premature infants. J. Pediatr. 109, 515–519.

Murray, E.L., Nieves, D., Bradley, J.S., et al., 2013. Characteristics of severe Bordetella pertussis infection among infants =90 days of age admitted to pediatric intensive care units – Southern California, September 2009-June 2011. J Ped. Infect. Dis. Published online January 10, 2013.

National Institute for Health and Care Excellence (NICE), 2015. Whooping Cough Management. www.cks.nice.org.uk.

Patel, A., Harrison, E., Durward, A., et al., 2000. Intratracheal recombinant human deoxyribonuclease in acute life threatening asthma refractory to conventional treatment. Br. J. Anaesth. 84 (4), 505–507.

Phipps, P., Garrard, C.S., 2003. The pulmonary physician in critical care. 12: Acute, severe asthma in the intensive care unit. Thorax 58, 81–88.

Pow, J., 1997. Methaemoglobinaemia: an unusual blue boy. Paediatr. Nurs. 9 (10), 24–25.

Resuscitation Council (UK), 2004. Acid–base balance: interpreting arterial blood gases. Advanced Life Support Manual, Appendix. Resuscitation Council (UK), London, p. 142.

Rettig, J.S., Smallwood, C.D., Wlsh, B.K., et al., 2015. High-frequency oscillatory ventilation in pediatric acute lung injury: a multicenter international experience. Crit. Care Med. 43 (12), 2660–2667.

Ross, P.A., Newth, C.J.L., Khemani, R.G., 2013. Accuracy of pulse oximetry in children. Pediatrics 133 (1), 22–29.

Schelvan, C., Copeman, A., Young, J., et al., 2002. *Paediatric Radiology for MRCPH/FRCR*. Royal Society of Medicine, London.

Serpa Neto, A., Cardoso, S.O., Manettta, J.A., et al., 2012. Association between use of lung protective ventilation with lower tidal volumes and clinical outcomes among patients without acute respiratory distress syndrome a meta-analysis. JAMA 308 (16), 1651.

Shann, F., 2017. *Drug Doses*, seventeenth edn. Department of Paediatrics. University of Melbourne, Parkville, Victoria.

Siemens Medical Engineering, 1993. System SV300. Life Support Systems, Sweden.

Taylor, M.B., Whitwam, J.G., 1986. The current status of pulse oximetry. Anaesthesia 41, 943–949.

ten Brink, F., Duke, T., Evans, J., 2013. High-flow nasal Prong oxygen therapy or nasophyngeal continuous positive airway pressure for children with moderate to severe respiratory distress? Pediatr. Crit. Care Med. 14 (7), e326–e331.

Teriz, N., Piquilloud, L., Roze, H., et al., 2012. Clinical review: update on neutrally adjusted ventilator assist- report of a round table conference. Crit. Care 16 (3), 225.

The Pediatric Acute Lung Consensus Conference Group, 2015. Pediatric acute respiratory distress syndroem: consensus recommendations from the Pediatric Acute Lung Injury Consensus Conference. Pediatr. Criti. Care Med. 16 (5), 428–439.

Tortora, G.J., Anagnostakos, N.P., 1984. *Principles of Anatomy and Physiology*, fourth ed. Harper, Sydney, NSW.

Turner, D.A., Arnold, J.H., 2007. Insights in pediatric ventilation: Timing of intubation, ventilator strategies, and weaning. Curr. Opin. Crit. Care. 13 (1), 57–63.

VandeKieft, M., Dorsey, D., Venticinque, S., et al., 2003. Effects of endotracheal cuff leak on gas flow patterns in a mechanical lung model during high frequency oscillatory ventilation. Am. J. Respir. Crit. Care Med. 167 , A178.

Ventre, K.M., Arnold, J.H., 2004. High frequency oscillatory ventilation in acute respiratory failure. Paediatr. Respir. Rev. 5, 323–332.

Wang, E.E., Law, B.J., Stephens, D., 1995. Pediatric Investigators Collaborative Network on Infections in Canada (PICNIC) Prospective study of risk factors and outcomes in patients hospitalised with respiratory syncytial viral lower respiratory tract infection. J. Pediatr. 126 (2), 212–219.

Young, D., Lamb, S.E., Shah, S., OSCAR Study Group, 2013. High Frequency oscillation for acute respiratory distress syndrome. N. Engl. J. Med. 368 (9), 806.

Zorc, J.J., Hall, C.B., 2010. Bronchiolitis: recent evidence on diagnosis and management. Pediatrics 125 (2), 342–349.

USEFUL WEBSITES

www.das.uk.com.
www.eme-med.co.uk.
www.maquet.com.
www.mediventintl.com.
www.viasysCriticalCare.com.

CARDIAC CARE

3

This chapter explains the normal heart, basic echocardiography terminology, congenital heart defects, acquired heart conditions, and surgery required to correct or palliate. Postoperative complications are discussed, as well as algorithms for managing abnormal rhythms and adjuncts such as pacing and extracorporeal membrane oxygenation (ECMO).

NORMAL HEART

Blood flow through the normal heart is shown in Fig. 3.1.

- Deoxygenated venous blood enters the right atrium (RA) via the superior vena cava (SVC) – from the head and the upper body – and the inferior vena cava (IVC) – from the lower body.
- Blood flows from the RA through a tricuspid valve into the right ventricle (RV).
- The RV pumps the blood through the pulmonary valve into the pulmonary artery (PA) and then to the lungs to be oxygenated. The main trunk of the PA divides into two – right and left PAs – to supply each lung separately.
- From the lungs the oxygenated blood flows to the left atrium (LA) via the pulmonary veins.
- From the LA the blood flows into the left ventricle (LV) through the mitral valve.
- The LV pumps the oxygenated blood through the aortic valve (AV) into the ascending aorta and from there to the systemic circulation.

NB If a neonate presents hypoxic without retaining CO_2, then congenital cyanotic heart disease is implied and a prostaglandin infusion (5–10 ng/kg/min) should be started until a definitive diagnosis is made.

NB The hyperoxia test – give fraction of inspired oxygen (F_iO_2) of 1.0 (100%) for 10 minutes to a cyanotic newborn and if the partial pressure of oxygen on an arterial blood gas does not increase to greater than 100 mm Hg or 20 KPa, then cyanotic congenital heart disease (right-to-left shunt) must be considered.

See Table 3.1 for signs, symptoms, and diagnosis of congenital heart disease.

Fig. 3.1 Blood flow through the normal heart. (With permission from Wilson, K.J.W., 1987. Ross and Wilson Anatomy and Physiology in Health and Illness, sixth ed. Churchill Livingstone, Edinburgh.)

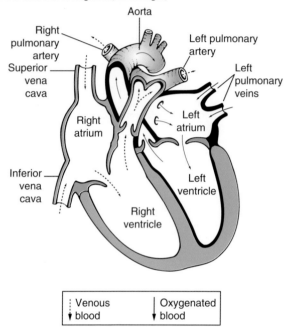

A detailed classification and explanation of congenital heart lesions is included later in this chapter.

Heart murmurs and shunt murmurs

See Fig. 3.2 for an illustration that provides a reference to auscultation positions for optimum identification for different heart and shunt murmurs.

Systolic murmurs are heard between the first and second heart sound, whereas diastolic murmurs are heard between the second sound and the first sound. Murmurs heard throughout systole are called pansystolic murmurs.

A shunt murmur is a continuous murmur that runs through systole and into diastole. Patent ductus arteriosus (PDA) murmur is best heard over the left subclavicular space, whereas a Blalock-Taussig (BT) shunt murmur may be best heard in the left infrascapular region.

Clinical signs that indicate congenital heart lesions

1. Presence of a murmur
2. Hypoxia that does not improve with oxygen
3. Difference in upper and lower limb blood pressure (arms higher blood pressure than legs)
4. Difference in preductal and postductal saturations
   NB Measure preductal saturations in the right hand and postductal saturations in either foot and not the left hand (Ruegger et al 2010).

Understanding basic echocardiogram terminology

Transthoracic echo is a useful tool for investigation of heart disease, but its limitations are implicit. Images are sometimes technically difficult to obtain, leading to inaccurate conclusions. It is important to know the structure and function of the heart, and a few technical terms and measurements are useful for all to understand.

AV concordance – atria and ventricles normally aligned

AV discordance – RA to anatomic LV and anatomic LA to RV

Situs solitus – normal anatomy (i.e., the anatomic RA is to the right and anterior)

Situs inversus – major visceral organs are reversed from their normal positions (mirror image) (e.g., the anatomic RA is on the left and posterior)

RA isomerism – both atria have anatomic features of RA

LA isomerism – both atria have anatomic features of LA

Dextrocardia – congenital cardiac malrotation in which heart is situated on the right side instead of the left

Ejection fraction – measures the percentage of blood that is pumped out of a ventricle when the heart contracts. Normal left ventricular ejection fraction (LVEF) ranges from 55% to 70%. Some children are admitted to intensive care with LVEF less than 15% and may be referred for assessment for transplantation.

Fig. 3.2 Heart and shunt murmur – position for auscultation.

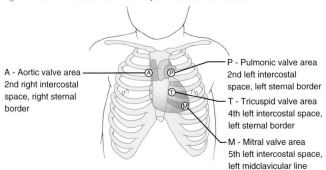

A - Aortic valve area
2nd right intercostal
space, right sternal
border

P - Pulmonic valve area
2nd left intercostal
space, left sternal border

T - Tricuspid valve area
4th left intercostal space,
left sternal border

M - Mitral valve area
5th left intercostal space,
left midclavicular line

Fig. 3.3 (A) Normal electrocardiogram trace (sinus rhythm). (B) Labelled portion of sinus rhythm.

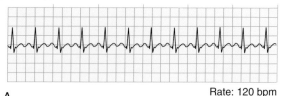

Rate: 120 bpm

A

B

Fractional shortening – measures the heart's muscular contractility. This measures and ratios the change in the diameter of the LV at the end of diastole and the end of systole. A normal range is approximately 20% to 45%.

Left ventricular end-diastolic z score – there is a calculator for left ventricular end-diastolic volume based upon the child's own height, weight, length, and body surface. There are apps available to calculate this (e.g., www.ubqo.com/cardioz).

NORMAL ELECTROCARDIOGRAM

An electrocardiogram (ECG) measures the electrical activity of the heart and records it on graph paper. This allows the sequence and magnitude of the electrical impulses generated by the heart to be analysed and evaluated (Fig. 3.3).

Information supplied by the ECG includes:

- Heart rate and rhythm
- Abnormalities of conduction
- Muscular damage (ischaemia)
- Hypertrophy
- Effects of electrolyte imbalance
- Influence of various drugs
- Pericardial disease

The contraction of any muscle is associated with electrical changes called depolarisation, and these changes can be detected by electrodes

Table 3.1	Signs, symptoms, and diagnosis of congenital heart defects								
Defect	Murmur	Heart failure	Cyanosis	Pulmonary blood flow	Blood pressure	Heart size	Chest x-ray	ECG	Comments/ presentation	Need prostin
Coarctation	Systolic murmur radiating to back between scapula	Yes	No	Pulmonary venous congestion	Higher BP readings in arms	May be enlarged	Cardiomegaly, signs of pulmonary oedema, venous congestion	Baby RVH, older child may have LVH	Grey, collapsed, acidotic, no femoral pulses, hepatomegaly	Yes
Tetralogy of Fallot	Yes	No	Yes	Reduced	Normal	Normal	Boot shaped heart with concave MPA segment	RAD, RVH	Often ↑ Hb and haematocrit	Yes if very blue
Ventricular septal defect	Yes	Possibly	No	Increased	Usually normal	May be enlarged	Cardiomegaly, pulmonary oedema	Large VSD – LAH, LVH	Delayed growth and development, repeated pulmonary infection, CHF may develop	No
Patent ductus arteriosus	Yes	Yes – if large duct	No	Increased pulmonary blood flow	Wide pulse pressure, low diastolic	May be enlarged if PDA large	If large PDA, cardiomegaly with LAE and increased PVM	CVH in large PDA, RVH if PVOD develops	If PDA large, CHF may develop	No
TGA	Yes if VSD, no if IVS	No	Yes-severe	Normal or minimally increased	Normal if VSD, lower with IVS	Narrow superior mediastinum	Egg-shaped heart	RAD, RVH	VSD present in 40% of cases	Yes

Continued

Table 3.1 Signs, symptoms and diagnosis of congenital heart defects—cont'd

Defect	Murmur	Heart failure	Cyanosis	Pulmonary blood flow	Blood pressure	Heart size	Chest x-ray	ECG	Comments/presentation	Need prostin
Truncus	Yes	Yes	Mild	Increased pulmonary blood flow	Wide pulse pressure	Enlarged	Cardiomegaly, pulmonary oedema	CVH	Cyanosis often noted immediately after birth	No
Hypoplastic left heart syndrome	No	Yes	Yes	May have pulmonary venous congestion	Normal or low	Enlarged	Pulmonary vascular congestion if restrictive ASD	RVH and RAD	Mild cyanosis, tachycardia, tachypnoea, metabolic acidosis	Yes
Obstructed total anomalous pulmonary venous drainage	No – but may have gallop rhythm	No	Severe	Pulmonary venous congestion	Normal or low	Normal or small because of decreased venous return to left heart	Pulmonary vascular congestion	RAD and RVH	Marked cyanosis and respiratory distress	Yes until echo
PA	No	No	Severe	Reduced	Normal	Normal or enlarged	RA enlargement, MPA segment concave with decreased PVMs	Normal QRS axis, RAH	Severe and progressive cyanosis from birth	Yes
TA	Yes	No	Severe	Reduced	Normal	Normal or slightly enlarged	'Boot-shaped' heart with concave MPA segment	Superior QRS axis, RAH or CAH and LVH	Severe cyanosis, poor feeding, tachypnoea – 50% have VSD and PS – 20% have TGA	Yes

| Critical AS | Yes – may be faint or absent in newborn | May develop | No | Normal or increased | Narrow pulse pressure | Normal or slightly enlarged | Usually normal | LVH | Weak, thready peripheral pulses | Yes |
| Ebstein anomaly | Yes | Yes | Yes – most are cyanosed | Reduced | Normal | Extreme enlargement | Extreme cardiomegaly, particularly RA and decreased PVMS | RBBB, RAH WPW syndrome, SVT and AV block sometimes present | Cyanosis of newborns may improve as PVR falls – SVT is common | Yes |

*NB In any presentation of a baby where a cardiac defect is suspected and the baby is cyanosed, Prostin should be started and then only discontinued on the advice of cardiologists or other specialists following echocardiogram.

ASD, Atrial septal defect; AV, atrioventricular; BP, blood pressure; CAH, combined atrial hypertrophy; CHF, congestive heart failure; CVH, common ventricular hypertrophy; IVS, intact ventricular septum; LAH, left atrial hypertrophy; LVH, left ventricular hypertrophy; MPA, main pulmonary artery; PDA, patent ductus arteriosus; PVM, pulmonary vascular marking; PVDD, pulmonary vascular obstructive disease; RA, right atrium; RAD, right axis deviation; RAH, right atrial hypertrophy; RBBB, right bundle branch block; RVH, right ventricular hypertrophy; SVT, supraventricular tachycardia; TGA, transposition of the great arteries; VSD, ventricular septal defect; WPW, Wolff–Parkinson–White.

Source: Adapted from Heese H de V 1992 Handbook of Paediatrics 4th edn. Oxford University Press. Cape Town; Park, M.K., 1997. The Pediatric Cardiology Handbook, second ed. CV Mosby, St. Louis, MO and Pearson, G., 2002. Handbook of Paediatric Intensive Care. WB Saunders, Edinburgh.

attached to the surface of the body. Although the heart has four chambers, from the electrical point of view it can be thought of as having only two because the atria contract together and then the ventricles contract together.

The electrical discharge for each cycle starts in the sinoatrial (SA) node in the RA. Depolarisation then spreads through the atrial muscle fibres. There is a delay while depolarisation spreads through the atrioventricular (AV) node (also in the RA). The conduction is then very rapid down specialised conduction tissue – first a single pathway, the bundle of His, then this divides in the septum between the ventricles into right and left bundle branches. The left bundle branch divides itself into two. Conduction spreads rapidly through the mass of the ventricular muscle through specialised tissue called Purkinje fibres. Repolarisation then takes place – the return of the ventricular mass to the electrical state (Hampton 1992).

- The P wave represents the contraction and depolarisation of the atria. Their muscle mass is relatively small, and the electrical charge accompanying their contraction is therefore also small.
- The PR interval represents the time taken for the impulse to spread from the SA node, through the atrial muscle and the AV node, down the bundle of His and into the ventricular muscle.
- The QRS complex represents ventricular depolarisation. Because the ventricles are large, there is a large deflection of the ECG when they contract.
- The T wave represents the return of the ventricular mass to the resting electrical state (repolarisation).

CARDIAC OUTPUT

Cardiac output is the amount of blood ejected by each ventricle (in litres or millilitres) per minute. Normal cardiac output is higher per kilogram of body weight in the child than in the adult.

- 400 mL/kg/min at birth
- 200 mL/kg/min within first weeks of life
- 100 mL/kg/min during adolescence (Hazinski 1992)

$$\text{Cardiac output} = \text{Stroke volume} \times \text{Heart rate}$$
$$\text{Preload} = \text{Afterload} \times \text{Contractility}$$

To obtain the 'normal' cardiac output for children of different ages and sizes, the cardiac index is calculated.

$$\text{Cardiac index} = \frac{\text{Cardiac output}}{\text{Body surface area } (m^2)}$$

Normal range = 3.5 to 5.5 L/min/m^2 body surface area (Shemie 1997)

Cardiac output is a prime determinant of haemodynamic function and in the critically ill child should be evaluated as either adequate or inadequate to meet the child's metabolic demands.

Preload is the amount of myocardial fibre stretch that is present before contraction and is related to the volume of blood in the ventricles prior to contraction, central venous pressure (CVP), and left atrial pressure (LAP) (Starling's law). Frank Starling's law observed that normal myocardium generates greater tension during contraction if it is stretched before contraction. However, fibre length is not readily measured and therefore preload or ventricular end-diastolic pressure is monitored as an indirect measurement.

Factors affecting preload: ventricular compliance, tachycardia.

Afterload refers to the resistance to ejection from a ventricle. Ventricular afterload is the sum of all forces opposing ventricular emptying. A decrease in afterload is often associated with an improvement in ventricular function. Because fibre shortening occurs only when the ventricle has generated sufficient tension to equal its afterload, an increase in ventricular afterload reduces contraction time and thus the stroke volume of the ventricle. It is also related to Poiseuille's law, which states that pressure is a product of flow and resistance:

$$\text{Pressure} = \text{Flow} \times \text{Resistance}$$

From this equation, an increase in resistance will be associated with a decrease in flow (stroke volume) unless pressure increases. Even a normal afterload may be excessive when myocardial function is poor.

Contractility refers to the strength and efficiency of contraction; it is the force generated by the myocardium, independent of preload and afterload. Contractility is reduced by many factors, including hypoxia, acidosis, excessive preload/afterload, hypocalcaemia, and nutritional deficiencies.

INVASIVE INTRAVASCULAR PRESSURE MONITORING

To monitor children accurately following cardiac surgery, various lines will be in situ to continuously monitor the child's cardiovascular status.

Intra-arterial pressure

Intra-arterial pressure monitoring is the only way to continuously measure the child's blood pressure. The systolic (higher) figure is the pressure when the ventricles contract, and the diastolic (lower) figure is the pressure when the ventricles are relaxing and filling. The normal arterial pulse contour has a sharp upstroke during rapid ejection, followed by slow ejection and subsequent decrease (Fig. 3.4). The dicrotic notch denotes the end of ejection and closure of the AV. Estimates can be made of cardiac output, based on the quality of the arterial pulse contour. Low cardiac output may show a narrowing pulse pressure.

Atrial pressure

Atrial pressure is an indirect measurement of ventricular preload. It should be remembered that interpretation of the measurements depends

Fig. 3.4 The arterial waveform. *BP*, Blood pressure. (From Chambers, D., Huang, C., Matthews, G., 2015. Arterial pressure waveforms, Figure 33.1, in Basic Physiology for Anaesthetists, © Cambridge University Press, pp. 150-152.)

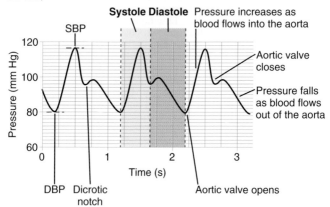

Fig. 3.5 The central venous pressure trace. A wave, due to atrial contraction. Absent in atrial fibrillation. Enlarged in tricuspid and pulmonary stenosis and pulmonary hypertension. C wave, due to bulging of tricuspid valve into RA. X descent, due to atrial relaxation. V wave, due to rise in atrial pressure before tricuspid valve opens. Y descent, due to atrial emptying as blood enters ventricle. Canon waves, large waves not corresponding to a,v, or c waves due to complete heart block or junctional rhythm. (From Anaesthesia UK, The central venous pressure trace. www.frca.co.uk.)

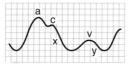

on the compliance of the ventricle and normal functioning of the AV valve.
- RA pressure can be directly measured via an RA line inserted during surgery; indirectly measured via a CVP line (Fig. 3.5). The RA pressure is usually low, with a mean of 5–10 mm Hg.
- LA pressure can be directly measured via an LA line inserted at time of surgery, which is also low, with a mean of 6–12 mm Hg and will be raised if there is left ventricular dysfunction or cardiac tamponade. The LA can be indirectly measured via pulmonary capillary wedge pressure, achieved through inflation of balloon tip of Swan-Ganz catheter.

Checking the position of a central venous catheter

After every neck central line insertion, the position of the line tip must be confirmed radiologically because if the line is too high, it can cause vessel wall erosion or if the tip is within the heart, it can cause arrhythmias, tamponade, cardiac perforation, or damage to the tricuspid valve (Stonelake & Bodenham 2006). This should also be confirmed by transducing the line to ensure that there has not been an accidental arterial cannulation.

The optimum position of a central line tip if placed via the internal jugular or subclavian route is controversial; the most common recommendation is that it should lie within the SVC, above its junction with the RA. The carina is a useful radiologic landmark because the central venous catheter should ideally lie just above the level of the carina (Melarkode & Latoo 2009).

NB The position of a central venous catheter tip will move as the patient changes position, so when a patient moves from a supine position to a sitting position, the catheter tip moves upwards in relation to the right atrium – up to 2–3 cm has been reported in the adult population (Vesely 2003).

TOP TIPS FOR POSTOPERATIVE CARDIAC MANAGEMENT

The goals of postoperative cardiac management are to optimise cardiopulmonary support, vigilantly monitor to identify complications quickly, and prevent secondary injury to the myocardium and other organs. It is also fundamental to provide effective analgesia and anxiolysis to minimise oxygen demand (Papo et al 1997).

Every centre that performs cardiac surgery will have its own guidelines for postoperative care; the following are intended as general reminders:

1. Ascertain preoperative anatomy and type of surgery performed. If cardiopulmonary bypass (CPB) was used, find out the duration of the bypass and cross-clamp time and whether there were any problems related to coming off bypass. It is important to check if there is any other relevant information from surgical/anaesthetic staff that you need to be aware of.

2. Assessment to include:

    A – Airway
    - Endotracheal (ET) tube size and length
    - Security of strapping
    - Equal breath sounds on both sides of chest on auscultation

    B – Breathing
    - Colour
    - *Saturations* (S_aO_2) – is this within an acceptable range given the procedure that has been performed? (Confirm S_aO_2 with blood co-oximetry measurement)

- Is nitric oxide (NO) being used?
- Chest movement, ventilation mode and settings
- Arterial blood gas analysis
- Chest x-ray will enable assessment of position of the ET tube, lung inflation, intravascular lines, drains, and pacing wire placement.

C – Circulation

- Heart rate and rhythm
- BP/CVP/right atrial pressure (RAP)/LAP/pulmonary artery pressure (PAP) and their wave forms; for example, does the BP waveform look flat or 'damp'? Is this caused by poor cardiac output or a problem with the line itself?
- Drugs – is the child receiving infusions of inotropes/vasodilators? If so, check the dosage, rate, and route and label lines clearly.
- If drains are present, confirm position (chest x-ray), label, and mark drainage on return from theatre. Most centres discard this total on fluid charts as drainage in theatre and calculate postoperative losses only. 'Milk' cardiac chest drains initially and at 15-min to hourly intervals thereafter, depending on drainage and local policy, to prevent blockage. Check drains are connected to thoracic suction at an appropriate pressure (10–20 cm H_2O).
- Are pacing wires in situ? If so, label (atrial/ventricular) and ensure that the metal ends are easily available should the child require pacing and that a pacing box is at the bedspace. By convention, atrial wires are placed on the right side of the chest and ventricular wires on the left.
- If the child is being paced, ascertain the underlying rate and rhythm and check with the surgeon/anaesthetist that the current settings on the pacing box are correct. A spare pacing box should be available.
- Full set of bloods to include full blood count and clotting screen – may need treating.
- Blood losses are usually replaced with whole blood or packed red cells, but what blood products has the patient received in theatre?
- Abnormal prothrombin or partial thromboplastin times are corrected with fresh frozen plasma and by keeping platelet count within normal limits.
- Low fibrinogen levels and other factor replacement can be corrected with cryoprecipitate.
- If bleeding is greater than 10 mL/kg/h despite blood and replacement for coagulation deficiencies, surgical exploration may be required to assess location of bleeding.

D – Disability (central nervous system)

- Assess and record pupil size and reaction to light.
- Administer analgesia as soon as child shows signs of waking from anaesthetic.
- Consider giving bolus and then infusion – usually of opiates (e.g., morphine/fentanyl); monitor effect.

- Muscle relaxants may be required to achieve synchrony with the ventilator (can also help to reduce the incidence of pulmonary hypertensive crisis).
- Near-infrared spectroscopy (NIRS) may be used to measure regional (left and right) cerebral tissue oxygen saturation – as a trend monitor with interventions to preserve cerebral saturation values close to individual baseline (Murkin & Arango 2009).

E – Electrolytes & metabolic status
- Arterial blood gas analysis, mixed venous saturations, and serum lactate to check the child is not hypoxaemic or hypercapnic and does not have a metabolic acidosis.
- Blood taken for an electrolyte screen will enable any necessary corrections to be made and allow assessment of ionised calcium, blood sugar, and magnesium levels.

F – Fluid management
- Maintenance fluids will be restricted (usually half to two-thirds maintenance), initially with added dextrose to prevent hypoglycaemia – check blood sugar level regularly.
- Assess urine output – note and discard urine in catheter bag from theatre (as with chest drains); aim for 0.5–1 mL/kg/h initially.
- To assess whether fluid management is effective:
  - Assess peripheral perfusion (pulses, capillary refill time)
  - Assess preload via CVP, LAP or both
  - Assess for adequate urine output
  - Assess urea and electrolytes, haemoglobin (Hb) and haematocrit, urine specific gravity
  - Assess ongoing fluid losses through drains
- Fluids are usually given in boluses of 5–10 mL/kg, monitoring preload and urine output.
- Nutritional support in the form of enteral or parenteral feeds is usually started within 48 hours of surgery.

CARDIOPULMONARY BYPASS

CPB is a mechanical means of circulating and oxygenating the patient's blood while diverting most of the circulation from the heart and lungs. During CPB the blood volume is circulated continuously between the patient and the bypass machine, where it is filtered, temperature regulated, and oxygenated.

The main factors involved in preventing complications of CPB are:
- Hypothermia – decreases tissue O_2 requirements, providing some protection against ischaemic injury
- Haemodilution – the patient's blood is diluted with a crystalloid solution via the bypass machine to reduce blood viscosity and consequent formation of microthrombi

- Anticoagulation – heparinisation of blood to prevent coagulation in the bypass machine
- Cold cardioplegia – provides local hypothermia when infused into the aortic root and coronary arteries after aortic cross-clamping to induce cardiac standstill
  The risks of surgery involving CPB include:
- Infection
- Bleeding
- Microemboli (e.g., fat, air)
- Platelet aggregation
- Cell haemolysis

IMPORTANT POSTOPERATIVE PROBLEMS

Cardiac tamponade

Cardiac tamponade after cardiac surgery is caused by fluid collecting within the pericardial sac, which impedes adequate diastolic relaxation and cardiac filling and impairs myocardial function. It occurs if mediastinal drainage is inadequate (hence the importance of meticulous management of chest drains) or if brisk bleeding related to poor coagulation occurs.

An acute manifestation of cardiac tamponade presents with a tachycardia, high CVP and LAP, and hypotension. Bradycardia is a late sign, which usually leads to cardiac arrest. Open pericardotomy is usually necessary to remove the fluid and therefore the pressure within the pericardium.

Pulmonary hypertensive crisis

Pulmonary hypertensive crisis is characterised by an acute rise in PA pressure followed by a reduction in cardiac output and a fall in arterial O_2 saturation. It occurs more commonly with certain cardiac defects (e.g., transposition of the great arteries [TGA], ventricular septal defect [VSD], atrioventricular septal defect [AVSD], truncus arteriosus). Management includes prophylaxis in those at risk by avoiding factors that lead to increased pulmonary vascular resistance, for example acidosis (partial pressure of carbon dioxide (P_{CO_2}) pH – aim for normal P_{CO_2} or mild alkalosis), pain (ensure effective analgesia and sedation is administered). NO may be used to improve pulmonary vasodilatation.

In the event of a pulmonary hypertensive crisis, treatment includes rapid hand bagging with 100% O_2 and boluses of intravenous (IV) sedation (e.g., morphine/fentanyl, together with muscle relaxants).

REMOVAL OF LEFT ATRIAL LINE

Each institution will have a different policy about who removes LA lines, and local guidelines must be followed. Use universal precautions and an aseptic technique:

- Check clotting results and discuss with bedside doctor (consider need to stop anticoagulants prior to procedure).

- Ensure blood is immediately available for the patient and stored nearby in case of need.
- LA line MUST be removed prior to removal of mediastinal drain (ensure that the drain is patent).
- Contact cardiothoracic team to inform them of the procedure and check they would be free to attend if required in an emergency.
- Prepare the child and family and ensure the child has an appropriate level of analgesia.
- Involve a play specialist, if available, to play with and distract the child.
- Inform paediatric intensive care unit (PICU) doctor and nurse in charge that the procedure is taking place to ensure it is an appropriate time according to unit needs.
- Remove dressing and clean area.
- If line has been stitched in, remove suture.
- Hold a piece of dry, sterile gauze at insertion site as you gently, with a continuous pressure, remove the LA line and then immediately apply firm pressure to site.
- Observe the chest drain closely (some centres advocate 'milking' the mediastinal drain, but others do not – follow local policy).
- Ensure the line is complete and undamaged.
- If resistance is felt, stop procedure and inform doctor.
- Cardiac tamponade does infrequently occur after removal of intracardiac lines. If there is significant bleeding from the mediastinal drain, or no drainage but cardiovascular instability (i.e., rising tachycardia with falling blood pressure), call for bedside doctor, cardiothoracic surgeon, and nurse in charge immediately, then milk the chest drain and resuscitate the child.

Care of chest drains

Check the following:
- Child has adequate analgesia.
- Drainage bottle must contain a specified amount of sterile water to ensure that the end of the chest drain tubing is underwater so the underwater sealed drainage acts as a one-way valve allowing air or fluid to escape.
- Ensure taping is secure, and all connections are tight. Maintain visibility of entry site to ensure intact and sterile system.
- Ensure correct placement by chest x-ray.
- Drainage bottle should be checked regularly, and the fluid level and thus the amount of fluid draining should be documented on the fluid chart.
- Drainage bottle must be kept below chest level to prevent fluid flowing back into the pleural space.
- Thoracic suction (low negative pressure) may be indicated and suction should be set at −10 to −20 cm H_2O (Munnell 1997).
- The drain should bubble (pneumothorax) or swing (effusion – changes in intrapleural pressure during inspiration and expiration cause the fluid level in the bottle to rise and fall).

- If there is no bubbling (possible that pneumothorax has resolved) or swinging, this could indicate tube blockage and this should be reported immediately to medical staff because there is a possibility that a tension pneumothorax could develop.
- Milking the tube with roller clamps can generate negative intrathoracic pressures of up to 400 cm H_2O and is not recommended to maintain patency or for drains sited for pneumothoraces or pleural effusion (Roskelly & Smith 2011).
- Check entry site for signs of leakage, redness, or infection and report any abnormal findings.
- Keep the dressing clean and dry.
- Chest drain should be removed during expiration using a two-person technique.
- Clamping chest drains is generally NOT recommended, but there are a few situations where it may be necessary to clamp for a brief period of time, for example:
  - If the tube becomes accidentally disconnected – until reconnection
  - Following significant and rapid drainage in the first hour following insertion and under guidance from a senior doctor
  - Following intrapleural fibriolytic instillation
  - Transferring a patient where the chest drain needs to be briefly raised to the level of the patient's chest
  - Clamps should be available at the patient's bedside.
- If you need to transfer a patient with a chest drain in situ, consider the use of a Heimlich valve, which may reduce the risk of tube dislodgement en route, but ensure the end of the Heimlich valve is not obstructed.

NB Potential complications related to chest drains include pneumothorax, surgical emphysema, infection, dislodgement, or a life-threatening tension pneumothorax, so patients with chest drains should be regularly monitored, looking at drain patency and site, assessed for pain and breathlessness and observed with regular observations of temperature, heart rate, blood pressure, respiratory rate, work of breathing, saturations and documentation for fluid loss and presence of bubbling, swing, and fluid loss. Report any concerns.

CLASSIFICATION OF CONGENITAL HEART DISEASE

When planning the care and management of children with congenital heart disease, it may be useful to categorise defects in terms of alteration to blood flow. Most cardiac defects fall into one of four categories:

Increased pulmonary flow (left-to-right shunt)
- PDA
- Atrial septal defect (ASD)
- VSD
- AVSD

Decreased pulmonary flow (oligaemia on chest x-ray)
- Pulmonary stenosis (PS)
- Pulmonary atresia (PA)
- Tetralogy of Fallot (TOF)
- Tricuspid atresia (TA)

Decreased systemic flow
- Coarctation of aorta (Coarct)
- Aortic stenosis (AS)
- Interrupted aortic arch (IAA)
- Hypoplastic left heart syndrome (HLHS)

Altered circulation (mixing of pulmonary and systemic blood flow)
- TGA
- Truncus arteriosus (Truncus)
- Total anomalous pulmonary venous drainage (TAPVD)
- Double-outlet right ventricle (DORV)

Defects with increased pulmonary blood flow
PATENT DUCTUS ARTERIOSUS
Persistence of this duct beyond the perinatal period – usually closes spontaneously within hours of birth. See Fig. 3.6.

Fig. 3.6 Patent ductus arteriosus.

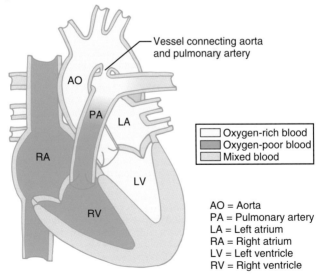

Vessel connecting aorta and pulmonary artery

AO

PA
LA

RA

LV

RV

Oxygen-rich blood
Oxygen-poor blood
Mixed blood

AO = Aorta
PA = Pulmonary artery
LA = Left atrium
RA = Right atrium
LV = Left ventricle
RV = Right ventricle

Effect: Blood flows from the aorta through the PDA to the PA – therefore there is increased flow to the lungs

Signs and symptoms: Generally asymptomatic but if large PDA with moderate to significant left to right shunt, the infant may present with tachypnea, difficulty in feeding, failure to thrive, pulmonary congestion, tachycardia, continuous murmur

Diagnosis: Echocardiography primarily

Management: Closed by cardiac catheter 'coil' procedure or surgically ligated – thoracotomy approach. In the preterm infant, indomethacin (prostaglandin synthetase inhibitor) may be used to close the PDA.

> With some complex cardiac defects, it is imperative that the ductus arteriosus is kept patent to maintain pulmonary blood flow (e.g., pulmonary atresia) or systemic blood flow (e.g., coarctation of aorta/hypoplastic left heart). A prostaglandin E_2 infusion will be set up to maintain a PDA (see Chapter 10).

Postoperative: Subacute bacterial endocarditis (SBE) prophylaxis for 6 months after successful surgery

ATRIAL SEPTAL DEFECT

A hole in the atrial septum, of which there are three major types:

- Secundum – defect in the middle of the atrial septum (most common type, and at least half of these defects close on their own)
- Primum – defect in lower section of the atrial septum (may involve valves)
- Sinus venosus – defect in upper section of atrial septum (rare)

Effect: Blood shunts left → right and if untreated can cause right heart failure, pulmonary hypertension, arrhythmia, or stroke.

Signs and symptoms: Depends of the size of the ASD because many children with ASD appear healthy with no symptoms. Large ASD may result in poor appetite, fatigue, poor growth, shortness of breath

Diagnosis: Heart murmur may be first indication (listen at upper left sternal border – pulmonic position), echo, chest x-ray, and ECG

Management: Closed by cardiac catheter 'umbrella' procedure or surgically – patch repair involving bypass surgery

Postoperative: Possibility of atrial arrhythmias

VENTRICULAR SEPTAL DEFECT

A hole in the ventricular septum that may be singular or multiple, may be small or large and are the most common congenital heart defect in children. A VSD may be:

- Membranous – defect located near heart valves
- Muscular – defect in lower part of septum
- Perimembranous VSD – in left ventricular outflow tract beneath the AV

- Outlet/infundibular
- Inlet septum

Of VSDs, 95% are not associated with chromosomal abnormalities but are common in patients with trisomies 13, 18, and 21.

Effect: Blood shunts left → right; therefore if large, greatly increased flow to lungs.

 NB If PS is present, flow may be right → left.

Signs and symptoms: Infants may present with CHF at 6–8 weeks of age as pulmonary vascular resistance (PVR) falls and left-to-right shunting increases. They may present with poor feeding, sweating, tachypnea, tachycardia and poor weight gain, harsh systolic murmur (listen at lower left sternal border – tricuspid position)

Diagnosis: Echocardiography, chest x-ray – may show cardiomegaly with large VSD (but if pulmonary hypertension may show large PA, oligaemic lung fields and normal heart size)

Management:
- Corrective – patch repair to VSD involving bypass surgery. If small, some centres may close VSD via cardiac catheter.
- Palliative – PA banding to restrict flow to the lungs. This procedure is reversed, band removed when the patient is old enough to have a full repair and the VSD closed.

Postoperative: Possibility of residual leak across patch, when SBE prophylaxis should be observed, bleeding, AV block.

ATRIOVENTRICULAR SEPTAL DEFECT

An AVSD is characterised by a common AV junction with deficient AV septum. There is a strong association with trisomy 21. There may be many other associated defects, of which subaortic stenosis, ventricular hypoplasia, atrial isomerism, or tetralogy of Fallot are the more common. An AVSD may be balanced (where the right and left sides of the heart are comparable in size) or unbalanced (where the AV junction is committed to either ventricle and there may be relative hypoplasia of the opposing ventricle).

Effect: Mixing of oxygenated and deoxygenated blood at both levels. May result in AV valve regurgitation, congestive cardiac failure, and left → right shunt with pulmonary hypertension.

Signs and symptoms: Mild cyanosis, congestive cardiac failure, systolic murmur due to increased flow through the pulmonary valve, may also have diastolic murmur due to increased flow through the tricuspid valve

Diagnosis: Cardiomegaly and increased pulmonary vascularity on chest x-ray, ECG – prolonged PR interval, partial right bundle branch block, superior QRS axis, echo

Management:
- Management of congestive cardiac failure with diuretics and captopril, possible need for nasogastric feeds

- Surgical repair of defect – bypass surgery to perform patch closures to ASD and VSD and reconstruct clefts of AV valves if necessary
- In unbalanced AVSD – may need single ventricle surgical approach

Postoperative: Possibility of arrhythmias (particularly supraventricular tachycardia [SVT] or complete heart block), degree of cardiac failure due to valve incompetence, pulmonary hypertension. SBE prophylaxis usually indicated.

Defects with decreased pulmonary blood flow

PULMONARY STENOSIS

Narrowing of the entrance to the PA due to either pulmonary valve or pulmonary outflow tract obstruction.

Effect: Reduced blood flow to the lungs. Usually asymptomatic with mild stenosis.

Signs and symptoms – Neonates with critical PS are cyanotic and tachypnoeic. Systolic murmur, delayed second heart sound with severe stenosis

Diagnosis: Echocardiogram because most children are diagnosed postnatally

Management: For neonates with critical PS and cyanosis, a prostaglandin E_2 infusion to reopen the ductus should be started. Stenosed area widened by cardiac catheter technique – balloon dilatation passed through narrowed area – or surgical correction – patch widening of the right ventricular outflow tract (RVOT). Valvotomy if the valve is the cause.

Postoperative: SBE may be indicated.

PULMONARY ATRESIA

An atretic pulmonary valve, resulting from its failure to develop. PA is commonly seen in children with 22q11.2 deletion (DiGeorge syndrome). There are two main types:

- PA with intact ventricular septum – where there is a small RV and PA (hypoplastic right heart)
- PA with a VSD

Effect: There is no blood flow from the RV to the lungs. The neonate is dependent on other defects (ASD, VSD, PDA) for survival. The size of the RV is variable and related to survival.

Signs and symptoms – There is severe and progressive cyanosis from birth, tachypnea, dyspnea, poor feeding, lethargy, pale, blue, murmur

Diagnosis – Chest x-ray, ECG, echo and cardiac catheterisation

Management:

- Palliative – maintain PDA with prostaglandin E_2 infusion
- Balloon atrial septostomy may be indicated to improve RA to LA shunting of blood in patients
- Radiofrequency perforation of the pulmonary valve and balloon dilatation of the artery if possible
- PDA stent
- May require BT shunt, Glenn shunt, and Fontan (if RV remains too small)

Postoperative: Most patients require close follow-up because none of the surgical procedures are curative. Arrhythmias and sudden death SBE prophylaxis if indicated.

MODIFIED BLALOCK-TAUSSIG SHUNT

This palliative surgery is used to improve pulmonary blood flow in duct-dependent cyanotic heart defects so that the PAs may grow before repair or further staged palliation takes place. A Gore-Tex conduit is stitched between the subclavian artery and the PA – the shunts can vary in size from 3.5 to 5 mm even in small babies because it is thought that the orifice of the subclavian artery acts to regulate blood flow through the shunt. The length of the conduit is adjusted so that it must lie straight without kinking. See Fig. 3.7.

There is a proclivity to underestimate the care and attention to detail required when caring for an infant or child undergoing a BT shunt, but neonatal mortality of 9% has been reported (Dirks et al 2013).

Postoperative complications:

- Shunt thrombosis – maintain good systemic arterial pressure through-out operation and postoperatively to ensure good flow through shunt (De Leval et al 1981).

Fig. 3.7 Blalock-Taussig shunt. *AO,* Aorta; *LA,* left atrium; *LV,* left ventricle; *PA,* pulmonary artery; *RA,* right atrium; *RV,* right ventricle.

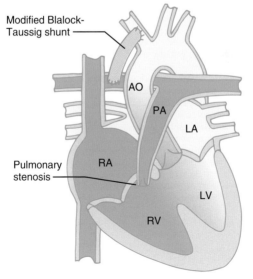

- Some centres use IV heparin initially then aspirin after extubation and once fed, for prophylaxis, but there is conflicting evidence around its use.
- Requirement of blood transfusion greater than 6 mL/kg found to be an independent predictor of mortality (Singh et al 2014).
- Look for signs of desaturation, listen for shunt murmur (continuous murmur in left infrascapular region), and if blockage suggested, this is an emergency (see later).
- Shunt kinking – many centres use thoracotomy approach, but this approach can cause PA distortion and unbalanced growth of branch PAs (Kandakure et al 2010), and it has been reported that it is 4 times more likely to fail if performed via thoracotomy rather than sternotomy (Odim et al 1995).
- Shunt too big – low systemic flow and low BP, and high saturations due to high pulmonary flow (review BP and watch diastolic pressure – if too low, this could compromise coronary flow and cause ischaemia)
- Shunt too small – low saturation and poor pulmonary blood flow, leading to hypoxia and poor oxygen delivery to tissues
- Excessive bleeding
- Low cardiac output

BLOCKED BLALOCK-TAUSSIG SHUNT

If a shunt is suspected of blocking with profound desaturation and absence of shunt murmur, this is an emergency. Follow local protocols, but the following information may be useful to consider:
- ABC resuscitation – bag/valve mask ventilate until intubation
- Hypotension will swiftly occur – consider fluid bolus and inotropic support; dopamine initially to maximise shunt perfusion pressure
- Request urgent echo
- Bolus heparin 50–100 units/kg (Giglia et al 2013)
- Restart prostin infusion in neonate
- Urgently inform cardiology and surgeon
- Consultants may consider use of recombinant tissue plasminogen activator (alteplase) but contraindicated if patient had recent surgery
- Consultant decision for cardiac catheter, balloon angioplasty, stent placement, thrombectomy, redo surgery, or ECMO

 NB Avoid dehydration in infants with shunts to minimise chance of shunt thrombosis (Fenton et al 2003).

FALLOT'S TETRALOGY (FIG. 3.8)

Four elements:
- VSD
- PS

Fig. 3.8 Blood flow through the heart with Fallot's tetralogy. (Adapted with permission from Whaley, L.F., Wong, D.L., 1991. Nursing Care of Infants and Children, fourth ed. CV Mosby, St Louis, MO.)

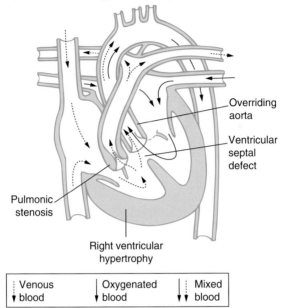

Venous blood	Oxygenated blood	Mixed blood

- Overriding aorta
- Right ventricular hypertrophy (RVH)

Effect: Degree of cyanosis depends on size of VSD and degree of PS, which affect direction of blood shunting through VSD.

Signs and symptoms: Cyanosis, fatigue, failure to thrive, poor feeding. Hypoxic 'spells' may occur, characterised by:
- Paroxysm of hyperpnoea (rapid and deep respiration)
- Irritability and prolonged crying
- Increasing cyanosis
- Decreased intensity of the heart murmur

A severe spell may lead to limpness, convulsions, cerebrovascular accident, or even death. Management is aimed at breaking the vicious cycle and includes positioning (squatting or knees to chest), IV morphine/ketamine, fluid bolus to increase RV preload reducing acidosis, and administering O_2.

Children with tetralogy of Fallot may have clubbing of the fingers. (Up to 34% of children with TOF may also have a right aortic arch. See vascular ring.)

Diagnosis: Physical examination, chest x-ray may show 'boot-shaped' heart, echo, ECG shows RVH, murmur may be heard at tricuspid position.

Management:

- Total correction bypass surgery involving VSD patch closure and patch widening of RVOT. This is the surgery of choice, usually repaired in infancy.
- Palliative if PS is severe, BT shunt (anastomosis between the subclavian artery and ipsilateral PA) prior to total correction to improve pulmonary blood flow.

Postoperative: Possibility of arrhythmias, particularly ventricular tachycardia (VT), and pulmonary hypertension. May require additional fluid to optimise preload because of RVH. Varying levels of activity limitation may be indicated. SBE prophylaxis may be indicated.

TRICUSPID ATRESIA

An atretic tricuspid valve resulting from its failure to develop. Three types of TA are described:

- TA with usual arrangement of the great vessels
- TA with D-transposition of the great arteries
- TA with L-transposition of the great arteries

Effect: No blood flow from RA to RV and therefore to the lungs. The neonate is dependent on other defects (e.g., PDA, ASD, VSD) for survival.

Signs and symptoms: Severe cyanosis, congestive cardiac failure, tachypnea, poor feeding, and failure to thrive are usual. May also see jugular venous distension and large liver and 80% will have a murmur. Some may present with bacterial endocarditis, headache, seizures, and neurologic deficits. Clubbing of fingers may occur after 3 months.

Diagnosis: Chest x-ray may show cardiomegaly with prominent right heart border (right atrial enlargement) with reduced pulmonary vascular markings (may be 'boot-shaped' heart), ECG – usually sinus rhythm although sometimes first-degree AV block, may have tall P waves due to atrial enlargement, cardiac catheterisation.

Management:

- Infants with decreased pulmonary blood flow – keep PDA patent with prostaglandin E_2 infusion and BT or Waterston shunt (anastomosis between the ascending aorta and right PA) to ensure blood flow to lungs.
- Infants with increased pulmonary blood flow (have an unrestrictive VSD and transposition) often present in severe congestive cardiac failure and require diuretics and PA banding to restrict pulmonary blood flow.
- Correction stage 1, bidirectional Glenn (BDG) shunt – SVC to right PA anastomosis with blood flow to both lungs. Stage 2, Fontan procedure – baffle (tunnel) of IVC flow through RA connecting directly to right PA where SVC is also directly connected.

A fenestration (hole) may be present in the baffle, allowing some escape into the RA if the pressure in the baffle becomes high.

Postoperative: For Glenn and Fontan procedures, extubate early (positive pressure ventilation impedes venous drainage). Possibility of pleural effusions due to high right-sided venous pressure. May need to be excluded from competitive sports and receive SBE prophylaxis.

Defects with decreased systemic blood flow

COARCTATION OF AORTA

Severe narrowing of a segment of the aorta.

This may be:

- Preductal narrowing proximal to ductus arteriosus. PDA allows blood to shunt from the PA to descending aorta.
- Postductal narrowing distal to ductus arteriosus. PDA allows blood to shunt from aorta to PA. Collateral circulation may supply blood from the subclavian arteries to the descending aorta.
- Periductal narrowing located at level of ductus arteriosus. Bidirectional shunting through the PDA may occur (proximal aorta → PDA; PDA → distal aorta).

Effect: Reduction in circulatory blood flow, signs of congestive heart failure and renal failure, which may lead to general circulatory shock.

Signs and symptoms: Usually in first few weeks of life, tachypnea, increased work of breathing, tachycardia, poor feeding, lethargy, congestive cardiac failure, absent femoral pulses, low cardiac output, often a systolic murmur (aortic position)

Diagnosis: Take four-limb BP and look for systolic pressure difference of 10–20 mm Hg between arms and legs may indicate coarctation. Echo, ECG, magnetic resonance imaging (MRI), cardiac catheterisation

Management: Surgical correction (not usually requiring bypass) in infancy if symptomatic – end-to-end anastomosis or subclavian flap repair (subclavian artery ligated so unable to obtain cuff BP in that arm).

 NB There is a risk of necrotising enterocolitis because of decreased mesenteric blood flow. If coarct is suspected, perform four-limb cuff BP to make comparisons.

Postoperative: Possibility of hypertension – infusion of vasodilator drugs (e.g., glyceryl trinitrate [GTN]) may be required. Necrotising enterocolitis/acute renal failure may develop, depending on the degree to which the blood supply was compromised. Recoarctation may occur. SBE prophylaxis may be indicated.

AORTIC STENOSIS

Obstruction to the blood flow between the LV and the aorta caused by stenosis (narrowing) of the AV at various locations:

- Valvular (most common) A bicuspid rather than tricuspid aortic valve is the most common form of AS.

- Subvalvular muscular obstruction below the AV; may be due to long, tunnel-like narrowing of the left ventricular outflow tract or another type of subvalvular stenosis, idiopathic hypertrophic subaortic stenosis, which is a primary disorder of the heart muscle (cardiomyopathy).
- Supravalvular aortic narrowing immediately above the valve, often associated with Williams syndrome (mental retardation, characteristic 'elfin face,' and PS).

Effect: Newborn infants with critical AS may develop congestive heart failure, with a clinical picture resembling sepsis with low cardiac output. Left ventricular hypertrophy may develop if the stenosis is severe. A poststenotic dilatation of the ascending aorta develops with valvular AS. Aortic regurgitation usually develops in subaortic AS.

Signs and symptoms: Congestive cardiac failure, tachycardic, tachypnea, low cardiac output, poor feeding, poor urine output, distress

Diagnosis: Examination – poor peripheral perfusion, reduced pulses, systolic murmur – listen in aortic position, echo, chest x-ray may show cardiomegaly with pulmonary venous congestion, MRI, ECG

Management:

- Palliative – in critically ill infants and children with congestive heart failure, O_2, diuretics and inotropes, possibly with prostaglandin infusion are indicated, with urgent need for surgery.
- Balloon valvuloplasty may be performed at cardiac catheterisation.
- Exercise restriction in children with moderate–severe form, good oral hygiene, and SBE prophylaxis are important.
- Surgical closed aortic valvotomy using calibrated dilators or balloon catheter without cardiac bypass, or the following procedures may be performed under cardiac bypass:
  - Artificial valve replacement with pulmonary valve autograft (Ross procedure – see later); valve replacement following aortic root enlargement (Konno procedure) for tunnel-like narrowing; excision of the membrane for discrete subvalvular stenosis; widening of the stenotic area using a diamond-shaped fabric patch for discrete supravalvular stenosis

Postoperative: Restriction from competitive sports recommended with children with moderate residual AS/regurgitation. SBE prophylaxis if indicated. Recurrence of discrete recurrent subaortic stenosis is frequent following surgical resection of the membrane.

Ross procedure: The Ross procedure is an AV replacement in which the patient's own pulmonary valve is transplanted to the AV position and the pulmonary valve is replaced with a homograft. An advantage for children is that the replaced AV retains growth potential and does not require anticoagulation therapy.

INTERRUPTED AORTIC ARCH

Interrupted is the absence or discontinuation of a portion of the aortic arch. There are three types, classified according to the site of the interruption (Fig. 3.9):

- Type A interruption occurs just beyond the left subclavian artery – approximately 30–40% reported cases

Fig. 3.9 Interrupted aortic arch – showing three types. *IAA*, Interrupted aortic arch; *PDA*, patent ductus arteriosus; *VSD*, ventricular septal defect. (From Everett, A.D., Lim, D.S., 2010. Illustrated Field Guide to Congenital Heart Disease and Repair, third ed. Scientific Software Solutions, Charlottesville, VA.)

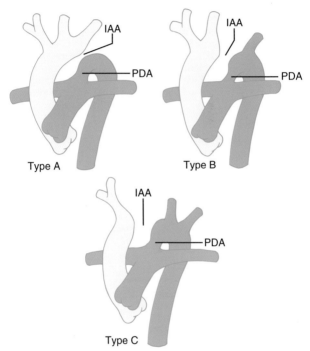

Type A

Type B

Type C

- Type B interruption occurs between the left carotid artery and the left subclavian artery: most common – approximately 53% reported cases
- Type C interruption occurs between innominate artery and left carotid artery – least common: approximately 4% reported cases (Cincinnati Children's Hospital Medical Center 2016)

Effect: PDA and VSD are almost always associated with this defect; patients with type B often have DiGeorge syndrome; bicuspid AV, mitral valve deformity, persistent truncus arteriosus, or subaortic stenosis may be present.

Signs and symptoms: Infants with PDA may appear asymptomatic or have normally saturated blood supplying upper body and then deoxygenated blood supplying the lower body with differential cyanosis.

The VSD presents left → right shunting, causing increased blood flow to the lungs and congestive heart failure. As the PDA closes, respiratory distress, cyanosis, and circulatory shock develop then death.

Diagnosis: Echo, ECG may show RVH and ST-T wave abnormalities, cardiac catheterisation to identify the site of arch interruption.

Management:

- Palliative prostaglandin E_2 infusion, intubation and ventilation, ascertain serum calcium and test for DiGeorge syndrome (i.e., chromosomal analysis for 22q deletion)
- Corrective surgical repair of interruption (primary anastomosis, vascular graft) and closure of a simple VSD are recommended if possible. If associated with complex defects, repair of the interruption and PA banding are performed initially with complete repair later.
- Yasui procedure (for systemic outflow tract obstruction [e.g., IAA plus left ventricular outflow tract obstruction [LVOTO] or AA or AS with VSD]) combines a Norwood stage 1 arch reconstruction (neo aorta to descending aorta with removal of PDA) and a Rastelli procedure to establish biventricular repair either in a two-stage or single-stage repair (Yasui et al 1987). See Fig. 3.10 for Yasui procedure.

Fig. 3.10 Yasui procedure. *LA*, Left atrium; *LV*, left ventricle; *RA*, right atrium; *RV*, right ventricle; *VSD*, ventricular septal defect.

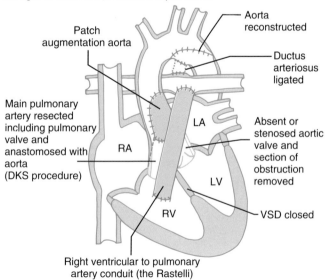

Patch augmentation aorta

Aorta reconstructed

Ductus arteriosus ligated

Main pulmonary artery resected including pulmonary valve and anastomosed with aorta (DKS procedure)

LA

RA

Absent or stenosed aortic valve and section of obstruction removed

LV

VSD closed

RV

Right ventricular to pulmonary artery conduit (the Rastelli)

HYPOPLASTIC LEFT HEART SYNDROME (FIG. 3.11)

A collection of complex defects on the left side of the heart:

- Underdeveloped LV
- Mitral valve stenosis/atresia
- Hypoplastic ascending aorta and aortic arch
- AS/atresia

Effect: Infant is reliant on PDA for systemic blood flow and patent foramen ovale (PFO) for mixing of blood at atrial level. Neonates present in hypotensive shock if ductus closure occurs, the inadequate systemic blood flow causing a profound metabolic acidosis. Fatal without surgical intervention.

Signs and symptoms: Cyanosis, tachypnea, respiratory distress, oliguria, poor peripheral perfusion, cardiogenic shock

Diagnosis: Clinical examination, echo, ECG, chest x-ray

Management: Parents are counselled in the antenatal period about treatment options for HLHS, and there is still a proportion of parents who decide to terminate pregnancy in light of this diagnosis,

Fig. 3.11 Blood flow through the heart in hypoplastic left heart syndrome. (Adapted with permission from Whaley, L.F., Wong, D.L., 1991. Nursing Care of Infants and Children, fourth ed. CV Mosby, St Louis, MO.)

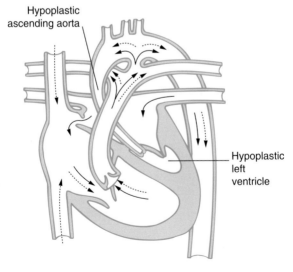

Hypoplastic ascending aorta

Hypoplastic left ventricle

| Venous blood | Oxygenated blood | Mixed blood |

or indeed opt to have their baby but decide not to take any surgical palliation. However, it is thought that approximately 70% of infants with HLHS who undergo palliation will reach adulthood (Feinstein et al 2012; Arnold et al 2014). Surgical options:

- Transplantation (not generally considered in the United Kingdom in neonates)
- Surgery – the Norwood 1 procedure or hybrid then a further two-stage surgery palliation to achieve separate systemic and pulmonary venous circulation with single ventricle physiology (Fontan)

Preoperative:
- Prostaglandin E_2 infusion to maintain PDA and therefore adequate systemic perfusion
- Aim for S_aO_2 75–85% to balance lungs versus systemic blood flow by using room air
- May need to intubate and ventilate – keeping PCO_2 at 5–6 kPa will increase pulmonary vascular resistance and help to keep S_aO_2 within desired range
- Correct acidosis

If the infant desaturates, increase F_iO_2, but if it is necessary to bag the infant, bag in **air**; remembering that O_2 is a pulmonary vasodilator, therefore use air to avoid unnecessary pulmonary vascular vasodilatation and subsequent pulmonary overcirculation. Consider also the effect of CO_2 (pulmonary vasoconstriction); hyperventilation will lower the CO_2 and again may cause pulmonary overcirculation. Use oxygen if the infant is profoundly desaturated or for resuscitation.

Stage 1 – Norwood procedure (Fig. 3.12):
Mean survival of Norwood 1 during time period 1980–2010 found to be 80% (Sistino & Bonilla 2012).
- Division of main PA and closure of distal stump
- Modified right BT shunt between subclavian artery and right PA to provide pulmonary blood flow. There will be continuous forward flow (in systole and diastole) into the BT shunt as the PVR is lower than the systemic vascular resistance – which can lead to low diastolic BP and coronary steal, which may result in reduced myocardial perfusion (Ohye et al 2004).
- PDA is ligated and atrial septum excised to allow mixing of blood across atria.
- Construction of new aortic arch between the main PA and ascending aorta and arch.

Postoperative:
Often chest left open to reduce risk of tamponade. High risk of low cardiac output, myocardial oedema, inflammatory stimuli from CPB. CPR required in up to 17% of babies. Arrhythmias common – SVT, JET, VT, and CHB (Wernovsky et al 2007). Commence heparin infusion within 1 hour of return to PICU (unless significant bleeding)

Fig. 3.12 Norwood procedure.

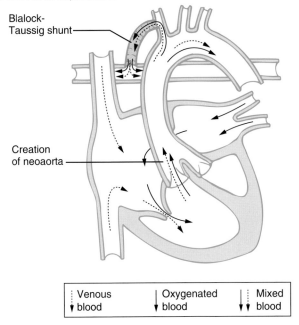

Blalock-
Taussig shunt

Creation
of neoaorta

| Venous blood | Oxygenated blood | Mixed blood |

to maintain the BT shunt but bleeding and coagulopathy common problems. Manipulate $P\text{CO}_2$ to balance the pulmonary versus systemic blood flow (e.g., keep $P\text{CO}_2$ at 5–6 kPa and aim for $S_a\text{O}_2$ 75–85%). Use regional saturation monitoring (NIRS) for cerebral and splanchnic saturations. Nil by mouth initially. (Each centre will have its own protocols and these should be used.)

Stage 1 – Sano shunt:
Pulmonary overcirculation through a systemic–pulmonary shunt (as earlier) has been documented as one of the major causes of early death after the Norwood procedure (Sano et al 2004). To avoid this an RV → pulmonary shunt known as the Sano shunt has been used in the first stage of palliation surgery. The important advantage of the Sano shunt is that flow occurs only during systole, with no competition between pulmonary and coronary blood flow during diastole, as is the case with the BT shunt. This is the most likely explanation for the much-improved stability of neonates which is seen following a Sano shunt (Jonas 2003). However, the effect on the growth of PAs is in question because on angiography prior to stage 2 palliation, infants who had a BT shunt had larger mid-branch PA diameter compared

Fig. 3.13 Sano shunt. (From Everett, A.D., Lim, D.S., 2010. Illustrated Field Guide to Congenital Heart Disease and Repair, third ed. Scientific Software Solutions, Charlottesville, VA.)

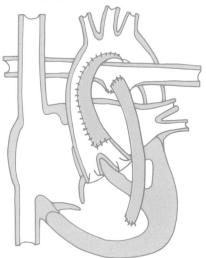

with infants with Sano shunts (Raja et al 2011; Aiyagari et al 2013). See Fig. 3.13 Sano shunt.

- Division of proximal main PA and closure of distal main PA
- Polytetrafluoroethylene (Gore-Tex) tube and cuff anastomosed to the distal end of the main PA
- Anastomosis of descending aorta to posterior wall of aortic arch. Entire aortic arch and ascending aorta reconstructed by direct anastomosis of proximal main PA. Small right ventriculotomy made in outflow tract for proximal anastomosis of RV–PA shunt.
- After completion of aortic reconstruction and atrial septectomy, proximal anastomosis of the RV–PA shunt was performed with the heart beating.

Postoperative: Similar principles to postoperative management of previous stage 1 Norwood except that pulmonary versus systemic balance of circulation is more stable, as described previously, and management is therefore reported to be more 'routine' (Jonas 2003).

Stage 1 – Hybrid procedure:

Some centres use hybrid procedure in 'high-risk' neonates (including low birth weight less than 2.5 kg, premature, poor ventricular function, restrictive atrial septum, aortic atresia, severe noncardiac abnormalities) (Bacha et al 2006).

- Banding of PAs to limit blood flow to lungs via sternotomy
- Stent to ductus arteriosus to maintain patency.

An advantage of this procedure is that it avoids CPB and cardioplegic arrest and thus reduces the risk of neurologic impairment that is associated with CPB in the critical neonatal period.

Postoperative: Potential problem of stent migration and the risk of poor perfusion due to unrepaired hypoplastic aortic arch.

Interstage mortality between stages 1 and 2 Norwood palliation has been reported between 2% and 16% (Feinstein et al 2012). These infants have poor cardiac reserve, and they will be on home monitoring programs.

Stage 2 – Hemi-Fontan (HF) OR BDG shunt:

- Performed at age of 3–6 months when there has been adequate growth of the PAs and there is low PVR
- Aim to reduce the work of the single ventricle

Hemi-Fontan operation: modified–BT shunt excised (or stented PDA excised and PAs debanded). The SVC is anastomosed to the right PA directing venous flow from the head and upper body to the lungs, and a patch is placed between the SVC and the RA to prevent flow from the SVC into the heart. HF may have an advantage over BDG because better caval offset avoids opposing blood streams from SVC and IVC competing after lateral tunnel completion (Talwar et al 2014).

See Fig. 3.14 for comparison of HF and BDG shunts.

Bidirectional Glen operation: modified–BT shunt taken down (or stented PDA excised and PAs debanded), the SVC is divided from the RA and sutured to the right PA, which directs deoxygenated blood passively from the head and neck directly to the lungs via the PAs.

Postoperative: Early extubation as positive pressure ventilation causes increased intrathoracic pressure which impedes passive blood flow from the head and neck to the lungs. Need to maintain adequate blood pressure as blood flow to lungs is passive from SVC. High venous pressures in head and upper extremities initially require heparin to prevent clots in new cavopulmonary connection; arrhythmias, phrenic nerve injury, and embolic episodes are also complications post stage 2 repair.

Stage 3 – Modified Fontan: Performed at age 2–3 years (Fig. 3.15):

- Aim is to separate pulmonary/systemic flow as long as pulmonary vascular resistance is sufficiently low.
- A tunnel is constructed (either extracardiac or a lateral atrial tunnel) to connect the IVC to the PA. A fenestration may be created between the tunnel and the RA that will act as a pop-off valve so that if right-sided pressures are high, small amounts of venous blood will be pushed through the fenestration.
- Systemic and pulmonary circulation will be separate after this surgery, so the child's saturations will be near normal.

Postoperative: Early extubation. Arrhythmias, particularly atrial tachycardia and fibrillation, and sinus node dysfunction. The long-term risk factor following a Fontan is the systemic ventricle that has right ventricular morphology and thus highly associated with heart failure and mortality (Feinstein et al 2012). Lymphatic circulation affected by high venous pressure and impaired thoracic duct drainage, obstructed lymphatic drainage may lead to interstitial pulmonary oedema and chylous pleural effusions.

Fig. 3.14 Hemi-Fontan compared with bidirectional Glenn shunt.

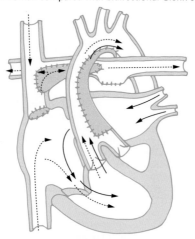

Hemi-fontan

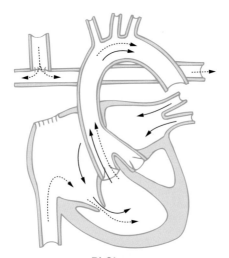

Bi-Glenn

⋮ Venous	↓ Oxygenated	⋮ Mixed
↓ blood	↓ blood	↓↓ blood

Fig. 3.15 Modified Fontan procedure.

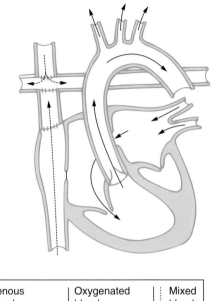

| : Venous | | Oxygenated | : Mixed |
| ▼ blood | ▼ | blood | ▼▼ blood |

Altered circulation

D-TRANSPOSITION OF THE GREAT ARTERIES

The aorta arises from the morphologic RV and the PA from the morphologic LV (Fig. 3.16). In approximately one-third of patients with TGA, there is also coronary artery abnormalities. It is important to note additional subtypes:

- TGA with intact ventricular septum
- TGA with VSD
- TGA with VDS and LVOTO
- TGA with VSD and pulmonary vascular obstructive disease

Effect: Systemic venous blood returns to the systemic arterial circulation and pulmonary – oxygenated – blood returns to the pulmonary circulation. Survival is impossible unless an additional defect (e.g., PFO, PDA, VSD) is present to allow mixing of oxygenated and deoxygenated blood.

Fig. 3.16 Transposition of the great arteries.

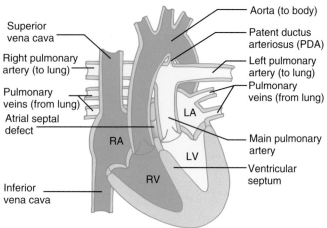

Signs and symptoms: TGA with intact ventricular septum and TGS with VSD and LVOTO will present within 24 hours with severe and progressive cyanosis. TGA with VSD may have mild cyanosis and may develop tachypnea, tachycardia, and failure to thrive in first few weeks of life.

Diagnosis: Use the hyperoxia test to establish whether cyanotic congenital heart disease of the newborn. Chest x-ray may show classic 'egg on a string' appearance in approximately one-third of patients with TGA, or it may appear normal or cardiomegaly with increased pulmonary markings if there is TGA and VSD. Echo is used for diagnosis, it is particularly important to note the origins of the coronary arteries. If there is uncertainty regarding the coronary arteries angiography or MRI may be necessary to delineate the vessels prior to surgery.

Management: Prostaglandin E_2 infusion to maintain PDA. Balloon atrial septostomy via cardiac catheterisation to improve mixing of blood if septum intact. Surgical options include:

• Jatene (arterial switch) procedure in the neonatal period, in which the PA and aorta are transposed and the coronary arteries are reimplanted into the aorta in its new location. Ideally surgery within first few weeks so that the LV is able to cope with systemic pressure postoperatively, having only been used to a low pressure and low resistance pulmonary circuit preoperatively for a limited period. See Fig. 3.17 Jatene arterial switch.

• PA band to increase LVOTO, thus 'training' the LV then a late arterial switch (watch for ↑LA pressure and LV dilatation after PA band because this could indicate poor tolerance of the band and impending collapse).

Fig. 3.17 Jatene arterial switch operation. (A) Transection of aorta (AO) and main pulmonary artery (PA). Removal of 'button' section of aorta with each coronary artery. (B) Coronary artery 'buttons' transferred to neo aorta. (C) Reconnection of the distal ascending aorta to main pulmonary artery. (D) Reconnection of the main pulmonary artery to the proximal aorta.

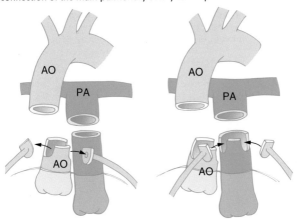

A Transection of aorta and main pulmonary artery.
Removal of "button" section of aorta with each coronary artery

B Coronary artery "buttons" transfered to neo aorta

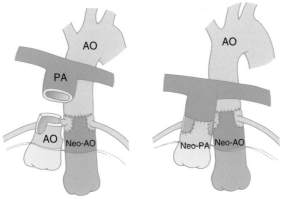

C Reconnection of the distal ascending aorta to main pulmonary artery

D Reconnection of the main pulmonary artery to the proximal aorta

Fig. 3.18 Rastelli operation. (A) The PA is divided from the LV, and the cardiac end is oversewn *(arrow)*. (B) An intracardiac tunnel *(arrow)* is placed between the large ventricular septal defect and the aorta. (C) The RV is connected to the divided PA by an aortic homograft or a valve-bearing prosthetic conduit. *Ao,* Aorta; *LA,* left atrium; *LV,* left ventricle; *PA,* pulmonary artery; *RA,* right atrium; *RV,* right ventricle. (Redrawn with permission from Park, M.K., 2003. The Pediatric Cardiology Handbook, third ed. CV Mosby, St Louis, MO.)

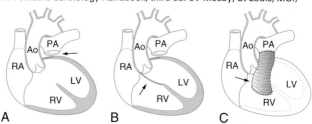

A   B   C

- Rastelli procedure – for TGA, VSD, and PS. A baffle is placed, closing the VSD and directing blood from LV to aorta. An RV-to-PA conduit is placed using a homograft (cadaver valved tissue) or Gore-Tex– or Dacron-containing bovine or porcine valve. See Fig. 3.18 Rastelli procedure.
- Nikaidoh procedure (Nikaidoh 1984) – for TGA, VSD, and PS. This was developed to avoid obstruction of the left and RVOTs. The main PA is divided just above the pulmonary valve, the valve is excised and the LVOT is widely opened. The aorta with attached coronaries is divided circumferentially with a wide rim of right ventricular free wall from the RV and sutured into place into the left ventricular outflow tract. The VSD will be closed via suture or patch. A pericardial patch is used to reconstruct the RVOT (or a homograft can be used). See Fig. 3.19 Nikaidoh procedure.

Postoperative: Possibility of coronary artery obstruction causing myocardial ischaemia/infarction/left ventricular dysfunction postarterial switch and ventricular dysrhythmias may occur. After Rastelli, watch for AV dissociation and other dysrhythmias and low cardiac output state. SBE prophylaxis may be indicated.

 Preoperatively, if it is necessary to bag the infant, use **air** if required because of the effect this will have on systemic flow (as discussed under HLHS).

Fig. 3.19 Nikaidoh procedure. *PS*, Pulmonary stenosis; *TGA*, transposition of the great arteries; *VSD*, ventricular septal defect.

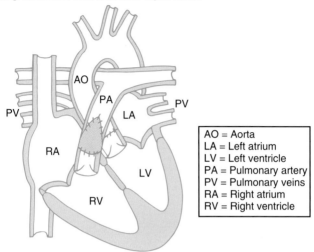

AO = Aorta
LA = Left atrium
LV = Left ventricle
PA = Pulmonary artery
PV = Pulmonary veins
RA = Right atrium
RV = Right ventricle

CONGENITALLY CORRECTED TRANSPOSITION OF THE GREAT ARTERIES

The atrial arrangement is normal (i.e., the RA is on the right of the LA; Fig. 3.20). However:

- The RA empties into the anatomic LV (identified as such by the presence of the bicuspid mitral rather than tricuspid valve).
- The LA empties into the anatomic RV (identified as such by the presence of the tricuspid rather than mitral valve).
- The great arteries are transposed, with the aorta arising from the RV and the PA arising from the LV. The aorta lies to the left of and anterior to the PA.
- The final result is a functional correction – oxygenated blood entering the LA flows to the anatomic RV and then out via the aorta.
- AV node is often divided causing rhythm disturbances – usually heart block.

Effect: Theoretically, no functional abnormalities exist, but most cases are complicated by associated defects: 60% have VSD with/without pyloric stenosis (PS) resulting in cyanosis; regurgitation of the systemic AV (tricuspid) valve; varying degrees of heart block; 20% have dextrocardia SVT.

Signs and symptoms: may be asymptomatic particularly in early childhood or

Fig. 3.20 Congenitally corrected transposition of the great arteries. *Ao*, Aorta; *LA*, left atrium; *LV*, left ventricle; *PA*, pulmonary artery; *RA*, right atrium; *RV*, right ventricle. (Redrawn with permission from Park, M.K., 2003. The Pediatric Cardiology Handbook, third ed. CV Mosby, St Louis, MO.)

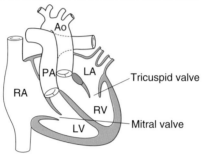

- Bradycardia
- Tachyarrhythmia
- Heart murmur due to associated VSD, PS, or tricuspid regurgitation
- Heart failure
- Pulmonary hypertension
- Cyanosis if has VSD

Diagnosis: Usually diagnosed in later childhood or as an adult with a failing RV, tricuspid regurgitation or heart block. Echo, cardiac MRI, ECG, and chest x-ray are used in diagnosis. ECG may show AV block, atrial arrhythmias, and abnormal ventricular activation due to ventricular bundle branch inversion.

Management:
- Palliative treatment of congestive heart failure and arrhythmias; SBE prophylaxis if indicated; PA banding if congestive heart failure is due to large VSD; systemic–pulmonary shunt for severe PS
- Corrective closure of VSD (total heart block common complication); relief of PS and/or valve replacement for significant tricuspid regurgitation; pacemaker implantation as indicated for complete heart block whether spontaneous or surgically induced.
- Double switch procedure – atrial switch (Senning or Mustard) and arterial switch may be used, but this may require LV preconditioning with a PA band to enable it to cope with systemic afterload. (See Fig. 3.21 Double switch procedure.) Intra-atrial baffles alter atrial blood flow, and the great vessels are transposed (see arterial switch in D-TGA). Conduction disturbances postoperatively are common due to interruption of the abnormally situated conduction pathway (commonly heart block). This is still considered experimental surgery.
- Cardiac transplantation may be required for a failing systemic RV.

Fig. 3.21 Double-switch operation. *PA*, Pulmonary artery; *VSD*, ventricular septal defect.

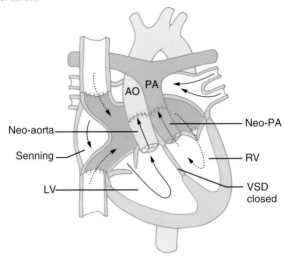

Postoperative: After VSD closure, tricuspid regurgitation can worsen due to septal shift and possible distortion of the AV valve annulus. Regular follow-up is needed for possible progression of AV block and for routine pacemaker care if implanted. Limitation of activity is indicated if haemodynamic abnormalities exist.

TRUNCUS ARTERIOSUS (COMMON ARTERIAL TRUNK)

Failure of normal septation and division of the common trunk into the PA and aorta. Fig. 3.22 shows truncus.

Effect: A single vessel arises from both ventricles, straddling a VSD and providing blood flow to pulmonary, systemic, and coronary circulation with a semilunar truncal valve. Four types:

- Type 1 – main PA arises from the truncus
- Type 2 – left and right PAs arise separately from the back of the truncus
- Type 3 – left and right PAs arise laterally from the truncus
- Type 4 – left and right PAs arise laterally from the descending aorta.

Signs and symptoms: Neonates may present in shock due to heart failure with significant pulmonary overcirculation (sepsis may be differential diagnosis). If there is profound truncal valve regurgitation, there will be signs of heart failure. In addition:

- Cyanosis (this may not be evident in very young babies who still have high PVR) but even older babies may have saturations in 90s

Fig. 3.22 Truncus arteriosus. (A) Type 1. (B) Type 2. (C) Type 3. (D) Type 4. (With permission from Park, M.K., 2003. The Pediatric Cardiology Handbook, third ed. CV Mosby, St Louis, MO.)

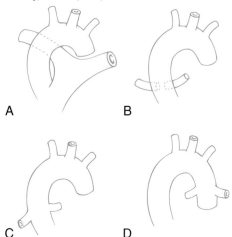

A   B

C   D

- Poor feeding
- Sweaty
- Tachypnea
- Pulmonary hypertension
- Heart failure (more pronounced when PVR falls and pulmonary overcirculation increases)
- IAA is a common anomaly associated with truncus, and these babies may present with cardiovascular collapse due to closure of the ductus arteriosus.
- Common association (approximately 20% of patients with truncus) with DiGeorge syndrome, so hypocalcaemia may be a finding (Momma 2010).
- Increased risk of necrotising enterocolitis (NEC) both preoperatively and postoperatively

Diagnosis: ECG shows sinus rhythm often with biventricular hypertrophy (if pulmonary overcirculation, LA enlargement may be identified). Chest x-ray may show cardiomegaly with increased pulmonary vascular markings. Echo can confirm truncus.

Management:
- Intravenous prostin should be commenced on any neonate with suspected congenital heart disease but will only be beneficial if the neonate with truncus has an associated IAA or coarctation.

- Primary repair – usually within first few months of life: PAs separated and conduit made from the RV to the pulmonary circulation with closure of the VSD.

Postoperative: Delayed sternal closure is often required, possibility of bleeding, truncal valve regurgitation, ventricular arrhythmias.

TOTAL ANOMALOUS PULMONARY VENOUS DRAINAGE

Failure of the pulmonary veins to join the LA; instead, they are abnormally connected to the systemic venous circulation via the RA or veins draining towards it (e.g., SVC).

Four types, classified according to the pulmonary venous point of attachment:

- Supracardiac (50% of TAPVD cases) – the common pulmonary vein drains into the SVC via the left SVC (vertical vein) and the left innominate vein with usually mild obstruction (Fig. 3.23 Supracardiac TAPVD)
- Cardiac (25%) – the common pulmonary vein drains into the coronary sinus or the pulmonary veins enter the RA separately through four openings
- Infracardiac (subdiaphragmatic) (25%) – the common pulmonary vein drains into the portal vein, ductus venosus, hepatic vein, then into the IVC and there will be obstruction requiring immediate surgical repair
- Mixed type – a combination of the other types

Effect: An interatrial communication is necessary for survival (PFO or ASD). If there is no obstruction to pulmonary venous return (most supracardiac and cardiac types), pulmonary venous return is large and there is only slight systemic arterial desaturation because there will be mixing of oxygenated and deoxygenated blood in the RA and right → left shunting from the RA through the ASD. If there is obstruction to pulmonary venous return (infracardiac type), pulmonary venous return is small and the infant is profoundly cyanosed.

Signs and symptoms: Depending on the type of TAPVD and level of obstruction, children present with varying degrees of cyanosis. Oxygen saturation may be in mid to high 80s in children without pulmonary venous obstruction and obviously can be much lower when obstruction is present. Other symptoms can include:

- Tachypnea and grunting
- ↑ work of breathing (e.g., recession)
- Murmur
- Signs of right heart failure
- Pulmonary oedema
- Pulmonary hypertension

Diagnosis: Depending on type of TAPVD, some or all symptoms may be present.

- Presence of a murmur, right heart failure, and cyanosis
- ECG – may indicate enlargement of right heart

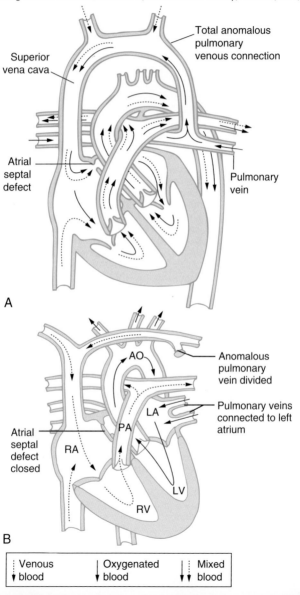

Fig. 3.23 (A) Blood flow through the heart with supracardiac total anomalous pulmonary venous drainage (TAPVD). (B) Repair of (TAPVD). *Ao*, Aorta; *LA*, left atrium; *LV*, left ventricle; *PA*, pulmonary artery; *RA*, right atrium; *RV*, right ventricle. ((A), Adapted with permission from Whaley, L.F., Wong, D.L., 1991. Nursing Care of Infants and Children, fourth ed. CV Mosby, St Louis, MO.)

- Chest x-ray – enlargement of right heart and increased blood flow to pulmonary vessels – classic 'snowman' sign (usually supracardiac TAPVD)
- Possible pulmonary oedema
- Echo – showing abnormal connection of pulmonary veins, identifying type of TAPVD, assessing also the blood flow across the ASD

Management: If obstructed, O_2, ventilation, and diuretics to manage pulmonary oedema, but emergency surgery is required. If there is a restrictive ASD, a balloon septostomy may be indicated. Surgical correction according to site of anomalous drainage – the aim is to channel pulmonary venous return to the LA, with closure of the ASD.

Postoperative: Possibility of atrial arrhythmias, may require extended period of ventilation postoperatively.

> In all cases of suspected congenital heart disease in a presenting cyanotic neonate, a prostin infusion should be commenced. However, the use of prostin in TAPVD could have positive or adverse effects. An increase in pulmonary flow could have a detrimental effect on oxygenation because it may aggravate the severity of obstruction. Conversely, prostin's dilatory effect on the ducti arteriosus and venosus has also been shown to decompress pulmonary vasculature and increase oxygenation by reducing ventilation–perfusion mismatch (Bullaboy et al 1984; Cirstoveanu et al 2012).

DOUBLE-OUTLET RIGHT VENTRICLE

The aorta and PAs arise side by side from the RV (Fig. 3.24) and may be normally related or transposed. The only outlet from the LV is a large VSD. The aortic and pulmonary valves are at the same level. DORV may be subdivided according to the position of the VSD and further by the presence of PS. Four main types have been defined by Association for Pediatric Cardiology (Franklin et al 2002):

- VSD type
- Fallot type
- TGA type
- DORV with noncommitted VSD

Effect:

- Subaortic VSD – oxygenated blood from the LV is directed to the aorta and desaturated systemic venous blood is directed to the PA producing mild or no stenosis. In the absence of PS the pulmonary blood flow is increased, resulting in congestive heart failure. The clinical picture resembles that of a large VSD with pulmonary hypertension and congestive heart failure.
- Fallot type – doubly committed VSD – in the presence of PS. The large interventricular communication is located immediately beneath both the aortic and pulmonary valves.
- TGA type – subpulmonary VSD oxygenated blood from LV is directed to the PA and desaturated blood from the systemic vein

Fig. 3.24 Double-outflow right ventricle with (A) subaortic ventricular septal defect (VSD), (B) subpulmonary VSD, (C) doubly committed VSD, (D) remote VSD. *Ao,* Aorta; *LA,* left atrium; *LV,* left ventricle; *PA,* pulmonary artery; *RA,* right atrium; *RV,* right ventricle. (Redrawn with permission from Royal Children's Hospital, 2005. Double Outlet Right Ventricle. Royal Children's Hospital, London. <www.rch.org.au/cardiology/defects>.)

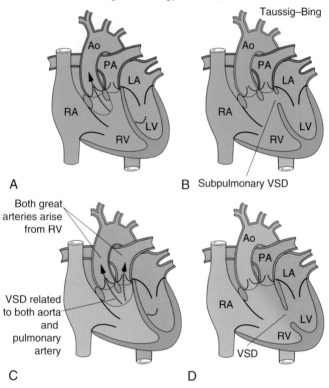

is directed to the aorta, producing severe cyanosis. Pulmonary blood flow increases with the fall of the PVR. Pulmonary vascular obstructive disease develops relatively early.

- Remote VSD – the most complex type; the VSD is remote as it opens into the RV beneath the tricuspid valve. Mild cyanosis is present and pulmonary blood flow is increased.

Signs and symptoms: A spectrum of symptoms is possible depending on the presence and degree of PS. If severe PS, then the neonate will be cyanosed or if there is unrestricted pulmonary blood flow, then signs of cardiac failure will be present.

Diagnosis: Chest x-ray shows cardiomegaly, ECG commonly shows RVH, right axis deviation and occasionally LVH, echo or cardiac MRI diagnostic.

Management:

- Medical: Use of prostin infusion initially for neonatal presentation with cyanosis. Treatment of congestive heart failure and SBE prophylaxis if indicated. For infants with large pulmonary blood flow and congestive heart failure, PA band may be required.
- Surgical:
  - VSD type – one-stage biventricular repair – creation of intra-ventricular tunnel between VSD and subaortic outflow tract by 6 months of age without PA banding
  - Fallot type – intraventricular tunnel procedure (VSD to aorta) plus relief of PS by patch graft at 6 months–2 years of age or homograft valved conduit between RV and PA at 4–5 years (but occasionally a BT shunt may be required as initial palliation)
  - TGA type – intraventricular tunnel between the subpulmonary VSD and aorta is desirable. If not possible an intraventricular tunnel between VSD and PA (turns it into TGA) plus arterial switch operation during the first month of life, or Senning operation (baffles to direct flow from SVC/IVC to RA and RV to PA; and from pulmonary veins to LA and LV to aorta)
  - Remote VSD: when possible an intraventricular tunnel procedure (VSD to aorta) is preferred. If not possible, either a Fontan-type operation or Senning operation plus closure of the VSD plus LV to aorta valved conduit placement is performed

Other complex congenital heart defects

ANOMALOUS LEFT CORONARY ARTERY FROM THE PULMONARY ARTERY

Anomalous left coronary artery from the pulmonary artery (ALCAPA) is a rare congenital coronary artery defect in which the left coronary artery arises from the PA instead of the aorta. In a structurally normal heart, the left main coronary artery divides into the left anterior descending artery and the circumflex artery which supply oxygen-rich blood from the aorta to the left side of the heart muscle. In ALCAPA the left coronary supplies oxygen-depleted blood from the PA to the left side of the heart, which can lead to myocardial ischaemia, poor function, dilated cardiomyopathy (DCM), and death if left untreated. See Fig. 3.25.

In the early neonatal period, ALCAPA may be well tolerated because high PA pressures equal systemic pressures and this leads to antegrade flow in both the left and normal right coronary arteries. When pulmonary arterial pressures decrease after birth, the flow in the anomalous left coronary artery will decrease, leading to myocardial ischaemia. This ischaemia will initially be transient, worse when crying or feeding due to increased myocardial demand, but further increases in myocardial

Fig. 3.25 Anomalous left coronary artery from the pulmonary artery. *Ao*, Aorta; *PA*, pulmonary artery.

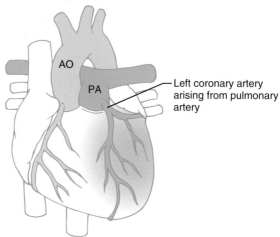

oxygen consumption can cause infarction of the anterolateral left ventricular wall, which can lead to mitral valve papillary muscle dysfunction and mitral valve insufficiency. Collateral vessels may then develop from the right coronary artery to the left coronary artery and a collateral circulation from right to left causes a retrograde flow into the pulmonary trunk due to low pulmonary vascular resistance (coronary steal).

Signs and symptoms:
- Usually present 2–6 weeks of age but can present later even into adulthood (usually as sudden death)
- Crying or sweating during feeding
- Pale
- Poor feeding
- Heart failure

Diagnosis of ALCAPA:
This will be diagnosed following:
- Chest x-ray – may show cardiomegaly with pulmonary congestion
- ECG – may show deep Q waves ≥3 mm with inverted T wave (Chang & Allada 2001) or ST changes
- Echocardiogram – shows poor LV function, mitral valve regurgitation, and collaterals flowing into ALCAPA
- Cardiac MRI
- Cardiac catheterisation

Management of ALCAPA:
Untreated ALCAPA has an estimated mortality of 90% in infancy (Wesselhoeft et al 1968).

Fig. 3.26 Vascular ring – showing double aortic arch.

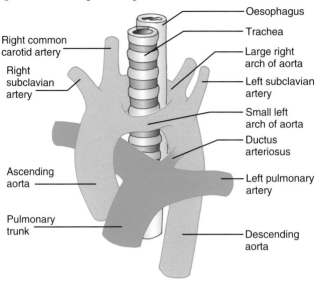

Surgical repair, preferably direct implantation of the left coronary
ostium in the left sinus of Valsalva in the aorta.

Postoperatively – may require inotropes due to preoperative poor
cardiac output. Possibility of cardiac dysrhythmias secondary to
preoperative myocardial ischaemia or infarction.

VASCULAR RING

A vascular ring is a congenital anomaly that occurs in early foetal development where some configuration of the great vessels forms a ring
around the trachea and oesophagus, causing compression. The most
common types are double aortic arch and right aortic arch with left
ligamentum arteriosum (Humphrey et al 2006). See Fig. 3.26.

Signs and symptoms: If the vascular ring is tight, the baby will present early in life with many of the following symptoms. If the degree
of constriction of the oesophagus or trachea is minimal, there may be
few or none of the following symptoms:

- Stridor
- Cyanosis
- Respiratory distress
- Wheeze
- Apnoea
- Dysphagia or difficulty in feeding

Some babies or children may also present with recurrent pneumonia or cough.

Diagnosis: Occasionally it may be possible to identify a right aortic arch on chest x-ray, particularly if there is tracheal compression. Bronchoscopy, echo, computerised tomography (CT), or cardiac MRI scans may also be used.

Management: Surgical division of the vascular ring often via a thoracotomy.

COR TRIATRIATUM

This is an extremely rare congenital anomaly in which either the LA or RA is divided into two compartments, thus literally making three atria (tri-atria). It is often associated with other cardiac anomalies such as TOF, DORV, partial anomalous pulmonary venous drainage (PAPVD). Signs and symptoms depend on the site of the extra accessory membrane and the number of openings in that membrane that may restrict ventricular inflow, as well as the presence of other congenital heart defects. Surgical resection of the membrane is a common approach.

CARDIOMYOPATHY

Cardiomyopathy means disease of the myocardium. There are five main categories (see next), but because the last three are very rare in the paediatric population, only the first two will be examined:
- DCM
- Hypertrophic cardiomyopathy (HCM) – obstructed on nonobstructed
- Restrictive cardiomyopathy
- Left ventricular noncompaction
- Arrhythmogenic right ventricular dysplasia

Causes:
In most cases the causes of cardiomyopathy are unknown; however, others may be caused by:
- Familial – where there are genetic changes
- Metabolic disorders
- Inherited muscle disorders
- Viral infection causing myocarditis, which can develop into cardiomyopathy
- Hormone deficiency
- Innate or acquired abnormal intramural coronary arteries

DILATED CARDIOMYOPATHY

DCM is the most common form of cardiomyopathy and cause of cardiac transplant in children (Towbin et al 2006). There can be genetic, infective, or environmental causes. It is estimated that between 20% and 30% of children diagnosed with DCM will have a relative with the same disease. Vitamin D deficiency causing hypocalcaemia and reversible DCM is being increasingly reported (Babu & Damda, 2013).

Signs and symptoms:

- May have no symptoms and be an incidental finding when treating a child for recurrent respiratory infections
- In babies – may present with irritability, poor feeding, failure to thrive, increased sweating, tachypnoea, wheeze, pallor
- Difficulty in breathing, symptoms of heart failure, cough, wheeze, decreased urine output, and oedema
- Rhythm disturbance, tachycardia, arrhythmia, syncope, seizure, or sudden death

Diagnosis of DCM:

Diagnosis of DCM can be made primarily using echocardiogram, after taking a history, and noting enlarged cardiac shadow on chest x-ray. A cardiac catheterisation may be used to biopsy myocardium to help distinguish between genetic and infectious causes.

Management of DCM:

There is no known cure for DCM; however, there are medical and supportive therapies available depending on severity of illness:

- Diuretics
- Inotropic agents – either oral or intravenous
- Angiotensin-converting inhibitors (e.g., captopril [after load reducing])
- β-blockers
- Anticoagulants
- Antiarrhythmic therapy
- Pacemakers
- Implantable defibrillators
- Cardiac assist devices
- Cardiac transplantation

 NB Children with DCM should not participate in competitive sports due to risk of increased heart failure, collapse, and sudden death.

HYPERTROPHIC CARDIOMYOPATHY

HCM is the presence of a hypertrophied, asymmetric, nondilated LV in the absence of any other disease and accounts for 42% of childhood cardiomyopathy (Colan 2010). The interventricular septum will be hypertrophied, but other abnormalities that may be interrelated to HCM include left ventricular outflow tract obstruction, diastolic dysfunction, mitral regurgitation, myocardial ischaemia, and arrhythmias (Almenar et al 1996). Approximately 75% of HCM are represented by familial HCM or an idiopathic cause, 9% with inborn errors of metabolism, 9% malformation syndromes, and 8% with neuromuscular disorders.

Signs and symptoms:

- Heart murmur
- Congestive heart failure, dyspnea
- Limited capacity for exercise, chest pain, palpitations, syncope

Children who have outflow tract obstruction are at a far greater risk for symptoms, progression to heart failure, and death (Maron et al 2003).

Exercise-induced outflow tract obstruction is also associated with a higher risk of symptoms, including arrhythmia and sudden death (Shah et al 2008).

Diagnosis of HCM:

Diagnosis of HCM can be made using an echocardiogram to measure ventricular wall thickness, ventricular size, systolic and diastolic function, outflow obstruction, and valve insufficiency but cardiac MRI may also be used. It is important to distinguish between physiologic ventricular hypertrophy that may occur in athletes and pathologic ventricular hypertrophy.

Management of HCM:

- Reduction in outflow tract obstruction is primary target
- β-blockers (propranolol or verapamil) – often help to relieve chest pain and dyspnea
- Calcium channel blockers
- Angiotensin-converting enzyme (ACE) inhibitors – (not in patients with LVOTO because it can reduce cavity size and increase outflow gradient) (Kyriakidis et al 1998)
- Alcohol septal ablation
- Surgical myectomy – surgical removal of part of septum that occludes LVOT
- Exercise restriction – no competitive sports
- Implantable cardioverter defibrillator

Diuretic therapy not thought to be beneficial as can lead to an increase in outflow gradient due to a reduced chamber volume and cardiac output can be decreased.

MYOCARDITIS

Myocarditis is an inflammatory disease of the myocardium, caused by viral infections, autoimmune diseases, environmental toxins, and adverse reactions to drugs. A causative pathogen is rarely identified (>10% of cases [Mason et al 1995]) but coxsackie B virus, adenovirus (Martin et al 1994), and recently parvovirus B19 are most commonly implicated (Molina et al 2013). Parvovirus B19 infects coronary endothelium, which leads to myocardial ischaemia and altered function, and causes significant mortality and morbidity (Molina et al 2013). There may be interruption in conduction pathways due to cytokine-mediated cell damage and oedema, which can lead to AV block, bundle branch block, intraventricular block, or sinus arrest (Chien et al 2008). Anecdotally, parents of children with acute myocarditis who present critically ill are informed that approximately one-third of children will recover, one-third will need long-term therapy/transplantation, and one-third will die. This is demonstrated in Molina's study, where approximately 32% of children survived without transplant, 42% had cardiac transplantation, and the remainder died (Molina et al 2013).

The incidence of myocarditis in children is unknown because many patients may be asymptomatic or only demonstrate a few symptoms and the diagnosis is made on presentation of a respiratory or gastrointestinal (GI) illness.

Signs and symptoms:
- Vomiting
- Dyspnea
- Viral prodrome which may include fever, frequently precedes onset of myocarditis (Mason et al 1995)
- Syncope
- Chest pain
- Tachycardia
- Arrhythmias
- Heart failure
- Sudden death

Diagnosis:

Diagnosis is made using a variety of tests that include:
- Bloods – cardiac enzymes, full blood count, erythrocyte sedimentation rate, C-reactive protein, rheumatology screening, viral antibody titres
- ECG – sinus tachycardia with nonspecific ST-T wave changes (Punja et al 2010), supraventricular and ventricular arrhythmias, prolonged QRS duration was an independent variable for transplantation or death (Ukena et al 2011), complete AV block
- Echo – to evaluate LV function. Common findings include global hypokinesis (generalised weakness of entire heart), reduced cardiac output, possible pericardial effusion
- Cardiac MRI
- Endomyocardial biopsy

Management:
- Heart failure therapy – diuretics, ACE inhibitors, β-blockers
- Inotropes
- Mechanical circulatory support (ventricular assist or ECMO) as bridge to transplant
- Pacemaker if AV block persists

The use of intravenous immunoglobulins is not routinely recommended for children with viral myocarditis (Robinson et al 2015).

 NB Children with acute myocarditis should not participate in strenuous physical activity for at least 6 months after onset of symptoms and only after evaluation of their heart function on exercise testing in a controlled environment (Pelliccia et al 2005).

ARRHYTHMIAS

Arrhythmias are deviations from the normal (sinus) rhythm of the heart. Arrhythmias that require immediate treatment in the child are those that significantly decrease cardiac output or systemic perfusion.

Fig. 3.27 Sinus bradycardia.

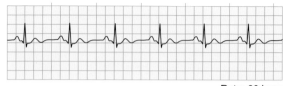

Rate: 60 bpm

Fig. 3.28 Junctional (nodal) rhythm.

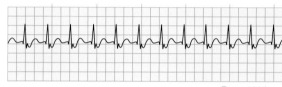

Rate: 120 bpm

There are three main classifications:
- Bradyarrhythmias – Too slow for the child's clinical condition
- Tachyarrhythmias – Too fast for the child's clinical condition
- Collapse rhythms – Ineffective conduction that is unable to sustain cardiac output.

Examples of bradyarrhythmias

SINUS BRADYCARDIA (FIG. 3.27)

Characteristics of sinus rhythm are present. Heart rate less than 80 beats per minute (bpm) in newborn infants and less than 60 bpm in older children may be significant.

Causes: Vagal stimulation, hypoxia, hypotension, raised intracranial pressure, hypothermia, hyperkalaemia, β-blocking drugs

Treatment: Treat underlying cause promptly

JUNCTIONAL (NODAL) RHYTHM (FIG. 3.28)

The P wave may be absent or QRS complexes are followed by inverted P waves. If there is persistent failure of the SA node, the AV node may act as the main pacemaker, with a relatively slow rate (40–60 bpm).

Causes: May occur in otherwise normal heart after cardiac surgery, digitalis toxicity, in conditions with increased vagal tone (e.g., raised intracranial pressure).

Significance: Slow heart rate may significantly decrease cardiac output and produce symptoms.

Treatment: No treatment is indicated if the child is asymptomatic. Treatment is directed to digitalis toxicity if this is the cause.

Fig. 3.29 First-degree heart block.

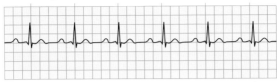

Rate: 60 bpm

Fig. 3.30 Second-degree heart block Mobitz type 1 (Wenckebach phenomenon). (With permission from Park, M.K., 1997. The Pediatric Cardiology Handbook, second ed. CV Mosby, St. Louis, MO.)

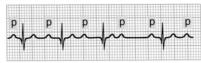

Heart (AV) block

This is a disturbance in conduction between the normal sinus impulse and the eventual ventricular response. It is classified according to the severity of the conduction disturbance.

FIRST-DEGREE HEART BLOCK (FIG. 3.29)

Abnormally prolonged PR interval due to a delay in conduction through the AV node.

Cause: Present in some healthy children, cardiomyopathies, congenital heart defects (e.g., ASD, Ebstein anomaly), following cardiac surgery, digitalis toxicity.

Significance: Usually no treatment indicated except in digitalis toxicity.

SECOND-DEGREE HEART BLOCK (FIG. 3.30)

Some but not all P waves are followed by QRS complexes (dropped beats). There are several types:

MOBITZ TYPE I (WENCKEBACH PHENOMENON)

The PR interval becomes progressively prolonged until one QRS complex is dropped completely.

Cause: Myocarditis, cardiomyopathy, myocardial infarction, congenital heart disease, cardiac surgery, digitalis toxicity; also affects otherwise healthy children.

Significance: The block is at the level of the AV node. Usually does not progress to complete heart block.

Treatment: Treat underlying cause.

MOBITZ TYPE II

The AV conduction is all or none; there is either normal AV conduction or the conduction is completely blocked.

Cause: As for Mobitz type I.

Significance: The block is at the level of the bundle of His. It is more serious than type I block because it may progress to complete heart block.

Treatment: Treat underlying cause. Prophylactic pacemaker therapy may be indicated.

TWO-TO-ONE (OR HIGHER) AV BLOCK

A QRS complex follows every second (third or fourth) P wave, resulting in 2:1 (3:1 or 4:1, respectively) AV block.

Cause: Similar to other second–degree AV blocks.

Significance: The block is usually at the AV nodal level and occasionally at the level of the bundle of His. It may occasionally progress to complete heart block.

Treatment: The underlying cause is treated. Electrophysiologic studies may be necessary to determine the level of the block. Occasional pacemaker therapy.

THIRD-DEGREE OR COMPLETE HEART BLOCK (FIG. 3.31)

Atrial and ventricular activities are entirely independent of one another. P waves and P–P intervals are regular at a heart rate reasonable for the child's age. QRS complexes are also regular but at a much slower rate than the P rate.

Causes: Maternal lupus erythematosus; congenital type may be isolated or associated with congenital heart disease (e.g., TGA). Acquired type is usually a complication of cardiac surgery. Rarely, severe myocarditis, mumps, diphtheria, tumours in the conduction system, overdose of certain drugs. May follow myocardial infarction. These causes produce either temporary or permanent heart block.

Significance: Congestive heart failure may develop in infancy, particularly if congenital heart defect is present. Children with isolated complete heart block can be asymptomatic in childhood.

Treatment: No treatment is indicated for asymptomatic congenital complete heart block. Temporary ventricular pacemaker is indicated for children with transient heart block. Permanent artificial ventricular pacemaker is indicated for children with surgically induced heart block and those who are asymptomatic or have congestive heart failure (Park 2003).

Consider:
- If increased vagal tone or primary AV block give atropine:
  - First dose: 0.02 mg/kg – may repeat
- Maximum dose for child: 1 mg
- Cardiac pacing

Fig. 3.31 Complete heart block.

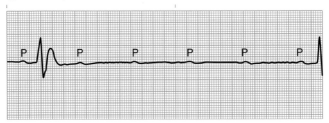

Rhythm	Regular, but atrial and ventricular rhythms are independent
Rate	Characterized by atrial rate usually normal and faster than ventricular rate
P wave	Normal shape and size, may appear within QRS complexes
PR Interval	Absent: the atria and vetricles beat independently
QRS	Normal, but wide if junctional escape focus
Notes	

Examples of tachyarrhythmias

SINUS TACHYCARDIA (FIG. 3.32)

The characteristics of sinus rhythm are present. A rate greater than 140 bpm in children and greater than 160 bpm in infants may be significant. The heart rate is usually less than 200 bpm.

Causes: Pain, anxiety, fever, hypovolaemia, circulatory shock, anaemia, congestive heart failure, myocardial disease

Significance: Increased cardiac work is well tolerated by the healthy myocardium.

Treatment: Treat the underlying cause.

SUPRAVENTRICULAR TACHYCARDIA (FIG. 3.33)

SVT in infants generally produces a heart rate of more than 220 bpm and often 250–300 bpm. Lower rates occur in children during SVT. The QRS complex is narrow, making differentiation between marked sinus tachycardia due to shock and SVT difficult, particularly because SVT may also be associated with poor systemic perfusion.

Fig. 3.32 Sinus tachycardia.

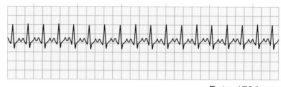

Rate: 170 bpm

Fig. 3.33 Supraventricular tachycardia. (With permission from Advanced Life Support Group, 2016. Advanced Paediatric Life Support: The Practical Approach, sixth ed. BMJ.)

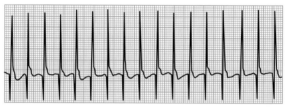

The following characteristics may help to distinguish between sinus tachycardia and SVT:

- Sinus tachycardia is typically characterised by a heart rate less than 200 bpm in infants and children, whereas infants with SVT typically have a heart rate greater than 200 bpm.
- P waves may be difficult to identify in both sinus tachycardia and SVT once the ventricular rate exceeds 200 bpm. If P waves are identifiable, they are usually upright in leads I and AVF in sinus tachycardia, whereas they are negative in leads II, III, and AVF in SVT.
- In sinus tachycardia, the heart rate varies from beat to beat and is often unresponsive to stimulation, but there is no beat-to-beat variability in SVT.
- Termination of SVT is abrupt, whereas the heart rate slows gradually in sinus tachycardia in response to treatment.
- A history consistent with shock (e.g., gastroenteritis or septicaemia) is usually present with sinus tachycardia (Advanced Life Support Group 2016).

Causes: No demonstrable heart disease present in many children. Some congenital cardiac defects (e.g., Ebstein anomaly, TGA) are more prone to this arrhythmia.

Significance: It may decrease cardiac output and result in congestive cardiac failure – if this develops, the infant's/child's condition can deteriorate rapidly. Cardiopulmonary stability during episodes of SVT is affected by the child's age, duration of SVT, and prior ventricular function and ventricular rate. If baseline myocardial function is impaired, SVT can produce signs of shock in a relatively short time.

Vagal manoeuvres

These include:
- Application of rubber glove filled with iced water over face – or wrapping infant in towel and immersing face in iced water for 5 seconds
- One-sided carotid sinus massage
- Valsalva manoeuvre (e.g., blowing hard through a straw)
- **Do not use ocular pressure in infants or children** because this may cause damage.

ALGORITHM FOR THE MANAGEMENT OF SUPRAVENTRICULAR TACHYCARDIA – SEE PAGE 13

Junctional ectopic tachycardia

Junctional ectopic tachycardia (JET) is an SVT which appears as a narrow QRS tachycardia with AV dissociation. (Normal QRS with retrograde P waves that may be observed in the terminal part of the QRS.) JET may be congenital or may occur postcardiac surgery.

Idiopathic chronic congenital JET – presumed to be present from birth but may not be detected initially, may result in cardiomyopathy, has a high mortality (up to 34%) secondary to congestive cardiac failure, ventricular fibrillation (VF), or atrio-ventricular block. Congenital JET may be treated with antiarrhythmic drugs, radiofrequency ablation, and pacemakers.

Postcardiac surgery – JET – the incidence of JET following cardiac surgery in paediatrics is thought to be approximately 10% (Andreasen et al 2008). It is associated with manipulation of the heart and thought to be secondary to trauma, inflammation of the conductive tissue, or infiltrative haemorrhage (Dodge-Khatami et al 2002). It often occurs when rewarming the patient and within 6–72 hours of cardiac surgery. It occurs more commonly after certain interventions:
- Tetralogy of Fallot repair – 21.9% of patients (Dodge-Khatami et al 2002)
- Fontan repair
- Arterial switch
- Long aortic cross-clamp times
- Use of dopamine and age younger than 6 months (Hoffman et al 2002)

General principles of treatment including checking and correcting any electrolyte imbalance, use of antiarrhythmic drugs (e.g., amiodarone following cardiology advice), controlled hypothermia, pacing, radiofrequency ablation. Postoperative JET is usually transient and often resolves within 36 hours, but it is considered one of the most refractory and lethal of the postoperative arrhythmias – does not respond to cardioversion, difficult to treat medically, results in the loss of AV synchrony in patients immediately after complex cardiac surgery, and so ECMO is provided if indicated.

Rhythm strip showing JET (Fig. 3.34)

Fig. 3.34 Junctional ectopic tachycardia. (With permission from Legras, M.D., 1997. Arrhythmias in the pediatric intensive care unit. In: Singh, N.L. (Ed.), Manual of Pediatric Critical Care. WB Saunders, Philadelphia, PA.)

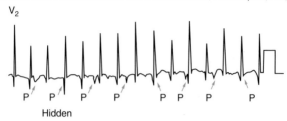

Fig. 3.35 Bigemini.

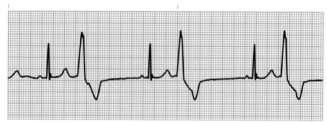

Rhythm	Irregular
Rate	The underlying rate
P wave	Absent
PR Interval	Not measurable
QRS	Wide (>0.10 sec), bizarre appearance
Notes	PVC appears every second beat

Bigemini

Bigemini is an arrhythmia in which premature ventricular contractions alternate with normal QRS complexes. The patient may be unaware of the arrhythmia. General principles of treatment include correcting electrolyte imbalance, avoiding stimulants, and ablation if the problem persists.

Rhythm strip showing bigemini (Fig. 3.35)

Fig. 3.36 Atrial fibrillation.

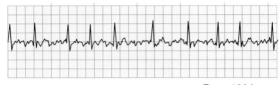

Rate: 100 bpm

Fig. 3.37 Ventricular fibrillation.

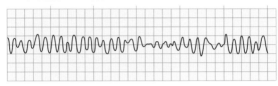

ATRIAL FIBRILLATION (FIG. 3.36)

Atrial fibrillation is characterised by an extremely fast atrial rate (flutter wave at 350–600 bpm) and an irregular ventricular response with normal QRS complexes.

Causes: Structural heart disease with dilated atria, myocarditis, previous surgery involving atria, digitalis toxicity

Significance: Rapid ventricular rate and the loss of coordinated contraction of the atria and the ventricles decrease cardiac output. Atrial thrombus formation may occur.

Treatment: Digoxin is given to slow the ventricular rate and propranolol may be added if necessary. Cardioversion may be indicated, but recurrence is common. Patients should preferably be anticoagulated for 3–4 weeks before and after cardioversion to prevent embolisation of atrial thrombus.

VENTRICULAR FIBRILLATION

VF is characterised by bizarre complexes at varying sizes and configuration. The rate is rapid and irregular. See Fig. 3.37.

Causes: Postoperative state, severe hypoxia, hyperkalaemia, digitalis, myocardial infarction, some drugs (e.g., anaesthetics)

Significance: Can be fatal because it results in ineffective circulation.

Treatment: See Algorithm (Advanced Life Support Group 2016) on page 7 for emergency treatment.

VENTRICULAR TACHYCARDIA (FIG. 3.38)

VT is characterised by rapid, wide QRS complexes (rate of 120–200 bpm) with an absence of P waves. The QRS complexes are slightly irregular and vary slightly in shape.

Fig. 3.38 Ventricular tachycardia.

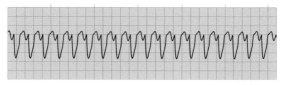

Rate: 180 bpm

Causes: Cardiomyopathy, cardiac tumours, preoperative or postoperative, congenital heart disease, digitalis toxicity, certain drugs including antibiotics, antihistamines, insecticides, and some anaesthetic agents

Significance: Usually signifies a serious myocardial pathology or dysfunction. Cardiac output may decrease notably and deteriorate to VF.

Treatment: Check whether pulse is present. If not, refer to algorithm on page 7. If pulse is present, synchronised cardioversion is required at 1 J/kg. See algorithm on page xxx.

Consider the following text for further clarification.

EARLY TREATMENT OF VENTRICULAR TACHYCARDIA (WITH PULSE) (ADVANCED LIFE SUPPORT GROUP 2016)

- Consult early consultation with paediatric cardiologist.
- May suggest use of amiodarone or procainamide – both can cause hypotension, which should be treated with volume expansion.
- Where VT has been caused by drug toxicity, sedation, anaesthesia, and DC shock may be the safest approach – use synchronised shocks initially because these are less likely to produce VF but, if they are ineffectual, subsequent attempts will have to be asynchronous if the child is in shock.
- The treatment of torsades de pointes VT is magnesium sulphate by IV infusion (50 mg/kg MM, max 2 g)
- Amiodarone 5 mg/kg may be given over a few minutes in VT if the child is in severe shock; however, as amiodarone depresses cardiac function, this should be given with full support available and consideration of a slower infusion.
- Seek advice.

ASYSTOLE (FIG. 3.39)

Asystole is characterised by a straight line on the ECG monitor, with P waves occasionally observed.

Causes: Respiratory arrest, myocardial infarction

Significance: Diagnosed by the absence of a palpable central pulse accompanied by apnoea, together with absent cardiac electrical activity

Treatment: Refer to APLS algorithm (Advanced Life Support Group 2016) on page 5.

Fig. 3.39 Asystole.

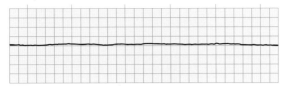

Fig. 3.40 Pulseless electrical activity. (Advanced Life Support Group, 2016. Advanced Paediatric Life Support: The Practical Approach, sixth ed. BMJ.)

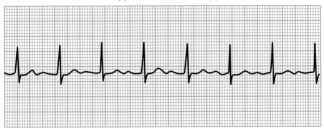

PULSELESS ELECTRICAL ACTIVITY (FIG. 3.40)

This was previously known as electromechanical dissociation. There are recognised complexes seen on the ECG monitor, but there is an absence of palpable pulses and inadequate cardiac output.

Causes: Include 4 Hs and 4 Ts:
- Hypovolaemia (most common cause)
- Hypothermia
- Hypoxaemia
- Hyperkalaemia
- Tamponade
- Tension pneumothorax
- Thromboembolism
- Toxicity (i.e., drug overdose [commonly tricyclic antidepressant])

Significance: The underlying cause of pulseless electrical activity (PEA) must be sought but PEA should be treated and managed like asystole until the specific cause has been identified and treated.

Treatment: See APLS algorithm (Advanced Life Support Group 2016) on page 5.

WOLFF–PARKINSON–WHITE SYNDROME (FIG. 3.41)

Wolff–Parkinson–White (WPW) syndrome is characterised by a short PR interval, and the QRS complex shows an early slurred upstroke called a delta wave.

Significance: Results from an anomalous conduction pathway between the atrium and the ventricle, bypassing the normal delay

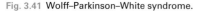
Fig. 3.41 Wolff–Parkinson–White syndrome.

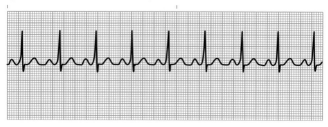

Rhythm	Regular, unless atrial fibrillation present
Rate	Nomal (60–100 bpm)
P wave	Normal
PR Interval	Can be short (<0.12 sec)
QRS	Usually wide (>0.12 sec)
Notes	Look for short PR interval and/or delta wave. A delta wave (positive or negative) distorts the early part of the QRS complex

of conduction in the AV node. Children with WPW syndrome are prone to sustained attacks of SVT (Park 1997).

LONG QT SYNDROME

Long QT syndrome may be hereditary or acquired but is characterised by an abnormally prolonged QT interval which can cause torsades de pointes and cardiac arrest. Congenital long QT is caused by transmembrane ion-channel protein disease, whereas acquired long QT may be caused by certain drugs, myocardial ischaemia, subarachnoid haemorrhage autonomic neuropathy, and human immunodeficiency virus (Khan 2002).

Signs and symptoms:
- Dizziness
- Syncope
- Seizures
- Sudden death

Diagnosis of long QT:
- ECG
- Medication stress test

- Genetic testing
- Probability based diagnostic criteria for long QT – see webpage (Schwartz et al 1993)

Management of long QT syndrome:
- β-blockers
- Potassium supplements in some cases
- Pacemaker of implantable cardioverter defibrillator
- Avoidance of medications that lengthen QT interval or lower potassium levels
- Avoid medicines that may trigger abnormal heart rhythms
- Avoid strenuous exercise and swimming

There is a long and ever-increasing list of medications that should be avoided in children with long QT syndrome, which can be found at www.torsades.org, but this requires payment because the list is continually updated.

ANAESTHESIA OF PATIENTS WITH LONG QT FOR EMERGENCY INTUBATION AND VENTILATION

There are scant and conflicting data regarding management of these patients, and no definitive guidelines are available. Drugs to be avoided in intubation and ventilation are shown later, but it is the responsibility of the clinicians caring for the child to ensure they have sought expert guidance prior to prescribing and inducing anaesthesia.

Anaesthetic agents NOT recommended in long QT because they prolong QT interval or induce torsades de pointes:

Atropine – lengthens QT interval (Annila et al 1993)
Sevoflurane – induces significant arrhythmias and other halogenated volatile agents prolong QT interval (Loeckinger et al 2003; Kenyon et al 2010)
Ketamine – sympathomimetic properties (Kies et al 2005)

Many inotropic drugs and vasoconstrictors prolong QT interval but, despite this, may be clinically indicated.

Sedation and anaesthetic agents that have been used in patients with congenital long QT syndrome:

Propofol (Kleinsasser et al 2000; Fazio et al 2013)
Thiopentone (Kies et al 2005; Drake et al 2007)
Atracurium (Fazio et al 2013)
Rocuronium (Wisely & Shipton 2002; Kies et al 2005)
Fentanyl (Medak & Benumof 1983; Chang et al 2008; Fazio et al 2013)
Morphine (Fazio et al 2013)
Midazolam (Michaloudis et al 1996; Owczuk et al 2009)

NB Children with long QT syndrome will have an increased risk of developing ventricular arrhythmias. Pain, anxiety, intubation, high-pressure ventilation, and many drugs may trigger torsades de pointes, so a defibrillator should be available at all times.

UNDERSTANDING CARDIAC PACING

Pacing in paediatrics is used mainly in congenital or postsurgical heart block, bradyarrhythmia, sinus node dysfunction following surgery (e.g., Fontan, switch) but may also be indicated with tachyarrhythmias and low cardiac output state. Pacing may be transcutaneous (pacing pads on a defibrillator), transoesophageal, transvenous, or via epicardial wires (atrial wires on right chest, ventricular wires on left side of chest even in dextra-cardia). Surgeons do not always put in both atrial and ventricular wires.

The most frequent indication for pacing is bradyarrhythmia. In children the fall in output with bradycardia is precipitate and dramatic. Even in older children and adults the ability to abruptly compensate by increasing stroke volume is limited. The indication for pacing a bradyarrhythmia is clinical evidence of a low cardiac output: altered conscious level, syncope, low urine output, poor peripheral perfusion, acidosis, or hypotension (Pearson 2002).

There are three basic concepts associated with pacing:
- Capturing – Whether the pacemaker is pacing the desired chamber(s).
- Sensing – Whether the pacemaker is sensing the patient's own (intrin-sic) contractions of the heart chambers. This is necessary so that the pacemaker avoids competition with the patient's own rhythm. The pacemaker only 'kicks in' when it cannot detect (sense) the patient's own effort.
- Threshold – The least amount of stimulus required to stimulate the myocardium or the least amount of voltage for the patient's own beats to be sensed (Horrocks 2002).

Pacing modes are described by a standard terminology that describes in sequence the chambers: paced, sensed, and the mode of pacing (Table 3.2).
Pacing boxes:
Transoesophageal
Single chamber – fixed or demand
Dual chamber – select mode

 NB ALWAYS consult the manufacturer's instruction manual before using a pacing box. If a child presents with an unknown pace-maker, an x-ray can identify the make on the circuit board. The internet can provide the manufacturer's telephone details which will be available 24/7/365 for model specific information. The fol-lowing information provides general, generic guidance only.

 NB NEVER put a magnet over a pacemaker because it may turn it off or alter the detection capability.

Table 3.2	Common pacing codes	
Code	**What it means**	**Uses**
AOO	Atrial fixed rate pacing, no sense, no inhibition	Requires functional AV conduction (AAI mode safer than AOO)
AAI	Atrial demand pacing	Sinus node dysfunction with normal AV conduction
VOO	Ventricular fixed rate pacing, no sense, no inhibition	Rarely used • Ventricular pacing regardless of the under-lying rhythm
VVI	Ventricular demand pacing	Ventricle will be paced if the patient's intrinsic ventricular rate is lower than the rate set on the pacemaker.
DOO	Dual pace, no sense, no inhibitions	Rarely used • Third-degree heart block
DVI	AV sequential pacing	Useful where there is supraventricular tachycardia
DDD	Dual pace, dual sense, dual inhibit/trigger	Used in AV block. A mode that can pace either or both A and V, sense and inhibit or trigger – commonly used
DDI	AV demand pacing	Used in sinus bradycardia or atrial arrhythmias (AF) – monitors both R atrium and R ventricle, maintaining minimum rate in each chamber

AF, Atrial fibrillation; *AV,* atrioventricular.

There is mainly a three-letter code that explains the pacing modality.
- First letter refers to the area paced (A = atria, V = ventricular, D = dual both atria and ventricular, O = none)
- Second letter refers to the area sensed
- Third letter refers to the response to a sensed event (T = triggered pacemaker output, I = inhibiting it, D = dual, or O = no response)

Atrial pacing – Pacing spike will precede the P wave.

Ventricular pacing – Pacing spike will precede the QRS complex. ST segments and T wave are discordant with the QRS complex (i.e., QRS complex is on opposite side of baseline from ST segment and T wave).

Baseline settings:

Select:
- Type of pacing – single chamber, fixed or demand, dual chamber mode
- Heart rate depending on age of child and clinical condition
- Atrial and/or ventricular sensitivity – the lower the setting, the MORE sensitive it is, so check the voltage at which the pacer is sensing cardiac activity and set the box just less than this level
- Atrial and/or ventricular pacing voltage – the higher the setting, the greater the voltage delivered to the epicardium to initiate myocardial contraction. Postoperatively, set the voltage at 2 volts higher than the threshold at which capture is obtained.

Troubleshooting:
- Seek urgent medical assistance if cardiac output falls in paced child.
- Check patient, leads, connections, pacing box.
- If failure to pace with absent pacing spike, check pacing rate and check sensitivity as may be set too high.
- If failure to capture with pacing spike present but no PQRS, increase voltage.
- If failure to sense with random pacing spike, increase sensitivity (lower mV setting).
- Change battery or pacing box.

Daily safety checks when paced:
- Ensure continuous ECG monitoring and check pulse.
- Check daily 12-lead ECG.
- A clinician with knowledge of physiology of the patient and the technology of the pacing box should assess the underlying rhythm and rate of the child by incrementally turning down the rate on the pacemaker, whilst monitoring cardiovascular parameters to consider ongoing requirements for pacing.
- The threshold should also be assessed (atrium and ventricle separately) by slowly turning down the voltage until loss of capture. The voltage should then be increased to 2 mV greater than the voltage threshold.
- Check pacemaker settings against documentation.
- Check all wire connections from patient to pacing box.
- Observe wire insertion site for signs of infection.
- Check that spare batteries and a spare functioning pacing box are to hand.
- Check limb perfusion if transvenous paced.

EXTRACORPOREAL MEMBRANE OXYGENATION

In ECMO, blood is drained from the vascular system, circulated outside the body by a mechanical pump, and then reinfused into the circulation. Outside the body the haemoglobin is saturated with oxygen and CO_2 is removed. Indications for ECMO can be divided into respiratory, cardiac, or both. ECMO was developed as treatment for severe respiratory failure in the 1970s. Initial trials of ECMO in adults with severe hypoxic failure had a very poor survival, which was not improved with ECMO (Zapol et al 1979). One of the main reasons for this may have been that the adults placed on ECMO had already suffered severe ventilator-induced lung injury (VILI) which could not be reversed (Maslach-Hubbard & Bratton 2013). However, in newborns, the spiral of hypoxia and acidosis resulting from severe pulmonary hypertension could be broken by the initiation of ECMO (Bartlett et al 1976). It was in neonates that the ECMO was initially driven forward. This development was supported by the establishment of the Extracorporeal Life Support Organization (ELSO). This is an international consortium of health care providers who contribute detailed data to a registry. This registry has supported the vast majority of ECMO clinical research.

		Survived extra corporeal life support (ECLS)		Survived to discharge (DC) or transfer	
	Total patients				
Neonatal					
Respiratory	28 723	24 155	84%	21 274	74%
Cardiac	6 269	3 885	62%	2 599	41%
ECPR	1 254	806	64%	514	41%
Paediatric					
Respiratory	7 210	4 787	66%	4 155	58%
Cardiac	8 021	5 341	67%	4 067	51%
ECPR	2 788	1 532	55%	1 144	41%

Table 3.3 Overall outcomes of neonatal and paediatric patients

ECPR, Extracorporeal cardiopulmonary resuscitation.
From ExtraCorporeal Life Support Organisation, 2016. The ELSO Registry: Benchmarking. <http://www.elso-swac2016.org> (accessed 02.10.17).

From this, ELSO develops standards and guidelines for the member programs and sponsors medical education. In the 2000s ECMO reemerged as a therapy for all patients with cardiorespiratory failure. The Cesar trial (Peek et al 2009) and the outbreak of swine flu were among the driving factors in the resurgence of ECMO. Advances in technology allowed adaptation of ECMO, and by 2013 it was increasingly seen as a standard therapy in critical care. ECMO, in all its forms, represents the most invasive form of life support. As with all complex therapies, ECMO requires a multidisciplinary team to manage it (Butt & MacLaren 2016). ECMO should be used only in centres where there is expertise in its initiation, maintenance, and discontinuation. See Table 3.3 and Fig. 3.42 for patient outcomes and numbers of patients and ECMO centres. ECMO does not modify underlying disease but acts as a supportive therapy to recovery or as a bridge to transplant. With improvements in technology, the duration of mechanical support is increasing. Indeed, in adults, patients are being discharged from hospital on MCS devices.

ECMO glossary:
Respiratory ECMO – ECMO initiated for severe respiratory failure.
Cardiac ECMO – ECMO initiated for circulatory support.
VV ECMO – venovenous ECMO. Blood is taken and returned to the venous circulation. This can be via two separate venous cannulae or via a double-lumen cannula in a single venous site. This form of ECMO is used for respiratory ECMO where cardiac function is adequate to maintain circulation.
VA ECMO – venoarterial ECMO. Blood is taken from the venous cannula and returned via an arterial cannula. This form of ECMO can be used in both cardiac and respiratory ECMO.
VAD – ventricular assist device. Can be to support the LV, RV, or both.
ECCOR – extracorporeal CO_2 removal.

Fig. 3.42 Extracorporeal membrane oxygenation centres and patient numbers. (ExtraCorporeal Life Support Organisation, 2016. The ELSO Registry: Benchmarking. <http://www.elso-swac2016.org> (accessed 02.10.17).)

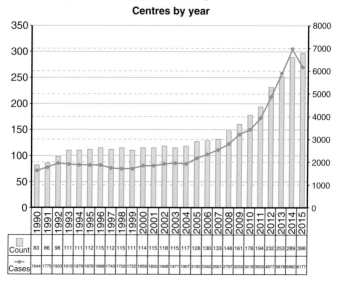

ECPR – extracorporeal cardiopulmonary resuscitation.
ELSO – Extracorporeal Life Support Organization
MCS – mechanical circulatory support describes any device that mechanically supports the circulation.

Respiratory extracorporeal membrane oxygenation
Indications include severe respiratory failure secondary to:

Acute respiratory distress syndrome
  Infective – bacterial or viral
  Meconium aspiration
Congenital diaphragmatic hernia
Asthma
Pulmonary haemorrhage or massive haemoptysis
Lung transplant
Primary graft failure
Bridge to transplant
Intraoperative extracorporeal membrane oxygenation
Pulmonary contusion
Smoke inhalation

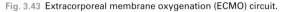

Fig. 3.43 Extracorporeal membrane oxygenation (ECMO) circuit.

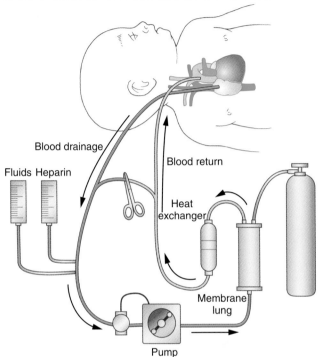

Although ECMO to treat severe respiratory failure took roots in the neonatal population, its use has been declining since 1992. This reflects an increased understanding of VILI and adoption of lung protective strategies. There has also been increased use of other less invasive therapies such as high-frequency oscillatory ventilation inhaled NO, surfactant and maternal antibiotic therapy (Maslach-Hubbard & Bratton 2013). The outcome from respiratory ECMO is related to the underlying pathology.

The use of ECMO for infants with congenital diaphragmatic hernias has remained more static in the intervening years, and unfortunately the mortality in this patient group still remains very high at 40–50%. Newer applications for respiratory ECMO include support of patients with chronic respiratory failure as a bridge to transplant and as cardiopulmonary support for organ donation in vivo and ex vivo (Magliocca et al 2005; Diso et al 2013; Butt & MacLaren 2016).

Cardiac extracorporeal membrane oxygenation

In 2013 the Pediatric Cardiac Intensive Care Society and ELSO issued a joint statement in which they stated that 'mechanical circulatory support is now standard in children with circulatory failure refractory to conventional support' (MacLaren et al 2013).

ECMO may be instituted for:

Congenital cardiac lesions
Preoperative or postoperative support
Congenital or acquired cardiomyopathy
Arrhythmias
Cardiac transplant
Bridge to transplant
Intraoperative extracorporeal membrane oxygenation
Primary graft failure
Sepsis

Contraindications to ECMO – absolute and relative

Unrecoverable heart and not a candidate for transplant or destination ventricular assist device therapy
Malignancy and immunodeficiency
Known severe brain injury or intracerebral haemorrhage
Unwitnessed cardiac arrest
Prolonged cardiopulmonary resuscitation without adequate tissue perfusion
Severe irreversible organ failure
Prematurity less than 35 weeks

Immunodeficiency is an identified risk factor for ECMO mortality. Survival rates in children on respiratory ECMO with underlying immunocompromised conditions ranged from 0% for haematopoietic stem cell transplant patients to 35% for solid organ transplants (Rehder et al 2013).

The work with neonates highlighted the importance of initiation of ECMO before irreversible organ injury developed and the risks of bleeding complications. Premature newborns with gestational age less than 35 weeks suffered high rates of severe of intraventricular haemorrhage (Hardart & Fackler 1999).

What does an extracorporeal membrane oxygenation circuit look like? See Fig. 3.43.

Access cannulae:

These may be single-lumen or double-lumen cannulae. The size of the cannula is determined by the size of the patient. Single-lumen cannulae are used in VA and VV ECMO. Double-lumen cannulae can be used as a single access in VV ECMO. Double-lumen cannulae may have less recirculation – which impairs oxygenation – and be better tolerated. However, complications with double-lumen catheters included right heart perforation (Hirose et al 2012). New cannulae are being developed with less resistance to flow or which are more biocompatible.

Pumps:

Traditionally, roller pumps were used, but the use of centrifugal pumps has increased significantly. They require shorter tubing and smaller priming volume but may be associated with increased haemolysis and renal injury in neonates. However, haemolysis can occur with both systems (Barrett et al 2012).

Oxygenators:

Polymethyl pentene nonporous hollow fibre oxygenators provide efficient gas exchange with smaller priming volumes and less resistance to flow.

Where do the cannulae go in the different types of extracorporeal membrane oxygenation?

- VA ECMO – Central
- Peripheral VA ECMO via internal jugular vein and carotid artery
- Peripheral VA ECMO via femoral vein and femoral artery (Fig. 3.44)
- VV ECMO (Fig. 3.45)

What are the differences between venovenous and venoarterial extracorporeal membrane oxygenation?

VA ECMO	VV ECMO
Provides support to assist the systemic circulation	Does not provide support to assist the systemic circulation
Requires both venous and arterial cannulation	Requires only venous cannulation
Bypasses the pulmonary circulation	Maintains pulmonary blood flow
Higher P_aO_2 achieved	Lower P_aO_2 achieved
Increased rate of systemic emboli causing stroke and seizures	Lower rate of systemic emboli
Increased coagulation requirements and increased risk of bleeding	Decreased rate of bleeding
Increased risk of infection especially if central cannulation used	Decreased risk of infection if percutaneous or single cannula used

ECMO, Extracorporeal membrane oxygenation; *VA*, venoarterial; *VV, venovenous.*

Fig. 3.44 Peripheral venoarterial extracorporeal membrane oxygenation via femoral vein and femoral artery. (Makdisi, G., I-wen, W., 2015. Extracorporeal membrane oxygenation (ECMO) review of a lifesaving technology. J. Thoracic. Dis. 7 (7), E166–E176.)

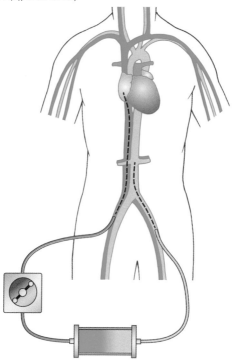

Managing the patient on extracorporeal membrane oxygenation

Sedation: Initially heavy sedation was used to manage patients on ECMO; however, as with all areas of intensive care, there is a growing realisation that sedation comes at a price. ELSO guidelines recommend that minimal sedation can be used if it is tolerated. Certainly in adult practice, patients who are on ECMO may not have any sedation at all and may be able to mobilise. However, in paediatrics, it is likely that sedation will be required while on ECMO. The aim should be to ensure a level of sedation to ensure patient safety and comfort while ideally allowing the patient to interact with family and staff (Frencker 2015).

Fig. 3.45 Venovenous ECMO: two-cannulation approach (A) *Left*: femoral vein (for drainage) and right internal jugular for infusion; *Right*: both femoral veins are used for drainage and perfusion. (B) Double-stage single cannular approach. *ECMO*, Extracorporeal membrane oxygenation.

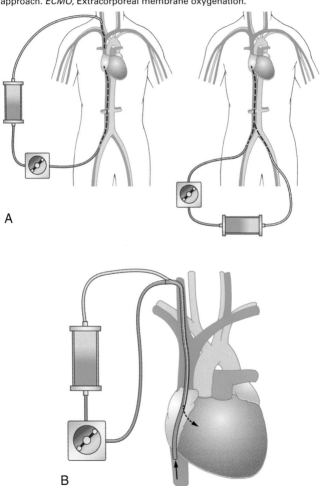

ECMO can be used to facilitate other treatments. This may include surgery or interventional procedures, chemotherapy, haemodialysis, rewarming in the case of hypothermia, or as a bridge to transplant or destination VAD therapy.

Positioning: As with any child in PICU, attention to detail with positioning and pressure areas is vital. This is particularly important in respect to the cannulas, which must be constantly monitored for bleeding, signs of infection, or dislodgement. Most ECMO units will have detailed protocols regarding monitoring of cannula position on x-ray and/or with echo. Any alterations in cannula position must be addressed urgently to avoid displacement, damage to vessels or to the heart itself, clot formation, or entraining of air.

Sepsis: Sepsis is a common complication of ECMO, and most units will have a surveillance policy involving routine testing of both patient and circuit. There will be a low threshold to treat, especially in patients with central cannulation.

Monitoring and transport: In view of the high incidence of intra-cranial haemorrhage and thrombosis, cranial ultrasound may be used in neonates and infants. It has the advantage of being performed at the bedside; however, it is limited in what it can view. For older patients and for more detailed imaging, CT may need to be performed. This may involve transporting the patient on ECMO to the CT scan. As well as transport within an institution, it may be necessary to transport a patient on ECMO to another hospital. Moving patients on ECMO is one of the areas for which the ECMO team and transport team will train and practice.

Nutrition: Ensuring adequate nutrition for the patient is part of the ongoing management of the patient on ECMO. Establishing enteral nutrition via an nasogastric or nasojejunal is the preferred option. Gut function may be impaired by the underlying condition and by the use of sedative drugs such as opiates. Anticoagulation leads to an increased incidence of GI bleeding.

Medication: Although there have been small studies looking at pharmacokinetics of drugs while on ECMO, particularly in neonates, there are still limited data in this area. The volume of distribution may be increased due to blood in the prime and/or adhesion of molecules to the circuit. However, many patients on ECMO develop renal impairment which affects clearance of drugs. Both of these factors can affect dosages on ECMO. Involvement of the pharmacy team may be very helpful to prevent underdosing or toxicity.

Complications on extracorporeal membrane oxygenation

Bleeding, thromboembolism, infection, and limb ischaemia are all recognised complications on ECMO. Each is affected by the mode of ECMO, the type and position of the cannula, and the choice and level of anti-coagulation used. VA ECMO requires higher levels of anticoagulation and has increased rates of stroke. Central cannulation has increased risk of bleeding and mediastinitis but allows you to use larger cannula and greater flow. This may be useful for children with sepsis where high flow rates are required. Neck cannulation is more likely to cause cerebral thromboembolic or bleeding complications and femoral cannulation is more likely to cause limb ischaemia (Makdisi & I-Wen 2015).

Mechanical complications can occur within the circuit. The most common of these is clot formation, which in the worst-case scenario can lead to obstruction of the pump head. When a patient is totally dependent on ECMO, the staff looking after that patient must be competent to change a component of or the whole ECMO circuit within a few minutes. They must also support the patient while a circuit change is ongoing. To achieve and maintain these skills the ECMO team must undergo a comprehensive training programme, which is maintained by ongoing medical education. ELSO recommends that each ECMO centre has a well-defined training programme for staff (Frencker 2015).

Anticoagulation must be strictly monitored on ECMO. Monitoring modalities may vary between units, with either anti-Xa or activated partial thromboplastin time used as per unit protocol. All ECMO circuits will have activated clotting time monitoring at the bedside.

VENTRICULAR ASSIST DEVICES

A ventricular assist device is a mechanical pump that supports the heart function. They may be used as a bridge to recovery post surgery, a bridge to heart transplant, or as a long-term solution if transplantation is not possible. A VAD consists of tubing that carries blood from the ventricles to a pump and returns blood to the circulation. A VAD has a power source and a control unit that monitors functions and alarms if there are problems with the circuit.

There are two basic types of VAD, left ventricular assist device (LVAD) and right ventricular assist device (RVAD). They may be used at the same time, creating a biventricular assist device. LVADs are most common. RVADs are usually only used for short-term support of the RV after surgery. VADs may be transcutaneous – where the VAD has its power source and pump outside the body. An example of this device would be the Berlin Heart. An implantable VAD has its pump located inside the body and a power source externally, which connects to the pump via a small hole usually in the abdomen. These devices are designed mainly for the adult patient; however, the technology is being continuously refined. Implantable VADs are a longer-term solution.

REFERENCES

Advanced Life Support Group, 2016. Advanced Paediatric Life Support: The Practical Approach. sixth ed. BMJ ©John Wiley & Sons, LTD.

Aiyagari, R., Rhodes, J.F., Shrader, P., et al., Pediatric Heart Network Investigators, 2013. Impact of pre-stage 11 hemodynamics and pulmonary artery anatomy on 12 month outcomes in the pediatric heart single ventricle reconstruction trial. J. Thoracic. Cardiovas. Surg. 148 (4), 1467–1474.

Almenar, L., Marti, S., Roldan, I., et al., 1996. Obstructive and non-obstructive hypertrophic cardiomyopathy: clinical, electricocardiographic and echo-cardiographic differences. Rev. Esp. Cardiol. 49 (6), 423–431.

Andreasen, J.B., Johnsen, S.P., Ravn, H.B., 2008. Junctional ectopic tachycardia after surgery for congenital heart disease in children. Intensive Care Med. 34 (5), 895–902.

Annila, P., Yli-Hankala, A., Lindgren, L., 1993. Effect of atropine on the QT interval and T wave amplitude in healthy volunteers. Br. J. Anaesth. 71, 736–737.

Arnold, R.R., Loukanov, T., Gorenflo, M., 2014. Hypoplastic left heart syndrome – unresolved issues. Front. Pediatr. 2, 125.

Babu, P., Damda, F., 2013. G77 A case of dilated cardiomyopathy due to nutritional vitamin D deficiency rickets. Arch. Dis. Child 98, A39–A40.

Bacha, E.A., Daves, S., Hardin, J., et al., 2006. Single-ventricle palliation for high-risk neonates: the emergence of an alternative hybrid stage 1 strategy. J. Thorac. Cardiovasc. Surg. 131, 163–171.

Barrett, C.S., Jaggers, J.J., Cook, E.F., et al., 2012. Outcomes in neonates undergoing extracorporeal membrane oxygenation using centrifugal versus roller pumps. Ann. Thorac. Surg. 94, 1635–1641.

Bartlett, R.H., Gazzaniga, A.B., Jefferies, M.R., et al., 1976. Extracorporeal membrane oxygenation (ECMO) cardiopulmonary support in infancy. Trans. Am. Soc. Artifi. Intern. Organs. 22, 80–93.

Bullaboy, C.A., Johnson, D.H., Azar, H., et al., 1984. Total anomalous pulmonary venous connection to portal system: a new therapeutic role for prostaglandin E1? Pediatr. Cardiol. 5, 115–116.

Butt, W., MacLaren, G., 2016. Extracorporeal membrane oxygenation 2016: an update [version1; referees: 3 approved] F1000Research 2016. 5(F100 Faculty Rev):750.

Chambers, D., Huang, C., Matthews, G., 2015. Arterial pressure waveforms, Figure 33.1, in Basic Physiology for Anaesthetists, © Cambridge University Press, pp. 150–151.

Chang, D.J., Kweon, T.D., Nam, S.B., et al., 2008. Effects of fentanyl pretreatment on the QTc interval during propofol induction. Anaesthesia 63, 1056–1060.

Chang, R.R., Allada, V., 2001. Electrographic and echocardiographic features that distinguish anomalous origin of the left coronary artery from pulmonary artery from idiopathic dilated cardiomyopathy. Pediatr. Cardiol. 22 (1), 3–10.

Chien, S.J., Liang, C.D., Lin, I.C., et al., 2008. Myocarditis complicated by complete atrioventricular block: nine years' experience in a medical center. Pediatr. Neonatol. 49 (6), 210–212.

Cincinnati Children's Hospital Medical Centre, 2016. Interrupted aortic arch – ventricular septal defect. Heart Institute Encyclopedia. www.cincinnatichildrens.org.

Cirstoveanu, C., Cinteza, E., Marcu, V., et al., 2012. Prostaglandin E1 on infradiaphragmatic type of total anomalous pulmonary venous connection – a case report. Maedica 7 (2), 167–172.

Colan, S.D., 2010. Hypertrophic cardiomyopathy in childhood. Heart Fail. Clin. 6 (4), 433–444.

De Leval, M.R., McKay, R., Jones, M., et al., 1981. Modified Blalock-Taussig shunt. Use of subclavian artery orifice as flow regulator in prosthetic systemic-pulmonary artery shunts. J. Thorac. Cardiovasc. Surg. 81 (1), 112–119.

Dirks, V., Pretre, R., Knirsch, W., et al., 2013. Modified Blalock-Taussig shunt: a not-so-simple palliative procedure. Eur. J. Cardiothorac. Surg. 44, 1096–1102.

Diso, D., Anile, M., Patella, M., et al., 2013. Lung transplantation for cystic fibrosis; outcome of 101 single-centre consecutive patients. Transplant. Proc. 45, 346–348.

Dodge-Khatami, A.1, Miller, O.I., Anderson, R.H., et al., 2002. Surgical substrates of postoperative junctional ectopic tachycardia in congenital heart defects. J. Thorac. Cardiovas. Surg. 123 (4), 624–630.

Drake, E., Preston, R., Douglas, J., 2007. Brief review: anesthetic implications of long QT syndrome in pregnancy. Can. J. Anaesth. 54, 561–572.

Extra Corporeal Life Support Organisation, 2016. The ELSO Registry: Benchmarking. www.elso-swac2016.org.

Fazio, G., Vernuccio, F., Grutta, G., et al., 2013. Drugs to be avoided in patients with long QT syndrome: focus on the anaesthesiological management. World J. Cardiol. 5 (4), 87–93.

Feinstein, J.A.1, Benson, D.W., Dubin, A.M., et al., 2012. Hypoplastic left heart syndrome: current considerations and expectations. J. Am. Coll. Cardiol. 59 (Suppl. 1), S1–S42.

Fenton, K.N., Siewers, R.D., Rebovich, B., et al., 2003. Interim mortality in infants with systemic to pulmonary artery shunts. Ann. Thorac. Surg. 76 (1), 152–156.

Franklin, R.C., Anderson, R.H., Daniels, O., et al., 2002. Report of the coding committee of the Association for European Paediatric Cardiology. Cardiol. Young 12, 611–618.

Frencker, B., 2015. Extracorporeal membrane oxygenation: a breakthrough for respiratory failure. J. Int. Med. 278, 586–598.

Giglia, T.M., Massicotte, M.P., Tweddell, J.S., et al., 2013. Prevention and treatment of thrombosis in pediatric and congenital heart disease. A Scientific Statement from the American Heart Association. Circulation 128, 2622–2703.

Hampton, J.R., 1992. The ECG Made Easy, fourth ed. Churchill Livingstone, Edinburgh.

Hardart, G.E., Fackler, J.C., 1999. Predictors of intracranial haemorrhage during neonatal extracorporeal membrane oxygenation. J. Pediatr. 134, 156–159.

Hazinski, M.F. (Ed.), 1992. Nursing Care of the Critically Ill Child, second ed. CV Mosby, St. Louis, MO.

Hirose, H., Yamane, K., Marhefka, G., et al., 2012. Right ventricular rupture and tamponade caused by malposition of Avalon cannula for veno-venous extracorporeal membrane oxygenation. J. Thorac. Surg. 7, 36.

Hoffman, T.M., Bush, D.M., Wernovsky, G., et al., 2002. Postoperative junctional ectopic tachycardia in children: incidence, risk factors and treatment. Ann. Thorac. Surg. 74 (5), 1607–1611.

Horrocks, F., 2002. Manual of Neonatal and Paediatric Heart Disease. Whurr, London.

Humphrey, C., Duncan, K., Fletcher, S., 2006. Decade of experience of vascular rings at a single institution. Pediatrics 117 (5), 903–908.

Jonas, R., 2003. Update on the Norwood procedure for hypoplastic left heart syndrome. Heart Views 4 (3), 5.

Kandakure, P.R., Dharmapuram, A.K., Ramadoss, N., et al., 2010. Sternotomy approach for modified Blalock–Taussig shunt: is it a safe option? Asian Cardiovasc. Thorac. Ann. 18, 368–372.

Kenyon, C.A., Flick, R., Moir, C., et al., 2010. Anaesthesia for videoscopic left cardiac sympathetic denervation in children with congenital long QT syndrome and catecholaminergic polymorphic ventricular tachycardia – a case series. Paediatr. Anaesth. 20, 465–470.

Khan, I.A., 2002. Long QT syndrome: diagnosis and management. Am. Heart J. 143 (1), 7–14.

Kies, S.J., Pabelick, C.M., Hurley, H.A., et al., 2005. Anesthesia for patients with congenital long QT syndrome. Anesthesiology 102, 204–210.

Kleinsasser, A., Kuenszberg, E., Loeckinger, A., et al., 2000. Sevoflurane but not propofol, significantly prolongs the Q-T interval. Anesth. Analg. 90, 25–27.

Kyriakidis, M., Triposkiadis, F., Dernellis, J., et al., 1998. Effects of cardiac versus circulatory angiotensin-converting enzyme inhibition on left ventricular diastolic function and coronary blood flow in hypertrophic obstructive cardiomyopathy. Circulation 97 (14), 1342–1347.

Loeckinger, A., Kleinsasser, A., Maier, S., et al., 2003. Sustained prolongation of the QTc interval after anaesthesia with sevoflurane in infants during the first 6 months of life. Anaesthesiology 98, 639–642.

MacLaren, G., Dodge-Khatami, A., Dalton, H.J., et al., 2013. Joint statement in mechanical circulatory support in children: a consensus review from the Pediatric Cardiac Intensive Care Society and the Extracorporeal Life Support Organization. Pedirat. Crit. Care Med. 14 (5), S1–S2.

Magliocca, J.F., Magee, J.C., Rowe, S.A., et al., 2005. Extracorporeal support for organ donation after cardiac death effectively expands the donor pool. J. Trauma 58, 1095–1101.

Makdisi, G., I-wen, W., 2015. Extracorporeal membrane oxygenation (ECMO) review of a lifesaving technology. J. Thorac. Dis. 7 (7), E166–E176.

Maron, M.S., Olivotto, I., Betocchi, S., et al., 2003. Effect of left ventricular outflow tract obstruction on clinical outcome in hypertrophic cardiomyopathy. Engl. J. Med. 348 (4), 295–303.

Maslach-Hubbard, A., Bratton, S.L., 2013. Extracorporeal membrane oxygenation for pediatric respiratory failure: history, development and current status. World J. Crit. Care Med. 2 (4), 29–39.

Mason, J.W., O'Connell, J.B., Herskowitz, A., et al., 1995. A clinical trial of immunosuppressive therapy for myocarditis. The Myocarditis Treatment Trial Investigators. Engl. J. Med. 333 (5), 269–275.

Martin, A.B., Webber, S., Fricker, F.J., et al., 1994. Acute myocarditis. Rapid diagnosis by PCR in children. Circulation 90 (1), 330–339.

Medak, R., Benumof, J.L., 1983. Perioperative management of hereditary arrhythmogenic syndromes. Br. J. Anaesth. 55, 361–364.

Melarkode, K., Latoo, M.Y., 2009. Pictorial essay: central venous catheters on chest radiographs. BJMP 2 (2), 55–56.

Michaloudis, D.G., Kanakoudis, F.S., Petrou, A.M., et al., 1996. The effects of midazolam or propofol followed by suxemethonium on the QT interval in humans. Eur. J. Anaesthesiol. 13, 364–368.

Molina, K.M., Garcia, X., Denfield, S.W., et al., 2013. Parvovirus B19 myocarditis causes significant morbidity and mortality in children. Pediatr. Cardiol. 34 (2), 390–397.

Momma, K., 2010. Cardiovascular anomalies associated with chromosome 22q11.2 deletion syndrome. Am. J. Cardiol. 105, 1617–1624.

Munnell, E.R., 1997. Thoracic drainage. Ann. Thorac. Surg. 63, 1497–1502.

Murkin, J.M., Arango, M., 2009. Near-infrared spectroscopy as an index of brain and tissue oxygenation. Br. J. Anaesth. 103 (Suppl. 1), 3–13.

Nikaidoh, H., 1984. Aortic translocation and biventricular outflow tract reconstruction. A new surgical repair for transposition of the great arteries associated with ventricular septal defect and pulmonary stenosis. J. Thorac. Cardiovasc. Surg. 88, 365–372.

Odim, J., Portzky, M., Zurakowski, D., et al., 1995. Sternotomy approach for the modified Blalock-Taussig shunt. Circulation 92, 256–261.

Ohye, R.G., Ludomirsky, A., Devaney, E.J., et al., 2004. Comparison of right ventricle to pulmonary artery conduit and modified Blalock-Taussig shunt hemodynamics after the Norwood operation. Ann. Thorac. Surg. 78, 1090–1093.

Owczuk, R., Twardowski, P., Dylczyk-Sommer, A., et al., 2009. Influence of promethazine on cardiac repolarisation: a double-blind, midazolam-controlled study. Anaesthesia 64, 609–614.

Papo, M.C., Hernan, L.J., Fuhrman, B.P., 1997. Postoperative cardiac care for congenital heart disease. In: Singh, N.L. (Ed.), Manual of Pediatric Critical Care. WB Saunders, Philadelphia, PA.

Park, M.K., 1997. The Pediatric Cardiology Handbook, second ed. CV Mosby, St. Louis, MO.

Park, M.K., 2003. The Pediatric Cardiology Handbook, third ed. CV Mosby, St Louis, MO.

Pearson, G., 2002. Handbook of Paediatric Intensive Care. WB Saunders, Edinburgh.

Peek, G.J., Mugford, M., Tiruvoipati, R., et al., CESAR Trial Collaboration, 2009. Efficacy and economic assessment of conventional ventilator support versus extracorporeal membrane oxygenation for severe adult respiratory failure (CESAR): a multicenter randomized controlled trial. Lancet 374, 1351–1363.

Pelliccia, A., Fagard, R., Bjørnstad, H.H., et al., Study Group of Sports Cardiology of the Working Group of Cardiac Rehabilitation and Exercise Physiology; Working Group of Myocardial and Pericardial Diseases of the European Society of Cardiology, 2005. Recommendations for competitive sports participation in athletes with cardiovascular disease: a consensus document from the Study Group of Sports Cardiology of the Working Group of Cardiac Rehabilitation and Exercise Physiology and the Working Group of Myocardial and Pericardial Diseases of the European Society of Cardiology. Eur. Heart J. 26 (14), 1422–1445.

Punja, M., Mark, D.G., McCoy, J.V., et al., 2010. Electrocardiographic manifestations of cardiac infectious-inflammatory disorders. Am. J. Emerg. Med. 28, 364–377.

Raja, S.G., Atamanyuk, I., Tsang, V.T., 2011. Impact of shunt type on growth of pulmonary arteries after Norwood stage 1 procedure: current best available evidence. World J. Pediatr. Congenit. Heart Surg. 2 (1), 90–96.

Rehder, K.J., Turner, D.A., Cheifetz, I.M., 2013. Extracorporeal membrane oxygenation for neonatal and pediatric respiratory failure: an evidence based review of the past decade (2002-2012). Pediatr. Crit. Care Med. 14 (9), 852–861.

Robinson, J., Hartling, L., Vandermeer, B., et al., 2015. Intravenous immunoglobulin for presumed viral myocarditis in children and adults. Cochrane Database Sys. Rev.. Issue 5. Art. No: CD004370. https://doi.org/10.1002/14651858.CD004370.pub3.

Roskelly, L., Smith, A.P., 2011. In: Dougherty, L., Lister, S. (Eds.), The Royal Marsden Hospital Manual of Clinical Nursing Procedures. Wiley and Son, Hoboken.

Royal Children's Hospital, 2005. Double Outlet Right Ventricle. Royal Children's Hospital, London. Available online at: www.rch.org.au/cardiology/defects.

Ruegger, C., Bucher, H.U., Mieth, R.A., 2010. Pulse oximetry in the newborn: is the left hand pre- or post-ductal? BMC Pediatr. 10, 35.

Sano, S., Ishino, K., Kado, H., et al., 2004. Outcome of right ventricle to pulmonary artery shunt in first stage palliation of hypoplastic left heart syndrome: a multi-institutional study. Ann. Thorac. Surg. 78, 1951–1958.

Schwartz, P.J., Moss, A.J., Vincent, G.M., et al., 1993. Diagnostic criteria for the long QT syndrome. An update. Circulation 88 (2), 782–784.

Shah, J.S., Esteban, M.T., Thaman, R., et al., 2008. Prevalence of exercise-induced left ventricular outflow tract obstruction in symptomatic patients with non-obstructive hypertrophic cardiomyopathy. Heart 94 (10), 1288–1294.

Shemie, S.D., 1997. Cardiovascular monitoring. In: Singh, N.L. (Ed.), Manual of Pediatric Critical Care. WB Saunders, Philadelphia, PA.

Singh, S.P., Chauhan, S., Choudhury, A., et al., 2014. Modified Blalock-Taussig shunt: comparison between neonates, infants and older children. Ann. Cardiol. Anaestheiol. 17 (3), 191–197.

Sistino, J.J., Bonilha, H.S., 2012. Improvements in survival and neurodevelopmental outcomes in surgical treatment of hypoplastic left heart syndrome: a meta-analytic review. J. Extra-Corpor. Technol. 44, 216–223.

Stonelake, P.A., Bodenham, A.R., 2006. The carina as a radiological landmark for central venous catheter tip position. Br. J. Anaesth. 96, 335–340.

Talwar, S., Nair, V.V., Choudhary, S.K., et al., 2014. The Hemi-Fontan operation: a critical overview. Ann. Pediatr. Cardiol. 7 (2), 120–125.

Towbin, J.A., Lowe, A.M., Colan, S.D., et al., 2006. Incidence, causes and outcomes of dilated cardiomyopathy in children. JAMA 296 (15), 1867–1876.

Ukena, C., Mahfoud, F., Kindermann, I., et al., 2011. Prognostic electro-cardiographic parameters in patients with suspected myocarditis. Eur. J. Heart Fail. 13 (4), 398–405.

Vesely, T., 2003. Central venous catheter tip position: a continuing controversy. J. Vascul. Interven. Radiol. 14, 527–534.

Wernovsky, G., Kuijpers, M., Van Rossem, M.C., et al., 2007. Postoperative course in the cardiac intensive care unit following the first stage of Norwood reconstruction. Cardiol. Young. 17, 652–665.

Wesselhoeft, H., Fawcett, J.S., Johnson, A.L., 1968. Anomalous origin of the left coronary from the pulmonary trunk. Its clinical spectrum, pathology and pathophysiology based on a review of 140 cases with seven further cases. Circulation 38, 403–425.

Wisely, N.A., Shipton, E.A., 2002. Long QT syndrome and anaesthesia. Eur. J. Anaesthesiol. 19, 853–859.

Yasui, H., Kado, H., Yonenaga, K., et al., 1987. Primary repair of interrupted aortic arch and severe aortic stenosis in neonates. J. Thorac. Cardiovasc. Surg. 93, 539–545.

Zapol, W.M., Snider, M.T., Hill, J.D., et al., 1979. Extracorporeal membrane oxygenation in severe acute respiratory failure. A randomized prospective study. JAMA 242, 2193–2196.

THE KIDNEYS AND RENAL REPLACEMENT

4

In the course of a day, the kidneys filter up to 180 liters (L) of plasma and then reabsorb more than 99% of the water, sodium, chloride, glucose, and amino acids. Acute kidney injury (AKI) is a common problem in paediatric intensive care with an incidence as high as 40% (Gupta et al 2016) and is an independent risk factor for increased morbidity and mortality (Alkandari et al 2011). AKI is characterised by the inability of the kidneys to concentrate urine, regulate electrolytes, excrete waste products, and maintain pH. The kidney is also responsible for the production of hormones that control the blood pressure (BP), red cell production, and calcium homeostasis.

Normal Ranges: It is useful to have a clear knowledge of the normal baseline ranges for serum electrolytes, urea, and creatinine when reviewing patients at risk of kidney injury. Ranges are listed in Table 4.1.

Blood pressure: The mercury sphygmomanometer was the original gold standard for BP measurement; however, these devices are no longer in regular use and have generally been replaced by oscillometric devices (e.g., Dinamap, Hewlett Packard). Noninvasive measurements with oscillometric devices have been validated with invasive arterial pressure measurements in infants (Chiolero et al 2010), but there is still a risk of over- and underestimation of BP. Continuous monitoring of BP via invasive arterial lines remains the most accurate method for measuring BP, which is preferred in cardiovascularly unstable patients and when treating hypertension in acute crisis situations.

KEY CONCEPTS

- **Hypertension:** A useful pocket guide to BP measurement was published by the National Heart, Lung & Blood Institute in the United States in 2007, which includes reference ranges for normal BP in children for each age and height range (NHLBI 2007). Hypertension is defined as a systolic blood pressure (sBP) greater than 95th percentile for age. Severe hypertension is defined as 20 mm Hg above the 95th percentile and is usually due to underlying disease. Hypertensive crisis is usually associated with BP 50% above normal or sBP >180 mm Hg.
- **Glomerular filtration rate (GFR)** is the rate at which the kidneys filter blood. Creatinine is waste product from muscle metabolism, which is exclusively filtered through the kidneys—in

Table 4.1 Normal values	
Urea (increase with age)	0.5–7.5 mmol/L
Creatinine (increase with age and muscle bulk)	10–90 µmol/L
Potassium	3.5–5 mmol/L
Sodium	135–145 mmol/L
Serum osmolality	280–300 mOsm/L

Fig. 4.1 Cross section of a kidney and close-up of the nephron.

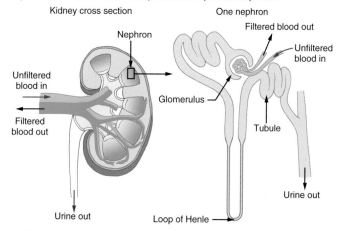

particular the glomerulus. Each kidney contains about 1 million nephrons (Fig. 4.1). Creatinine may be underestimated in children who are malnourished or have liver failure, and biomarkers such as Cystatin C may be more useful in these situations. The most accurate way to measure GFR is using radioactive substances with Inulin currently being the gold standard. However, in practice, GFR is usually estimated using an equation that takes account of the serum creatinine levels, age, and length of the child (Schwartz formula: height x constant [most universal is 40/creatinine]). As kidney function is proportional to the size of the kidney and the person, adjustment for body surface area is necessary to compare GFRs of different sized individuals. The average body surface area of a young adult is 1.73 m^2, therefore GFR is measured as millilitres/minute/1.73 m^2. A normal GFR ranges from 80–120 mL/min/1.73 m^2 for anyone over 2 years and is easy to explain to parents that a GFR should be 100% (100 mL/min/1.73 m^2). A low GFR (<60 mL/min/1.73 m^2) reflects a significant reduction in the number of functioning nephrons. Doses of medication may need to be adjusted in children with very low GFRs (<15 mL/min/1.73 m^2); advice can be obtained from pharmacists or local formularies.

NEW BIOMARKER

- Neutrophil galactinase-associated lipocalin (NGAL) is a protein secreted into the urine that is very sensitive to kidney injury. It is released into the tubular lumen very soon after kidney injury and the level rises in proportion to the degree of injury. Changes in urine NGAL can be detected 1 or 2 days before a rise in serum creatinine is noted. As it is secreted by the renal tubules, it is a marker of intrinsic renal problems rather than just low perfusion to the kidney. Only 1 mL of urine is necessary for laboratory testing. Urinary NGAL levels of less than 50 ng/mL suggest a very low risk; above 150 ng/mL the risk is increased, and above 300 ng/mL there is a very high risk of kidney injury.

ACUTE KIDNEY INJURY

AKI is the sudden loss of kidney function characterised by a decrease in the GFR and a progressive rise of serum creatinine and urea. This may be accompanied by oliguria (<1 mL/kg/h) or occasionally polyuria. There are more than 30 definitions of AKI, but the two most popular are the paediatric RIFLE and KDIGO (Kidney Disease: Improving Global Outcomes). Details of these definitions can be found in Table 4.2.

Causes of AKI can be described as prerenal (low perfusion to kidney reducing effective glomerular filtration), intrarenal (inflammation and injury directly to the nephrons), or postrenal (obstruction to flow of urine from kidneys or bladder). Examples from each category are listed in Table 4.3. It is important to identify the potential cause in order to start the correct treatment. Prerenal and postrenal are associated with intrinsically normal kidneys, which can regain function if the haemodyamics are restored and the obstruction is relieved. In the case of intrinsic renal causes, it is important to initiate early renal support and stop any nephrotoxic therapies (e.g., aminoglycosides, contrast).

The reasons for initiating renal replacement therapy in the paediatric intensive care unit (PICU) are:

- Fluid overload
- Isolated electrolyte abnormalities
- Combination of fluid and electrolyte derangements
- Symptomatic uraemia (high urea causing encephalopathy, pericarditis, bleeding)
- Persistent severe metabolic acidosis
- Metabolic abnormality (e.g., hyperammonaemia)
- Drug intoxication or overdose
- To allow greater fluid and nutrition intake.

Table 4.2   Diagnostic criteria for acute kidney injury

pRIFLE

	eCCI	Urine output
Risk	Decrease by 25%	<0.5 mL/kg/h for 8 h
Injury	Decrease by 50%	<0.5 mL/kg/h for 16 h
Failure	Decrease by 75% or <35 mL/min/1.73 m^2	<0.3 mL/kg/h for 24 h OR anuric for 12 h
Loss	Persistent renal failure >4 weeks	Not applicable
End stage	Persistent renal failure >3 months	Not applicable

KDIGO

	SCr	Urine output
Stage 1	Increase 1.5–1.9 × baseline or increase ≥27 µmol/L	<0.5 mL/kg/h for 6–12 h
Stage 2	Increase 2–2.9 × baseline	<0.5 mL/kg/h for ≥12 h
Stage 3	Increase >3 × baseline OR SCr ≥354 µmol/L OR Initiation of RRT OR eGFR <35 mL/min/1.73 m^2	<0.3 mL/kg/h for ≥24 h OR anuric for ≥12 h

Both pRIFLE and KDIGO classification systems stratify AKI into levels of severity, which are determined by changes in serum creatinine (SCr)/estimated creatinine clearance (eCCI), and changes in urine output. AKI severity strata can be reached through fulfilling criteria for either changes in SCr/eCCI or changes in urine output.

AKI, Acute kidney injury; *eGFR,* estimated glomerular filtration rate; *KDIGO,* Kidney Disease: Improving Global Outcomes; *pRIFLE,* paediatric Risk or renal dysfunction, Injury to the kidney, Failure of kidney function, Loss of kidney function, and End-stage renal disease; *RRT,* renal replacement therapy.

McCaffrey, J., Dhakal, A.K., Milford, D.V., Webb, N.J., Lennon, R., 2016. Recent development in the detection and management of acute kidney injury. Arch. Dis. Child. 0, 1–6.

Methods of providing renal replacement therapy in intensive care are:
- Peritoneal dialysis (PD)
- Continuous veno-venous haemofiltration (CVVH)
- Continuous veno-venous haemodiafiltration (CVVHD)
- Haemodialysis

See Table 4.4 for the advantages and disadvantages of types of treatment.

Table 4.3 Causes of acute kidney injury

Type of kidney injury	Aetiology (case)
Prerenal	Reduced intravascular volume (e.g., diarrhoea, blood loss, shock)
	Reduced effective intravascular volume (e.g., heart failure, coarctation of the aorta)
Intrinsic renal disease	Acute tubular necrosis (vasomotor nephropathy)
	Hypoxic ischaemic insult
	Drug induced
	Toxin mediated (e.g., myoglobin, ethylene glycol, methanol)
	Tumour lysis syndrome
	Renal vein thrombosis
	Glomerulonephritis
	Interstitial nephritis
	Cortical necrosis
	Haemolytic uraemic syndrome
	Idiopathic
Postrenal (obstruction)	Obstruction to single kidney
	Bilateral ureteral obstruction
	Urethral obstruction (e.g., posterior urethral valves)

Table 4.4 Advantages and disadvantages of various modalities of renal replacement therapy for acute renal failure

Type	Complexity	Use in hypotension	Efficiency	Volume control	Anticoagulation
Peritoneal dialysis	Low	Yes	Moderate	Moderate	No
Intermittent dialysis	Moderate	No	High	Moderate	Yes
Continuous veno-venous haemofiltration	Moderate	Yes	Moderate	Good	Yes
Continuous veno-venous haemodiafiltration	High	Yes	High	Good	Yes

Strazdins, V., Watson, A., Harvey, B., 2004. Renal replacement therapy for acute renal failure in children: European guidelines. Pediatr. Nephrol. 19, 199–207.

PERITONEAL DIALYSIS

PD is usually the first choice of renal support in the critically ill child but may be contraindicated by an acute surgical abdomen, access difficulties, or catheter malfunction.

PD involves the introduction of dialysis fluid (called dialysate) into the peritoneal cavity through a catheter placed in the lower part of the abdomen. The peritoneum serves as the dialysis membrane. Fluid is held in the abdomen for a prescribed dwell time and then drained out into a sterile container. During the dwell time solutes and waste products (e.g., potassium, urea, and creatinine) move from an area of high concentration (blood) to lower concentration (dialysate) until equilibrium is reached or the fluid is drained out; this is called **solute removal by diffusion.**

An osmotic pressure gradient is applied by the addition to the dialysis fluid of an osmotic agent, glucose, which draws water from the blood across the peritoneal membrane into the dialysate. The movement of water molecules across a membrane to the side with more osmotically active particles is called **osmosis.**

When the dialysis fluid is drained from the abdominal cavity, it contains waste products and excess fluid extracted from the blood.

Fluid and solute removal in PD is controlled by:

- Glucose concentration
- Dwell time
- Volume
- Peritoneal membrane characteristics

Some solutes are transported in the opposite direction (i.e., from the dialysis fluid to the blood) during dialysis, which is why the PD fluid needs to contain sufficient amounts of a buffer (e.g., bicarbonate or lactate) to balance the pH. There is evidence that bicarbonate or a combination of bicarbonate and lactate buffered solutions are better tolerated and more effective than lactate buffered solutions alone (Wang 2001).

The following details need to be prescribed for PD:

1. **Exchange volume** 20–30 mL/kg is generally effective. It will take a longer time for the concentration gradient to decline in a large volume of fluid. In the critically ill child, it may be necessary to start with a smaller volume (10 mL/kg) because of cardiovascular instability and emergency catheter placement. PD can also be of value when used for cooling purposes in the critically ill child with a pyrexia that is unresponsive to other antipyretic therapy with dialysate that can be either cooled or at room temperature.

2. **Fill time, dwell time, and drain time** fluid removal rate is highest at the beginning of each exchange cycle, when the glucose concentration difference between the blood and the fresh dialysate solution is at its greatest. After a peak is reached, the removed volume falls as fluid and is transported in the reverse direction; that is, from the dialysis fluid back to the blood. If the dialysis solution is kept in the abdominal cavity long enough, the patient will gain rather than lose fluid. In the PICU setting, short cycles of 30–60 minutes are initially applied with a dwell time of 10–40 minutes to rapidly clear waste and other molecules.

3. **Composition of the dialysate standard** solutions are available with variable glucose concentrations: for example, 1.36%, 2.27%,

or 3.86%. The higher the concentration of glucose, the larger the osmotic pressure, resulting in more fluid removal. It is possible to use a combination of these different solutions, either by giving 50% of each for every cycle (use burette) or by alternating the different strengths so each is given only on alternate cycles.

4. **Heparin** (500 IU/L) is usually added to the dialysate to prevent fibrin formation and clotting in the catheter.

5. **Potassium** may also be added to maintain a normal serum potassium level. Most PD solutions do not contain any potassium at all; once serum potassium levels approach the normal range (<6 mmol/L) it is important to add potassium to the PD fluid to avoid hypokalaemia.

PD performed in the PICU is continuous, and is maintained until the child is able to pass adequate volumes of urine and the kidney function is improving.

 Aim to use the minimum concentration of glucose dialysate when possible—prolonged use of a high concentration glucose solution can result in sclerosis of the peritoneum, making further PD impossible.

Problems

Technical problems with PD are mostly related to catheter malfunction:
- If fill time takes longer than 10 minutes it usually indicates catheter obstruction.
- If less than 80% of the previous fill volume returns during the full drainage period, then drainage is inadequate.

Causes

- External kinks
- Fibrin or blood clot plugging
- Poor position or migration of catheter
- Obstruction by omentum
- Leaks around catheter site.

Action

- Reposition patient
- Alert medical colleagues, as catheter may benefit from careful flushing with sterile saline; abdominal x-ray will confirm the position of catheter in abdomen
- Fibrin clotting may require urokinase infusion into catheter
- Leaks around the catheter site will increase the risk of infection in addition to impairing the dialysis process; therefore medical staff may have to introduce a new catheter or optimise the seal of the present catheter.

Peritonitis remains a constant threat, especially if there has been a lot of manipulation of the catheter. Cloudy PD fluid, abdominal tenderness, or redness at the catheter insertion site require urgent attention (Warady 2000). Management may include antibiotics administered via the PD catheter, or possibly catheter removal. Removal of the catheter will necessitate sutures to close the skin, and tunnelled catheters may need to be removed in theatre.

CONTINUOUS VENO-VENOUS HAEMOFILTRATION

Haemofiltration = ultrafiltration + convection + fluid replacement.
- **Ultrafiltration** – the movement of fluid (water) down a pressure gradient; that is, from a region of high pressure on one side of the membrane to a region of low pressure on the other.
- **Convection** – the movement of solutes with a water flow (solvent drag); for example, the movement of membrane-permeable solutes with ultrafiltered water. Although the convection associated with ultrafiltration results in some solute transfer, this is primarily by passive diffusion.

CVVH is the removal of fluid via a semipermeable membrane (haemofilter) using a circuit with a pump. The blood is obtained and returned to the venous circulation; this is an uninterrupted process.

Indications for use of CVVH:
- When PD is contraindicated or has failed
- Hypervolaemia that does not require haemodialysis because of improving renal function (urea, creatinine, and other electrolytes assessed)
- To ensure that adequate nutrition can be given in suitable volumes by removing equivalent volume

CONTINUOUS VENO-VENOUS HAEMODIAFILTRATION

Haemodiafiltration = ultrafiltration + convection + fluid replacement + diffusion.

CVVHD is the removal of excess fluid and biochemical waste products via a semipermeable membrane (haemofilter). Dialysis is performed by infusing dialysate fluid using a countercurrent flow through the haemofilter. The circuit has a pump. The blood is obtained and returned to the venous circulation; this is an uninterrupted process.

Indications for the use of CVVHD:
- When PD is contraindicated or has failed
- To ensure that parenteral nutrition can be given in suitable volumes, to help decrease or prevent catabolism, ensuring that the equivalent volume can be removed
- When electrolytes are seriously deranged, particularly potassium
- In certain metabolic disorders (e.g., hyperammonaemia)
- When the child is not cardiovascularly stable enough to tolerate haemodialysis

HAEMODIALYSIS

Haemodialysis = ultrafiltration + diffusion.

Haemodialysis is the removal of excess fluid and biochemical waste products via a semipermeable membrane (haemofilter). Dialysis is performed by infusing dialysate fluid using a countercurrent flow through the haemofilter. The circuit has a pump. The blood is obtained from and returned to the venous circulation.

Haemodialysis is an intermittent treatment; it can be used as a 'follow-on' treatment for children who, when critically ill, were receiving CVVHD, and whose condition is now stable enough to tolerate larger volumes of fluid and solute removal being undertaken on an intermittent basis (e.g., once daily).

FLUIDS FOR CONTINUOUS VENO-VENOUS HAEMOFILTRATION / CONTINUOUS VENO-VENOUS HAEMODIAFILTRATION

The purpose of predilution fluid is to achieve high ultrafiltration rates (UFRs) without additional risk of haemofilter thrombosis. There are a variety of types of replacement fluid manufactured for CVVHD, which can be changed according to the patient's requirements and are categorised basically according to the inclusion/exclusion of potassium and buffer, which may be either bicarbonate or lactate. Other electrolytes may also need to be prescribed according to patient requirements.

The following are some examples:

- Potassium-free lactate-buffered fluid – Lactosol
- Potassium-free bicarbonate-buffered fluid – Hemosol BO
- Potassium 4 mmol/L lactate-buffered fluid – Hemolactol
- Potassium 4 mmol/L bicarbonate-buffered fluid – Prismasol 4

Hemosol BO is considered by some centres to be the fluid of choice for the majority of haemofiltered patients, and the following points related to its use may be helpful:

- Buffered with bicarbonate (32 mmol/L) and does not require any additional bicarbonate infused into the patient
- Potassium free – add potassium according to guidelines. Never add more than 4 mmol/L of potassium
- The only relative contraindication to its use is metabolic alkalosis (pH >7.5)
- This solution does not contain sufficient lactate to cause or mask hyperlactaemia and should still be used in these patients

To prepare Hemosol BO solution for use, the separate bicarbonate bag provided should be mixed in with it, as instructed by the manufacturer immediately before use.

 Do not add calcium or phosphate into this solution as it may precipitate. Always supplement Ca, Mg, or phosphate directly to the patient.

A predilution fluid should not contain more than 4 mmol/L of potassium regardless of how low the plasma potassium level may be. It is better to give intravenous potassium if hypokalaemia does not correct on haemofiltration.

ANTICOAGULATION

The aim of anticoagulation is to prevent clotting of the extracorporeal circuit with minimal risk to the patient. Various methods of anticoagulation are used.

Heparin

Heparin acts by inhibiting the conversion of prothrombin to thrombin and neutralises the actions of thrombin. Some authors advise an initial bolus of heparin (maximum 50 IU/kg) at the time of connection to the extracorporeal circuit followed by a continuous infusion of 0–30 IU/kg/h (Strazdins et al 2004). Rate of infusion should be adjusted according to local guidance.

Record the amount of heparin infused hourly to ensure that the heparin pump is infusing correctly and the correct dose is being given.

Some centres prefer to leave heparin infusing until treatment is discontinued to ensure that patency of access is maintained after treatment is discontinued.

 You may need to give a bolus of heparin if blood products are administered, as the transfusion will increase the viscosity of the blood, which can lead to a decrease in the ultrafiltration, or solute removal, and clotting problems may occur in the circuit.

Epoprostenol/prostacyclin

An infusion of prostacyclin may be used instead of heparin when the child has a low platelet count, to prevent or stop heparin-induced thrombocytopenia (Nevard & Rigden 1995).

Dose range: 2–8 ng/kg/min (Deep et al 2017). Activated clotting time (ACT) monitoring is unhelpful because of prostacyclin's action in inhibiting platelet aggregation. Unlike heparin, boluses of prostacyclin should **not** be given when blood products are administered.

Citrate

Regional anticoagulation with citrate is favoured by some centres (Mehta et al 1991, Chadha et al 2000). Sodium citrate chelates ionised calcium necessary for the coagulation cascade and systemic anticoagulation is avoided by infusing calcium through a separate central line. Appropriate (calcium-free) dilution fluids must be selected for use with citrate. The disadvantages include the possibility of various acid base and electrolyte disturbances including hypernatraemia, hypocalcaemia, and metabolic alkalosis (Strazdins et al 2004).

Monitoring

Opinions vary as to the most effective way of monitoring anticoagulation, so local guidance should be followed.

Although local guidelines must be adhered to, the following may be helpful:

- In patients with normal coagulation (international normalised ratio [INR] <1.5 or partial thromboplastin time [PTT] <2.0 and platelets >50):
  - Use a fixed rate of 24 IU/kg/h heparin
  - If PTT at 8 hours greater than 2.0 reduce heparin dose to 10 international units/kilogram/hour (IU/kg/h)
  - If PTT persistently greater than 2.0 on 5 IU/kg/h **stop** anticoagulation
- In patients with coagulopathy (INR >2.0, PTT >2.0 or platelets <50) or high risk of bleeding (defined as ongoing active bleeding/ major bleed in last 48 hours or surgery in last 24 hours) no anticoagulation may be the safest option
- ACT has the advantage of a rapid bedside test and may be used as a guide but is less accurate than PTT and should not be used alone, particularly in patients at a high risk of bleeding or thrombosis
- If a filter clots in less than 24 hours, the most likely problem is inadequate Vas-Cath size or position

The following should also be observed:

- Fibrin and clot deposition in venous bubble trap as clots build up in greater areas of stasis
- Rising venous pressure may indicate clot formation in the venous side of vascular access or venous bubble trap
- Rising transmembrane pressure (TMP) may indicate clot formation in the filter
- Darkening blood circuit may indicate clotting
- Continuous decrease in the rate of ultrafiltration
- Observe the haemofilter for clots, dark streaks, or areas of gravity separation of the blood into plasma and cells

Brief written observations on the condition of the circuit, recorded hourly on the appropriate chart, may be helpful.

 Patients may cool rapidly on continuous veno-venous haemofiltration as heat is lost across the haemofilter surface—monitor core temperature continuously and consider active warming measures. Some machines have the capacity to prewarm predilution fluid—use according to manufacturer's instructions and local policy.

Priming the circuit

When priming lines during setting up filter circuit, heparinised saline (5000 IU heparin to 1 L 0.9% saline) is generally used. Where the circuit volume exceeds 10% of the child's extracorporeal blood volume and/or the child is anaemic, it is advisable to transfuse the volume of packed cells sufficient to correct the anaemia/provide the deficit in extracorporeal blood volume prior to starting haemofiltration. Some centres recommend priming the circuit with blood for neonates.

Checklist for continuous veno-venous haemofiltration/HD

1. Record patient weight
2. Place large bore Vas-Cath (preferably neck veins)
3. Confirm position of Vas-Cath prior to use (above diaphragm and not crossing midline)
4. Select predilution fluid (add potassium according to guideline if potassium free fluid)
5. Consider blood prime if patient <10 kg
6. Select filter size according to weight
7. Choose optimal blood flow rate
8. Set UFR
9. Prescribe desired fluid balance (i.e., how much fluid to be removed per hour)
10. Anticoagulation as per regime
11. Monitor arterial/venous line pressure and TMP
12. Monitor patient temperature
13. Calculate filtration fraction and recirculation rates if the CVVH does not appear to be effective.

TROUBLESHOOTING CONTINUOUS VENO-VENOUS HAEMOFILTRATION/CONTINUOUS VENO-VENOUS HAEMODIAFILTRATION: GENERAL REASONS

Problems that may be encountered include:
- Access difficulties
- Filter clotting
- Infections

FOR ALARMS

Alarm: Intermittent arterial pressure alarm
Cause: Catheter intermittently sucking against vessel wall
Action: Turn down pump speed, but not below three-quarters of the maximum rate; consider rotating the catheter 180 degrees
   Remember: the arterial sensor measures negative pressure. An increasingly negative arterial pressure reading indicates that it is becoming more difficult to pull blood out from the 'arterial' line. The catheter could be wedged against vessel/occluded/clotted.

Alarm: Arterial pressure alarm followed by venous pressure alarm

Cause: Restriction of blood flow pre-pump causing arterial pressure alarm and stopping pump, causing venous pressure to drop and alarm

Action: Correct kinked line and poor position of catheter, for example. Press venous pressure button to start blood pump and keep pressing until light goes out. If arterial pressure alarm comes on again, turn off blood pump and rotate catheter 180 degrees. Restart pump.

Alarm: High venous pressure alarm

Cause: Restriction of blood flow going back to the patient:
- Clotting in venous drip chamber
- Kinked line
- Poor catheter position

Action: Check for kinks. Consider clots—try to wash back circuit; that is, run saline through filter and venous bubble trap to aid visibility. Clots in venous line/filter may need to change them. Recheck catheter position on chest x-ray and echocardiogram if necessary.

Alarm: Air detector alarm and venous pressure alarm

Cause: Level of blood in drip chamber fallen/frothing of blood in drip chamber

Action: The pump will stop; raise the level in the drip chamber by removing air with a syringe. Restart pump.

The suggestions above are for general guidance only and are not intended to replace instructions in the operator's manual of individual machines.

PLASMA EXCHANGE

Plasma exchange is a treatment that is used to treat diseases that are plasma-mediated or plasma-borne, including diseases that involve the immune system. The aim of the treatment is to remove autoantibodies, pathogenic immune complexes, and inflammatory mediators. The treatment rapidly removes these substances, thereby reducing the effects of the disease processes.

Diseases that have been *treated* with plasma exchange include:
- Haemolytic uraemic syndrome (where there is neurologic involvement)
- Guillain–Barré syndrome
- Systemic lupus erythematosus
- Renal transplant rejection
- Myasthenia gravis
- Henoch–Schönlein purpura
- Immune mediated encephalitis

A plasma filter is used for the procedure, and this removes the child's circulating plasma (albumin, antibodies and immune complexes, and clotting factors). During the procedure, the child is given albumin 4.5% to replace that removed. Fresh frozen plasma (FFP) is also given to replace clotting factors lost. Therefore, only the circulating antibodies and immune complexes are removed.

The PICU nurse's responsibilities include:
- Accurate measurement of fluid input and output
- Monitoring patient's haemodynamic status and altering fluid balance accordingly
- Prewarming replacement fluid and monitoring the patient's temperature
- Titration of heparin infusion to maintain optimal clotting times
- Regular assessment of blood gases and biochemistry
- Maintenance of asepsis with the catheter site and the blood circuit
- Maintenance of the blood circuit—acting as a 'troubleshooter'
- Source of information and reassurance to the patient and family

RENAL DISEASE

Two renal diseases that may require the admission of a child to a PICU are nephrotic syndrome and haemolytic–uraemic syndrome (HUS).

Nephrotic syndrome

Nephrotic syndrome is a symptom complex characterised by oedema, marked proteinuria, hypercholesterolaemia, and hypoalbuminaemia. Although there are many types of the disease, minimal change nephrotic syndrome is the most common in children.

The syndrome may be classified as primary (associated with a primary glomerular disease) or secondary (resulting from a wide variety of disease states or nephrotoxic agents).

- For unknown reasons the glomerular membrane, usually impermeable to large proteins, becomes permeable
- Protein, especially albumin, leaks through the membrane and is lost in the urine
- Plasma proteins decrease as proteinuria increases
- The colloidal osmotic pressure, which holds water in the vascular compartments, is reduced as a result of the decreased amount of serum proteins. This allows fluid to flow from the capillaries into the extracellular space, producing oedema. Accumulation of fluid in the interstitial spaces and peritoneal cavity is also increased by an overproduction of aldosterone, which causes retention of sodium.
- There is increased susceptibility to infection because of decreased gammaglobulin

Management is aimed at:
- Restoration or maintenance of adequate circulating blood volume and systemic perfusion
- Maintenance of fluid and electrolyte balance
- Minimising glomerular damage and maximising renal function
- Ensuring patient comfort and preventing infection

Most cases respond to steroid therapy, which appears to affect the basic disease process in addition to controlling the oedema. Those who are not steroid-responsive or who lose steroid responsiveness may respond to cytotic therapy.

Urine specific gravity will be falsely elevated in the presence of proteinuria with the administration of osmotic diuretics. Urine osmolality is believed to be the best indicator of renal function because it reflects renal concentrating ability and is not affected by the presence of large molecules in the urine (Brunner & Suddarth 1991).

Haemolytic–uraemic syndrome

HUS is the association of an acute haemolytic anaemia, thrombocytopenia, and acute renal failure. This syndrome is one of the most common causes of acute renal failure in children. It often follows a gastrointestinal illness or, in younger children, respiratory illness.

The most common cause of diarrhoea positive HUS is *Escherichia coli* O157; and an important diarrhoea negative infective cause is Pneumococcus (often with a primary respiratory tract infection):

- The main site of injury is believed to be the endothelial lining of the small arteries and arterioles, particularly in the kidney
- The intravascular deposition of platelets and fibrin results in partial or complete occlusion of the small arterioles and capillaries in the kidney
- As a result of passing through these vessels, it is believed that erythrocytes are damaged, removed from the circulation by the spleen, and their life span reduced, resulting in a severe, progressive anaemia
- Thrombocytopenia may be present, possibly caused by the aggregation, consumption, or destruction of platelets within the kidney
- HUS is associated with damage to the glomerular endothelial cells. As a result, renal blood flow and GFR can be reduced in a degree proportional to the glomerular injury
- Cortical necrosis may be produced by renal ischaemia, and renal tubular damage may be seen. While much of this damage is reversible, recurrences can occur or progressive renal failure may develop
- Central nervous system involvement may be evident. Irritability, seizures, abnormal posturing, hemiparesis, or hypertensive encephalopathy may develop. It is believed that the development of neurologic symptoms, particularly coma, is associated with a poor prognosis.
  Management is aimed at:
- Achieving and maintaining correct fluid and electrolyte balance
- Blood transfusions with caution, avoiding plasma rich products such as FFP
- Treatment of anuria or oliguric renal failure that may require peritoneal or haemodialysis
- Management of hypertension

- If the child has bloody diarrhoea and/or abdominal distension with decreased gut motility, it may be necessary to be nil by mouth with the provision of parenteral nutrition
- Recognition and treatment of any neurologic complications, which may be an indication for plasmapheresis
- Informing and supporting the child and family (adapted from Hazinski 1992)

HYPERTENSIVE CRISIS

A hypertensive crisis is defined as a sudden and abrupt elevation in BP (Chandar & Zilleruelo 2012). If the hypertension is associated with end-organ injury, such as encephalopathy, cardiac failure or renal failure, it requires urgent reduction of the BP by 25–30% over 6–8 hours. Hypertensive crisis can occur in patients with known hypertension or as a new presentation. A list of causes and associated signs can be found in Table 4.5. Initial treatment is usually via intravenous (IV) therapy, in order to titrate the dose carefully and avoid a precipitous drop in BP (list of management Table 4.6). If IV access cannot be obtained, oral treatment with nifedipine using very low doses can be started. However, this should be administered with extreme caution as a sudden drop in BP may cause significant myocardial strain.

Table 4.5 Causes and presentation of hypertensive emergencies

Age group	Aetiology	History	Physical examination
Newborn	Renal artery and venous thrombosis Autosomal recessive polycystic kidney disease Coarctation of the aorta Congenital nephrotic syndrome (diffuse mesangial sclerosis) Other renal parenchymal disease Renal artery stenosis Tumor Iatrogenic Mydriatics Theophylline overdose Caffeine overdose	Umbilical artery catheterisation Oligohydramnios Prolonged mechanical ventilation Family history of renal disease Medications	Pulse volume and BP in four extremities Signs of congestive heart failure Abdominal mass and bruit Ambiguous genitalia

Table 4.5	Causes and presentation of hypertensive emergencies—cont'd		
Age group	**Aetiology**	**History**	**Physical examination**
Infancy to 12 years	Renal parenchymal disease Polycystic kidney disease Renovascular disease Tumor Endocrine causes Coarctation of the aorta	Poor feeding Failure to gain weight History of UTI History of low birth weight Family history of renal disease Headache, palpitation, blurred vision Medications Accidental ingestion Excessive weight gain	Heart rate, BMI, pulse volume, and BP in four extremities Cardiovascular/pulmonary examination Abdominal mass and bruit Skin rash Peripheral oedema Retinal examination Ambiguous genitalia
Adolescence	Essential hypertension Metabolic syndrome Renal parenchymal disease Iatrogenic Anabolic steroids Substance abuse Decongestants Renovascular disease Coarctation of the aorta Endocrine causes	History of fever and/or joint pain History of UTI History of low birth weight Family history of hypertension and renal disease Medications Drug overdose Headache, palpitation, blurred vision	Heart rate, BMI, pulse volume, and BP in four extremities Cardiovascular pulmonary examination Thyroid examination Abdominal mass and bruit Skin rash Peripheral oedema Retinal examination

BMI, Body mass index; *BP,* blood pressure; *UTI,* urinary tract infection.
Chandar, J., Zilleruelo, G., 2012. Hypertensive crisis in children. Pediatr. Nephrol 27, 741–751.

RENAL TRANSPLANT

The major indications for renal transplant in infants are:
- Congenital abnormalities of the urinary tract
- Congenital nephrotic syndrome
- Neonatal cortical necrosis due to thrombosis
- Autosomal recessive polycystic kidney disease
  And in older children (Sharma et al 2013) are:
- Congenital anomalies
- Obstructive uropathies
- Focal segmental glomerulosclerosis

Living related donors (LRD) account for 74% of infant renal transplants and 50% of paediatric transplants. There are several advantages to LRD transplants, such as being able to plan the time of surgery, the donor age is often low (<35 years), and the cold-ischemia time is minimised, which improves graft survival. Early transplant is generally favoured in children with end-stage renal disease to improve growth, development and avoid the complications of dialysis, such as peritonitis and venous access problems.

Table 4.6 Drugs used in management of acute hypertensive emergencies

Drug used in therapy	Class	Route	Dose	Adverse effects
Hypertensive emergency				
Labetalol	α and β blocker	IV infusion bolus	0.25–1.5 mg/kg/h 0.2–1 mg/kg/dose Maximum 20 mg/dose	Use with caution in hyperkalemia and CHF
Esmolol	β blocker	IV	Bolus 100–500 μg over 1 min; 25–100 μg/kg/min; can increase to 500 μg/kg/min	Can cause CHF, bradycardia, and bronchospasm; contraindicated in cocaine toxicity
Phentolamine	α blocker	IV	0.1–0.2 mg/kg/dose	Orthostatic hypotension, tachycardia, gastrointestinal disturbances
Fenoldapam	Dopamine receptor agonist	IV	0.8–3 μg/kg/min	Tachycardia; increased intracranial pressure
Hydralazine	Vasodilator	IV	0.1–0.5 mg/kg/dose every 4–6 h	Tachycardia, flushing, lupus-like syndrome
Sodium nitroprusside	Vasodilator	IV	0.5–0.8 μg/kg/min	Thiocyanate toxicity with decreased renal function
Enalaprilat	ACE inhibitor	IV	0.005–0.01 mg/kg/day	Acute renal failure and hyperkalemia
Hypertensive urgency				
Furosemide	Diuretic	IV/PO	1–2 mg/kg/dose	Electrolyte disturbances
Isradipine	Ca++ channel blocker	PO	0.05–0.1 mg/kg/dose up to 5 mg/dose	Tachycardia; headache
Nifedipine	Ca++ channel blocker	Sub-lingual/PO	0.1–0.25 mg/kg/dose	Precipitous drop in blood pressure; tachycardia; headache
Clonidine	Central α agonist	PO	0.05–0.3 mg	Rebound hypertension; sedation
Minoxidil	Vasodilator	PO	0.1–2 mg/kg/dose	Pericardial effusion

ACE, Angiotensin-converting enzyme; *CHF*, congestive heart failure; *IV*, intravenous; *PO*, orally.
Chandar, J., Zilleruelo, G., 2012. Hypertensive crisis in children. Pediatr. Nephrol. 27, 741–751.

Paediatric transplantation may be intraperitoneal with a midline incision, and the donor renal vein and artery are anastomosed directly onto the recipient inferior vena cava and aorta, respectively. In this situation, the adult-sized kidney can occupy the entire right side of the abdomen leading to bowel dysfunction and ileus in the early postoperative period. The alternative is extraperitoneal placement with an incision above the groin; in this case the renal vessels are anastomosed onto the common iliac artery and vein. The available space for an adult-size kidney may also present problems and to avoid pressure and perfusion problems, the fascia may be left open for a few days after the initial operation (Jalanko et al 2016).

Following paediatric renal transplant, the important short-term issues that may need to be addressed in PICU are:

- Abundant fluid administration to ensure adequate renal blood flow. High cardiac output and volume overload may be required to adequately perfuse the adult graft. It may be necessary to maintain a central venous pressure (CVP) of 10 cm H_2O for good perfusion. A combination of fluid replacement and inotropes are necessary to achieve these targets in the early postoperative phase.
- Regular ultrasound scan to confirm good renal circulation and detect any fluid collections.
- Careful monitoring and electrolyte supplementation. Polyuria is common in the first few postoperative days; increased fluid replacement may be required to avoid dehydration. Regular weight and BP monitoring is necessary; some degree of fluid overload and hypertension (systolic >100 mm Hg) are tolerated and anticipated in the early phase. Hyerkalaemia (K 5–6 mmol/L) is common in the first few postoperative days and does not usually require treatment. However, low Na, Mg, and Ca should be supplemented. Oral magnesium, phosphate, and calcium supplements may be required for months after transplantation.
- Early detection and treatment of any infections. Antibiotic prophylaxis is usually continued while a urinary catheter is in situ. Co-trimoxazole for *Pneumocystis jirovecii* and ganciclovir for CMV are routinely used for 3–6 months. Serum monitoring (polymerase chain reaction [PCR]) for CMV, Epstein–Barr virus (EBV), and polyomaviruses is highly recommended. The management of EBV and polyomaviruses is complex as there is no specific therapy, and reduction of immunosuppression may be necessary to facilitate an appropriate host response.
- Needle biopsy may be necessary if any signs of rejection are detected.
- Monitoring of all immune suppression, the specific immune suppression regimen will be determined by local practice.

REFERENCES

Alkandari, O., Eddington, K.A., Hyder, A., Gauvin, F., Ducret, T., Gottesman, V., Zappitelli, M., 2011. Acute kidney injury is an independent risk factor for pediatric intensive care mortality, longer length of stay and prolonged mechanical ventilation in critically ill children: a two center retrospective cohort study. Crit. Care 15 (3), R146.

Brunner, L., Suddarth, D.S., 1991. The Lippincott Manual of Pediatric Nursing, fourth ed. Chapman & Hall, London.

Chadha, V., Warady, B., Blowey, D., et al., 2000. Tenckhoff catheters prove superior to Cook catheters in pediatric acute peritoneal dialysis. Am. J. Kidney. Dis. 35, 1111–1116.

Chandar, J., Zilleruelo, G., 2012. Hyertensive crisis in children. Pediatr. Nephrol. 27, 741–751.

Chiolero, A., Paradis, G., Lambert, M., 2010. Accuracy of oscillometric devices in children and adults. Blood Press 19 (4), 254–259.

Deep, A., Zoha, M., Kukreja, D., 2017. Prostacyclin as an anticoagulanat for continuous renal replacement therapy in children. Blood Purif. 43, 279–289.

Gupta, S., Sengar, G.H., Mehti, P.V., Beniwal, M., Kumawat, M., 2016. Acute kidney injury in pedaitric intensive care unit. Indian. J. Crit. Care Med. 20 (9), 526–529.

Hazinski, M.F. (Ed.), 1992. Nursing Care of the Critically Ill Child, second ed. C V Mosby, St Louis, Missouri.

Jalanko, H., Mattila, I., Holmberg, C., 2016. Renal transplantation in infants. Pediatr. Nephrol. 31, 725–735.

McCaffrey, J., Dhakal, A.K., Milford, D.V., Webb, N.J., Lennon, R., 2016. Recent development in the detection and management of acute kidney injury. Archi. Dis. Child. 0, 1–6.

Mehta, R., McDonald, B., Ward, D., 1991. Regional citrate anticoagulation for continuous arteriovenous hemodialysis: an update after 12 months. Contrib. Nephrol. 93, 210–214.

National High Blood Pressure Education Working Group on High Blood Pressure in Children & Adolescents, 2007. A pocket guide to blood pressure measurement in children. US Department of Health and Human Services, National Heart and Lung Institute Publication 07-5268, May 2007.

Nevard, C.F., Rigden, S.P., 1995. Haemofiltration in paediatric practice. Curr. Paediatr. 5, 14–16.

Sharma, A., Ramanthan, R., Posner, M., Fisher, R., 2013. Pediatric kidney transplantation: a review. Transpl. Res. Risk Manag. 5, 21–31.

Strazdins, V., Watson, A., Harvey, B., 2004. Renal replacement therapy for acute renal failure in children: European guidelines. Pediatr. Nephrol. 19, 199–207.

Wang, T., Lindholm, B., 2001. Peritoneal dialysis solutions. Perit. Dial. Int. 21 (3), S89–S95.

Warady, B.A., on behalf of the International Society of Peritoneal Dialysis Advisory Committee on Peritonitis Management in Pediatric Patients, 2000. Consensus guidelines for the treatment of peritonitis in pediatric patients receiving peritoneal dialysis. Perit. Dial. Int. 20, 610–624.

LIVER FUNCTION AND FAILURE

5

UNDERSTANDING LIVER FUNCTION

The liver is a vital organ, which plays an active role in many body functions. In order to be effective the liver uses up to one-quarter of the body's total metabolic demand, rendering the liver vulnerable to injury from low perfusion states (e.g., after cardiac surgery or during sepsis). The liver receives 75% of its blood supply from the portal vein and only 25% of the blood supply from the hepatic artery. The portal vein and hepatic artery converge in the liver and empty into sinusoids, which bathe the hepatocytes and then drain into a central vein leading to the hepatic vein. Due to this sinusoidal architecture of the liver, if it is injured the liver can be a source of massive bleeding, which can be difficult to control.

Key functions performed by the liver include:

- **Metabolism** The liver regulates the amount of glucose, protein, vitamins, minerals, and fat that are either stored or released into the bloodstream. The liver also plays a central role in the metabolism of most drugs and the excretion of waste products such as ammonia (from protein metabolism) and bilirubin (haemoglobin breakdown).
- **Production** Many plasma proteins, such as alpha and beta globulins, albumin, prothrombin, and fibrinogen are formed in the liver. Albumin is important as it serves as a vehicle for the transport of drugs, bilirubin and hormones, and it plays an important role maintaining oncotic equilibrium. Clotting factors (I, II, V, VII, IX and X) and anticoagulants (protein C, protein S, and antithrombin II) are also synthesised in the hepatocytes.
- **Detoxification and filtration** Kupffer cells make up approximately 10% of all cells in the liver. Their principal functions include phagocytes of particulate matter, detoxification of endotoxin, processing of antigens, and mediation of various immune responses. The liver is also responsible for the clearance of toxins and the drugs that are consumed.
- **Vascular storage** The liver is able to expand to increase the volume of blood and plasma stored in the sinusoids. In an adult, up to 600 mL of blood may be stored on the liver at any one stage. (Adapted from Siconolfi 1995)

The function of the liver can be assessed using a combination of tests:

- **Clinical findings**: Jaundice, easy bruising and bleeding, oedema, and a fluctuating level of consciousness may indicate impaired liver function.

Table 5.1   Liver function tests (adult American values have been replaced by commonly accepted British values)

Specific test	Normal range	Levels elevated because of:
Alanine transferase (ALT)	0–55 U/L	Hepatitis, hepatotoxic drugs, cholestasis
Alkaline phosphatase (ALP)	145–320 U/L	Biliary obstruction, primary liver tumour
Gamma glutamyl transferase (GGT)	8–78 U/L	Hepatitis, cirrhosis, cholestasis
Lactate dehydrogenase (LDH)	286–580 U/L	Myocardial infarction, haemolytic anaemia
Serum ammonia	<40 μmol/L	Urea cycle defects, hepatic encephalopathy, coma
Bilirubin – total	0–22 μmol/L	Hepatitis, jaundice, neonatal jaundice, obstruction of bile flow, infection
Prothrombin time (PT) or INR	0.8–1.1 s	Vitamin K deficiency, DIC, salicylate intoxication
Activated prothrombin time (APTT) Fibrinogen	0.8–1.2 s 2.02–4.24 g/L	Clotting factor deficiencies, DIC

DIC, Disseminated intravascular coagulation; *INR,* international normalised ratio.
Adapted and used with permission from Siconolfi, L.A., 1995. Clarifying the complexity of liver function tests. Nursing 25 (5), © Springhouse Corporation/www.springnet.com.

- **Biochemical tests**: Glucose, lactate, protein, albumin, C-reactive protein (CRP), and ammonia are all regulated by the liver and may be early indicators of impaired liver function. Raised liver enzymes particularly alanine transaminase (ALT) and aspartate aminotransferase (AST) indicate hepatocyte injury and necrosis. Coagulation tests (e.g., activated prothrombin time [APTT], international normalised ratio [INR], and fibrinogen) indicate the liver's ability to produce coagulation products.
- **Radiology**: The structure and blood flow of the liver and portal vein can be assessed with imaging studies such as ultrasound scans, computerised tomography (CT), and magnetic resonance imaging (MRI).
- **Histology**: Liver biopsy is the gold standard test to identify the cause of liver disease.

A summary of the test used to assess liver function can be found in Table 5.1.

THE JAUNDICED BABY

Hyperbilirubinemia

Jaundice is the discolouration of skin and sclera caused by abnormally high blood levels of the pigment bilirubin, which is a product of haemoglobin breakdown (Fig. 5.1). There are two types of bilirubin: unconjugated and conjugated.

Fig. 5.1 The normal metabolism of bilirubin. (With permission from McCance, K.L., Heuther, S., 1992. Pediatric gastrointestinal disorders. In: Hazinski, M.F. (Ed.), Nursing Care of the Critically Ill Child, second ed. CV Mosby, St Louis, MO.)

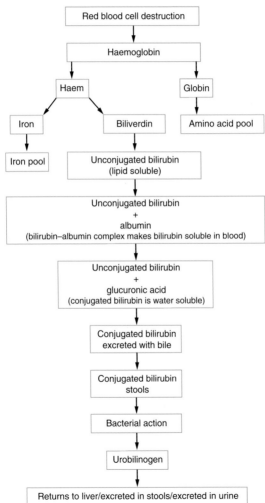

The National Collaborating Centre for Women's and Children's Health was commissioned by NICE (National Institute of Clinical Excellence) in the United Kingdom to create guidance for the management of neonatal jaundice. This guidance contains treatment charts on which the age/gestation of the infant is plotted, together with the weight and the unconjugated bilirubin level, in order to assess if phototherapy is indicated; this can be found on the NICE website (www.nice.org.uk/guidance/cg98).

Kernicterus is yellow (bilirubin) staining of the basal ganglia in the brain of neonates due to high levels of unconjugated bilirubin. The symptoms include lethargy, uncontrolled jerky movements, and hearing loss. A serum bilirubin level greater than 340 mmol/L in babies with a gestational age greater than 36 weeks or a rapidly rising bilirubin level (8.5 mmol/L/h) increases the risk of developing kernicterus. This is a serious condition with a mortality of up to 10% and 70% risk of long-term morbidity. A surge in the incidence of kernicterus has been associated with early postnatal discharge and a relaxation in the attitude to neonatal jaundice.

Phototherapy

Phototherapy is the use of blue/ultraviolet light on neonates, which causes bilirubin oxidation and destruction. The infant is kept unclothed to maximise the surface area exposed to the light; appropriate measures are required to prevent heat loss (e.g., covered incubator). Protective patches are placed over the infant's eyes. Insensible water loss is increased during phototherapy and the fluid allowance should be increased accordingly.

Unconjugated bilirubin

- Lipid soluble
- Toxic to the brain if high or rapidly rising level – kernicterus
- Responds to phototherapy
- High levels can be caused by:
  - Excessive turnover of blood cells, which is the rapid breakdown of red cells after birth releasing too much bilirubin for the immature liver to conjugate, a common cause of neonatal jaundice.
  - Abnormality in the liver preventing the conjugation of bilirubin (rare inherited conditions)

Conjugated bilirubin

- Water soluble
- Excreted in stool/urine/bile: pale stools and jaundice indicate a serious liver disorder, which must be urgently investigated
- High levels can be caused by:
  - Obstruction to flow of bile from liver; for example, biliary atresia

- Abnormally small and/or reduced number of bile ducts inside the liver
- Liver disease causing damage to liver cells; for example, infection, genetic disease

A 'split' bilirubin level test measures serum levels of unconjugated and conjugated bilirubin. Jaundice in any baby aged 14+ days or conjugated jaundice must always be investigated.

BILIARY ATRESIA

Biliary atresia is the most common cause of conjugated hyperbilirubinemia in infants. Biliary atresia is due to narrowed, obstructed, or absent bile ducts which can be at the level of the common bile duct, common hepatic duct, or most commonly at the proximal bile ducts (Fig. 5.2). A variety of potential causative factors have been investigated including genetic, autoimmune, and viral infections but no unifying cause has been identified. Patients usually present with jaundice in the first 6 weeks of life. The diagnosis is made with a combination of blood tests and diagnostic imaging, such as an ultrasound scan. Early surgery is necessary to prevent the progression towards cirrhosis and ultimately liver failure. A hepatoportoenterostomy, also known as a Kasai operation, was first described by Kasai in 1959; it involves the drainage of bile from the portal system into the jejunum using a loop of bowel (40–50 cm Roux limb). The Kasai operation facilitates improvement in jaundice in 47–65% of cases. An appropriate fall in the serum bilirubin within 3 months is a good indicator of potential recovery (Zagory et al 2015). However, despite surgery, many patients with biliary atresia will still ultimately progress to chronic liver failure and portal hypertension, and will require a liver transplant.

ACUTE LIVER FAILURE

Acute liver failure is a multisystem disease with a fluctuating course: encephalopathy and raised intracranial pressure indicate life-threatening disease (D'Agostino 2012). In the absence of encephalopathy, the severity of liver impairment is best assessed by the severity of coagulopathy (Bhaduri & Miele-Vergani 1996, p 349).

There are a wide variety of causes of liver failure in children that can be categorised in an age-dependent manner. In neonates and infants, metabolic disorders and infective agents are the most common causes identified. In children older than 1 year of age, aetiologies are similar to adults; however, a large proportion are cases where the cause remains unknown (Cochran & Losek 2007).

Aetiology

Under 1 year of age:
- Inherited/metabolic; for example, galactosaemia, urea cycle disorder, neonatal hemochromatosis (Cochran & Losek 2007)

Fig. 5.2 Images of the Kasai classification of biliary atresia demonstrating the various levels of bile duct obstruction or narrowing. *CBD,* Common bile duct.

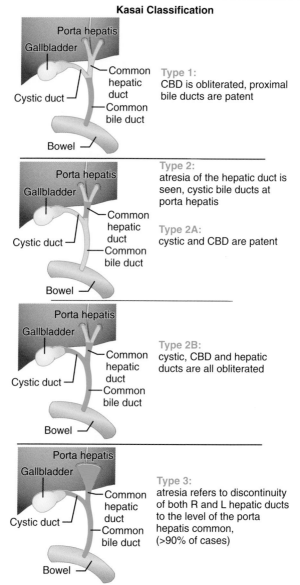

Kasai Classification

Type 1:
CBD is obliterated, proximal bile ducts are patent

Type 2:
atresia of the hepatic duct is seen, cystic bile ducts at porta hepatis

Type 2A:
cystic and CBD are patent

Type 2B:
cystic, CBD and hepatic ducts are all obliterated

Type 3:
atresia refers to discontinuity of both R and L hepatic ducts to the level of the porta hepatis common, (>90% of cases)

Table 5.2	Classification of acute liver failure			
	Interval of jaundice to encephalopathy	Cerebral oedema	Prognosis	Leading cause
Hyperacute	7 days	Common	Moderate	Virus A, B paracetamol
Acute	8–28 days	Common	Poor	Non-A/B/C; drugs
Subacute	29 days–12 weeks	Poor	Poor	Non-A/B/C; drugs

Adapted from O'Grady, J., Schalm, S., Williams, R., 1993. Acute liver failure: redefining the syndromes. Lancet 342, 275.

- Infective; for example, cytomegalovirus, Epstein–Barr virus (EBV), adenovirus, hepatitis A and B (Braccio et al 2017)

Older children:

- Infective (viral hepatitis A, B, non-A, non-B) and other infections (e.g., malaria)
- Autoimmune diseases
- Infiltrative (e.g., leukaemia)
- Toxic or drug related (e.g., paracetamol, cytotoxic drugs). Ischaemic, for example, due to sepsis/shock (Mowat 1994)

In the paediatric intensive care unit (PICU) liver failure may more commonly result as part of multiorgan failure. It is important to note that the clinical presentation of liver failure can be missed, especially if jaundice is not present, and it should be considered in patients with a fluctuating level of consciousness or deranged coagulation tests.

Prognosis

Subgroups of hyperacute, acute, and subacute liver failure reflect the different clinical patterns of the illness, aetiology, and prognosis (Table 5.2). These universal classifications originate from O'Grady et al (1993) based on a retrospective analysis of 539 cases.

In children, encephalopathy is an uncommon and ominous sign. The presentation of a child with an INR above 4 at any time is associated with a high mortality rate and is currently the criterion used for emergency transplant listing, although each case is assessed individually. No specific diagnosis is possible before orthotopic liver transplantation in 40–50% of cases, which should not delay the procedure. Neonates with a coagulopathy have a particularly bad prognosis (Lee 1993; Baker et al 1998; Riordan & Williams 1999).

In the event that liver failure is not part of overall multiorgan failure, extensive laboratory investigations may be necessary to find the cause and to determine whether any specific treatment is indicated. Several types of extracorporeal liver support systems (ELSS) can be divided into artificial liver support (ALS) and bioartificial liver support (Jain & Dhawan 2017). Most of the research in ELSS is adult focused with very little evidence from paediatric studies. ALS is most commonly in the form of albumin dialysis devices, such as MARS (molecular absorbent recirculating system, Baxter) or Prometheus (Fractionated Plasma Separation and Adsorption system, Baxter). Transplantation is the only life-saving procedure, and centres that perform this surgery have certain criteria for assessing whether or not it is indicated. Transfer to specialist centres should therefore be arranged in this instance, together with the incorporation of their recommendations for the management of the child prior to and during transfer (De Jaeger & Lacroix 1997).

Goals of management

In the PICU setting the first aim is to restore the intravascular volume and support systemic perfusion to prevent further injury to the liver and other organ systems (Bernal & Wendon 2013).

Management includes the following considerations:

- Endotracheal intubation and ventilation for airway protection and to ensure oxygen and carbon dioxide levels are well controlled
- Appropriate cardiovascular support to ensure adequate systemic circulation by restoring circulating volume and using vasopressors, such as noradrenaline
- Intravenous (IV) glucose (25–50% infusions may be necessary) to prevent hypoglycaemia, which may be profound in liver failure. Maintenance fluids should not be stopped in liver failure
- Only treat coagulation defects if the patient is bleeding or invasive procedures are planned. Recombinant factor VII can be used to correct refractory coagulopathy and facilitate invasive procedures, such as a liver biopsy, and it is favoured due to the low volume required. Naturally occurring factor VII has the shortest half-life of all the vitamin–K-dependent clotting factors and is therefore the first to be depleted in liver failure (Chuansumrit et al 2001).
- Haemodialysis or haemodiafiltration is often necessary to support renal function and reduce ammonia levels
- Infection is a major cause of morbidity and mortality in liver failure. Children with liver failure may not show the typical signs of infection such as fever, raised CRP, or white cell count due to their altered immune status. Careful monitoring for signs of infection (regular blood cultures) and a low threshold for prescribing antibiotics and antifungal treatment is necessary

Encephalopathy

Encephalopathy and cerebral oedema are important and life-threatening complications of liver failure. The severity of the encephalopathy can be graded 1–4 (Table 5.3); children with grade 3 and 4 encephalopathy are likely to require liver transplantation. The cause of the encephalopathy in liver failure is not clear; however, a wide range of neurotoxic substances including ammonia accumulate in the circulation in liver failure and play a central role. There is a close relationship between sustained levels of ammonia (150–200 mmol/L) and the development of encephalopathy with the risk of raised intracranial pressure. Ammonia

Table 5.3	Hepatic encephalopathy grading
Grade 0	Clinically normal mental status but minimal changes in memory concentration, intellectual function, and coordination
Grade 1	Mild confusion/anxiety, disturbed or reversal of sleep rhythm, shortened attention span, slowing of ability to perform mental tasks (simple addition or subtraction). In young children, irritability, altered sleep pattern, unexplained bursts of excessive crying
Grade 2	Drowsiness, confusion, mood swings with personality changes, inappropriate behaviour, intermittent disorientation of time and place, gross deficit in ability to perform mental tasks. In young children, excessive sleepiness, inability to interact with or recognise parents, lack of interest in favourite toys and activities
Grade 3	Pronounced confusion, delirious but arousable, persistent disorientation of time and place, hyperreflexia with a positive Babinskis sign
Grade 4	Comatose with or without decerebrate or decorticate posturing, response to pain present (IVa) or no response to pain (IVb)

is cerebrally metabolised to intracellular glutamine, which affects neurotransmitter release and mitochondrial function causing altered cerebral function and brain swelling (Desjardins et al 2012). In patients with established encephalopathy the risk of cerebral oedema can be reduced with osmotherapy (hypertonic saline), plus limiting cerebral metabolism through sedation and avoiding hyperthermia.

PORTAL HYPERTENSION

Portal hypertension is the presence of increased pressure in the hepatic portal system, which drains blood from the intestines, stomach, and pancreas to the liver. This can be detected by Doppler ultrasound scan to assess flow in the portal and hepatic vessels as well as the liver architecture. Usually the pressure in this system is very low (<5 mm Hg). Increased resistance can be due to a problem at the prehepatic, intrahepatic, or posthepatic level (Table 5.4). Prehepatic portal hypertension can be caused by extrahepatic portal vein obstruction (EHPVO) due to umbilical catheters and severe dehydration; however, in up to 50% of cases no clear cause is identified. EHPVO can be treated by creating a shunt between the splanchnic vein (draining the intestines) and the portal vein at the recessus of Rex, known as a meso-Rex bypass. In other forms of portal hypertension, the only successful long-term treatment is a liver transplant.

The signs of portal hypertension include ascites, splenomegaly, and varices of the oesophagus, anterior abdominal wall, and anorectal region. The diagnosis can be confirmed by ultrasound, CT scan, or MRI demonstrating an enlarged portal vein.

Ascites

Ascites is excessive accumulation of fluid in the peritoneal space. Large volumes are obvious but even a small volume can be detected by

Table 5.4	Causes of portal hypertension in children
Prehepatic	Extrahepatic portal vein obstruction (EPVO)
	Congenital stenosis of the portal vein
	Extrinsic compression of the portal vein
	Arterioportal fistulae
Intrahepatic	Cirrhosis
	Biliary atresia
	Hepatoportal sclerosis
	Granulomatous disease (e.g., tuberculosis)
Posthepatic	Hepatic vein thrombosis (Budd Chiari syndrome)
	Congenital malformation or thrombosis of the inferior vena cava (IVC)
	Constrictive pericarditis

Grimaldi, C., de Ville de Goyet, J., Nobili, V., 2012. Portal hypertension in children. Clin. Res. Hepatol. Gastroenetrol. 36, 260–261.

ultrasound scan. Fluid enters the peritoneal space due to a combination of high levels of circulating antidiuretic hormone and low serum albumin causing leakage from the splanchnic capillaries and liver sinusoids in patients with cirrhosis and portal hypertension. Needle aspiration is recommended if there is any concern about infection (peritonitis). Spontaneous bacterial peritonitis can aggravate encephalopathy and cause pyrexia and abdominal pain. A third-generation cephalosporin (e.g., cefotaxime) is a good starting agent for treatment until a particular organism is identified. Spironolactone and frusemide should be used in combination to reduce the fluid overload state. There is evidence from a meta-analysis of four randomised controlled trials that albumin infusions reduce mortality and the incidence of renal failure in these patients (Salerno et al 2013).

Variceal haemorrhage

Portal hypertension may be clinically silent, and present suddenly, with hematemesis or a large gastric bleed, due to oesophageal and gastric varices (Bloom et al 2015). In adults, treatment with propranolol may reduce bleeding from the varices, but there is not enough evidence to recommend this treatment in children. Aspirin and nonsteroidals should be avoided as they increase the risk of bleeding from gastric varices. There is a high incidence of variceal haemorrhage in children with biliary atresia, even after a portoenterostomy (Kasai) procedure.

- Almost half of the acute variceal bleeds will stop spontaneously, which is probably due to hypovolaemia and splanchnic vasoconstriction.
- Blood transfusion should be cautious, aiming for a haemoglobin of 80 g/L to avoid aggravating the bleeding.
- Targeting a platelet count of 70×10^9/L also reduces bleeding.
- Trying to correct the INR with clotting products such as fresh frozen plasma (FFP) can be challenging as the volume required may increase

- the portal pressure and cause rebleeding; therefore do not aim to fully correct INR but treat empirically to limit ongoing bleeding.
- Antibiotics have been shown to reduce the rate of rebleeding and improve survival.
- Urgent endoscopy (<15 hours) is strongly associated with a better outcome (Hsu et al 2009). If the bleeding is controlled the patient should be admitted to the intensive care unit for careful observation and complete a 5-day course of antibiotics.
- Should rebleeding occur, endoscopy may be repeated but these patients often require a surgical shunt.
- If the bleeding cannot be controlled by endoscopy, a Sengstaken-Blakemore tube may be used to stabilise the patient.

SENGSTAKEN-BLAKEMORE TUBE

A Sengstaken-Blakemore tube is a rubber tube that has two inflatable balloons at the lower end, one of which when inflated exerts direct pressure on the oesophagus while the other maintains the position of the tube. Correctly positioned in the oesophagus, this tube can stop the bleeding of varices by applying direct pressure of the inflated balloon on the submucosa. This technique is only usually undertaken by a senior member of the surgical/intensivist medical team under IV sedation. A Sengstaken-Blakemore tube should not be left in place for longer than 24 hours as this may begin to cause local pressure injuries.

LIVER TRANSPLANT

Paediatric transplants account for about 10% of all liver transplant cases. Indications for liver transplant include chronic liver failure, acute liver failure, primary hepatic malignancy, and inborn errors of metabolism (Bramhall et al 2001). Improved understanding of both donor and recipient factors has led to increasing survival posttransplant, which is reported as greater than 85% 5-year survival (Nacoti et al 2016). Paediatric liver transplant is usually only performed in highly specialised centres. Each centre will provide specific local guidelines for immediate and long-term postoperative management. Patients should be referred to transplant centres when major complications, such as cirrhosis, variceal haemorrhages, and encephalopathy or hepatorenal syndrome (HRS), occur to ensure early assessment for liver transplant and appropriate treatment is commenced (EASL guidelines 2016).

One of the biggest challenges regarding paediatric liver transplant was the availability of suitable size-matched donors. However, surgical advances – such as reduced size liver transplant, split-liver transplant in which a whole deceased donor liver is partitioned into two separate grafts creating a left lateral segment for a paediatric recipient and extended right lobe graft for an adult recipient, and finally living donor transplant, which involves transplanting a segment of living-donor adult liver into a child (Emre et al 2012) – have improved the availability of grafts for children.

Postoperative care

- Patients usually require postoperative ventilation.
- Gradual reintroduction of oral feeding occurs.
- Prophylactic antimicrobial treatment should include antibiotics, antifungal, and antiviral agents.
- Immunosuppression involves mainly calcineurin inhibitors (tacrolimus or cyclosporine) and corticosteroids to suppress T cells. The highest risk period for rejection is within the first 3 months posttransplant.
  - Intensive induction prevents acute rejection, specific therapies (e.g., thymoglobulin), which are only used for the first month after transplant.
  - Maintenance immunosuppression may include mycophenolate mofetil (MMF), which can be combined with tacrolimus to suppress T and B cells and to improve graft survival and reduced nephrotoxicity. Sirolimus may be introduced later, after wound healing is complete and the risk of thrombosis is reduced, to allow dose reduction of tacrolimus or cyclosporine in order to improve renal function.
  - The long-term aim of immunosuppression is to sustain a graft with the lowest level of treatment in order to limit the side effects. This phase focuses on the reduction of treatment – especially the high-dose steroids.

Complications posttransplant

- Hepatic artery thrombosis is the primary cause of early graft failure and retransplantation within 30 days of surgery, and can occur despite prolongation of standard coagulation test (Nacoti et al 2016). Clinical signs include acute liver failure, increasing bilirubin, and altered mental state. Patients should be urgently evaluated by ultrasound with Doppler imaging and spiral CT to assess arterial flow. Surgical revascularisation, biliary interventional radiology, or retransplantation may be necessary to ensure survival (Kling et al 2004).
- Bile leaks and anastomosis strictures are a common postoperative problem. They can be diagnosed with ultrasound, MRI, percutaneous transhepatic cholangiography, or endoscopic retrograde cholangiography (ERCP). Early leaks often require surgical reintervention. Strictures may be managed nonoperatively with stent placement or tube drainage.
- Infections: bacterial infections are the most common problem in the early postoperative phase. In the following 2 weeks, fungal infections predominate. After 6 weeks patients are at increased risk of viral infections.
- Lymphoproliferative disorders: long-term immunosuppression increases the risk of cancers. Posttransplant lymphoproliferative disorder (PTLD) affects 2–6% of posttransplant patients. This risk is highest during the first 2 years and has been attributed to EBV. Treatment generally focuses on reducing the level of immunosuppression. Rituximab (monoclonal antibody against CD20) may also play a role.

- Psychosocial: specific risk factors may lead to poor compliance with immunosuppression increasing the risk of graft rejection. Therefore a formal psychosocial assessment of patient and their family is necessary to evaluate their ability to comply with the regimen prior to listing the patient for a transplant.

HEPATORENAL SYNDROME (HRS)

Paediatric patients with cirrhosis and other causes of chronic liver failure occasionally develop acute renal failure (HRS I) or a gradual decline in renal function (HRS II) despite a normal appearance of the kidneys. HRS is characterised by oliguria, low urinary sodium (<20 mmol), and hyponatremia (Wadei et al 2006). In most cases the renal failure resolves following liver transplantation; however, the early mortality in this group of patients is high. HRS is due to renal vasoconstriction, which is unresponsive to fluid resuscitation. Haemodialysis is required to support patients while awaiting a liver transplant.

HEPATOPULMONARY SYNDROME

Hepatopulmonary syndrome is characterised by cyanosis, liver failure, and dilatation of pulmonary vessels. Children with this condition are more breathless sitting up and may have clubbed fingers or toes. This is a rare complication of liver disease and portal hypertension due to small arteriovenous connections inside the lung attributed to high circulating levels of vasodilators such as nitric oxide and endothelin-1. The only definitive treatment is liver transplant. Even with liver transplantation, the 5-year survival in this group is lower than patients without this condition. Portopulmonary syndrome is pulmonary hypertension that develops in patients with portal hypertension without any other identified cause. These patients respond to traditional treatment for pulmonary hypertension but are only cured by a liver transplant.

REFERENCES

Baker, A., Dhawan, A., Heaton, N., 1998. Who needs a liver transplant? (New disease specifications). Arch. Dis. Child. 79, 460–464.

Bernal, A., Wendon, J., 2013. Acute liver failure. Engl. J. Med. 369, 2525–2534.

Bhaduri, B.R., Miele-Vergani, G., 1996. Fulminant hepatic failure: pediatric aspects. Semin. Liver Dis. 16, 349–355.

Bloom, S., Kemp, W., Lubel, J., 2015. Portal hypertension: pathophysiology, diagnosis and management. Int. Med. J. 45, 16–26.

Braccio, S., Irwin, A., Riordan, A., et al., 2017. Acute infectious hepatatitis in hospitalized children: a British Paedaitric Surveillance Study. Arch. Dis. Child. 102, 624–628.

Bramhall, S.R., Minford, E., Gunson, B., et al., 2001. Liver transplantation in the UK. World J. Gastroenterol. 75 (5), 602–611.

Chuansumrit, A., Treepongjaruna, S., Phuapradit, P., 2001. Combined fresh frozen plasma with recombinant factor VIIa in restoring haemostasis for invasive procedures in children with liver diseases. Thromb. Haemost. 85, 748–749.

Cochran, J., Losek, J., 2007. Acute liver failure in children. Pediatr. Emerg. Care 23 (2), 129–135.

D'Agostino, D., Diaz, S., Sanchez, M.C., et al., 2012. Management and prognosis of liver failure in children. Curr. Gastroenterol. Reports 14, 262–269.

De Jaeger, A., Lacroix, J., 1997. Hepatic failure. In: Singh, N.C. (Ed.), Manual of Pediatric critical care. WB Saunders, Philadelphia, PA.

Desjardins, P., Du, T., Jiang, W., et al., 2012. Pathogenesis of hepatic encephalopathy and brain edema in acute liver failure: role of glutamine refined. Neurochem. Int. 60, 690–696.

Emre, S., Umman, V., Cimsit, B., et al., 2012. Current concepts in pedaitric liver transplantation. Mt. Sinai J. Med. 79, 199–213.

European Association for the Study of the Liver (EASL), 2016. Practice guidelines for liver transplantation. J. Hepatol. 64 (2), 433–485.

Hsu, Y.C., Chung, C.S., Tseng, C.H., et al., 2009. Delayed endoscopy as a risk factor for in-hospital mortality in cirrhotic patients with acute variceal haemorrhage. J. Gastroenterol. Hepatol. 24, 1294–1299.

Jain, V., Dhawan, A., 2017. Extracorporeal liver support systems in pedaitric liver failure. J. Pediatr. Gastroenterol. Nutr. 64 (6), 855–863.

Kling, K., Lau, H., Colombani, P., 2004. Biliary complications of living related paediatric liver transplant patients. Pediatr. Transplan. 8 (2), 178–184.

Lee, W., 1993. Acute liver failure. N. Engl. J. Med. 329, 1862–1870.

Mowat, A.P., 1994. Liver Disorders in Childhood, third ed. Butterworth Heinemann, Oxford.

Nacoti, M., Corbella, D., Fazzi, F., et al., 2016. Coagulopathy and transfusion therapy in pediatric liver transplantation. World Gastroenterol. 22 (6), 2005–2023.

O'Grady, J., Schalm, S., Williams, R., 1993. Acute liver failure: redefining the syndromes. Lancet 342, 275.

Riordan, S.M., Williams, R., 1999. Cause and prognosis in acute liver failure. Liver Transplan. Surg. 5, 86–89.

Salerno, F., Navickis, R.J., Wilkes, M.M., 2013. Albumin infusion improves outcomes of patients with spontaneous bacterial peritonitis: a meta-analysis of randomised control trials. Clin. Gastroenetrol. Hepatol. 11, 123–130.

Siconolfi, L.A., 1995. Clarifying the complexity of liver function tests. Nursing 25 (5).

Wadei, H.M., Mai, M.L., Ahsan, N., et al., 2006. Hepatorenal syndrome: pathophysiology and management. Clin. J. Am. Soc. Nehrol. 1, 1066–1079.

Zagory, J.A., Nguyen, M.V., Wang, K.S., 2015. Recent advances in pathogenesis and management of biliary atresia. Curr. Opin. Pediatr. 27, 389–394.

USEFUL WEBSITES

www.bspghan.org.uk.
www.aasld.org.
www.vivo.colostate.edu useful information about anatomy and physiology
of the liver.
www.nice.org.uk/guidance/cg98.

NEUROLOGY – ASSESSMENT AND MANAGEMENT

6

In the paediatric intensive care unit (PICU) environment, health professionals are likely to encounter a variety of causes of neurologic deficit, requiring careful assessment and management.

GUIDELINES FOR NEUROLOGIC ASSESSMENT

A variety of neurologic assessment tools are suitable for use in children. Many are derivatives of the Glasgow Coma Scale (GCS) (Teasdale & Jennett 1974) or the Adelaide Scale (Simpson & Reilly 1982). The need for the tool to be age-appropriate (i.e., for the neurologic immaturity of the child to be taken into consideration) has been recognised to improve the accuracy and validity of the assessment.

An example of an age-appropriate GCS chart is illustrated in Fig. 6.1.

- The chart should be used as part of an overall assessment, including vital signs, assessment of the fontanelle, if appropriate, and the child's reaction to his/her surroundings and, in particular, to family/caregivers.
- Care must be taken to ensure that the pain application, where required, is appropriate and applied for a sufficient length of time to allow the best response to be elicited – until the patient responds, or a minimum of 15 and a maximum of 30 seconds is recommended (Lower 2002).
- The effects of drugs that are being administered or have been administered must be acknowledged.
- Continuity of interpretation of neurologic observations is improved if, during handover between shifts, a joint neurologic assessment is executed (e.g., agreement on pupil size).
- A careful explanation of all procedures to be used during a neurologic assessment must be given to relatives/visitors to minimise distress.

COMPONENTS OF THE GLASGOW COMA SCALE

Eye opening

The ability to obey commands is dependent upon the age and compliance of the child.

Fig. 6.1 Example of neurologic assessment charts: Glasgow Coma Scale and Children's Glasgow Coma Scale (under 5 years).

Glasgow Coma Scale (4–15 years)		Child's Glasgow Coma Scale (<4 years)	
Response	Score	Response	Score
Eye opening		**Eye opening**	
Spontaneously	4	Spontaneously	4
To verbal stimuli	3	To verbal stimuli	3
To pain	2	To pain	2
No resoponse to pain	1	No response to pain	1
Best motor response		**Best motor response**	
Obeys verbal command	6	Spontaneous or obeys verbal command	6
Localises to pain	5	Localises to pain or withdraws to touch	5
Withdraws from pain	4	Withdraws from pain	4
Abnormal flexion to pain (decorticate)	3	Abnormal flexion to pain (decorticate)	3
Abnormal extension to pain (decerebrate)	2	Abnormal extension to pain (decerebrate)	2
No response to pain	1	No response to pain	1
Best verbal response		**Best verbal response**	
Orientated and converses	5	Alert, babbbles, coos, words to usual ability	5
Disorientated and converses	4	Less than usual words spontaneous irritable cry	4
Inappropriate words	3	Cries only to pain	3
Incomprehensible sounds	2	Moans to pain	2
No response to pain	1	No response to pain	1

If the child does not open her eyes spontaneously, assess her response to speech by calling her name, first quietly and then loudly if there is no initial response. If the child is of preschool age and above, ask her to open her eyes. To elicit the best response, ask the child's parents, if present, to call her name. If there is no response, use a graded sequence of stimulation as recommended by Lower (2002) – shout, shake, pain. The interpretation of 'shake' is intended as a rousing stimulus rather than an actual physical shaking action, prior to the application of a pain stimulus (details below under motor response) to a child who may simply be drowsy.

To assess pupils, unless the eyes are open, open both carefully and assess the size of the pupils together; it is easier to see differences when both are viewed simultaneously. The use of a pupil size chart beside the child's face can promote accurate measurement of pupil size. Also consider the lighting in the child's bed space; if it is either very bright or dimmed, this could affect the pupil size when assessed. Interpretation can also differ between assessing individuals.

Each pupil's response to light is recorded appropriately with a + or − sign, and an H for hippus response, which occurs when the pupil constricts then dilates to light. Note whether the pupils respond briskly or sluggishly. If in doubt, get a colleague to check.

Eyes that are closed by swelling can be indicated by C; if the chart you are using does not specify the above, you could formulate a 'key' for clarification. Note also the position of the pupils (e.g., they may be divergent, or 'sunsetting' in appearance). Pupils resemble a setting sun because of downward deviation caused by pressure on cranial nerve III, the oculomotor nerve. This is a concerning sign indicating increasing intracranial pressure (ICP).

Verbal response

Charts will vary in the age-appropriateness of this category. In the charts shown, while 'orientated and converses' indicates the best response from the 5-year-old, 'babbles, coos, words to usual ability' is the best response from babies and children under this age. 'Cries to pain' is an appropriate response in the youngest infants (0–6 months). Again, involve the parents where possible and take into consideration the child's own stage of development. Has the child reached developmental milestones or are there known delays/deficits? The inability to produce a verbal response because of an endotracheal or tracheostomy tube is documented as T.

Motor response

If the child obeys commands (e.g., by squeezing your fingers or wriggling his toes when asked) he also may be able to lift his hands and feet off the bed, or push against you with them. This enables you to assess any differences in strength/weakness between the child's left and right sides. Ensure that the *best* motor response is charted, as well as differences; involve the parents where possible.

Painful stimuli should be central to avoid eliciting a spinal or reflex response. This approach may include:

- Pressing the superior orbital ridge
- Sternal rub
- Trapezius squeeze (children aged 5 years and above only, because there is insufficient development of muscle before this age).

 Consider other injuries/surgical procedures, for example:
- Avoid orbital ridge if facial injuries are present
- Avoid sternal rub if the patient has chest injuries or a recent sternotomy

As stated, administer for a sufficient time to allow the best response to be elicited: until the patient responds, or a minimum of 15 and maximum of 30 seconds (Lower 2002).

The application of a peripheral pain stimulus is appropriate on certain occasions; for example, when all limbs except one respond to central pain stimulus and it is necessary to test whether that limb is capable of moving. Press a pencil against a nail bed for the time as stated previously and monitor the reaction (Lower 2002).

A child aged 6–24 months is deemed capable of localising pain, but from 0 to 6 months the maximum response is flexion to pain. In contrast to appropriate flexion there is also abnormal posturing:

- Decorticate posturing: abnormal flexion of limbs to centre of body and rigid extension of legs
- Decerebrate posturing: rigid extension of all four limbs.

Also, consider cough and gag reflexes (endotracheal tube and using a Yankauer suction tip at the back of the throat, respectively, could be used to test these).

- Posturing: Does the child appear to move normally or abnormally?
- Motor responses: Any change is likely to be on the opposite side of the problem
- Pupillary responses: Changes usually occur on the same side as the lesion; for example, if a brain tumour is on the left side, the pupil changes will be on the left and the motor changes will be on the right.

Pupil constriction can be caused by drugs (e.g., fentanyl or morphine). Bilaterally dilated pupils may indicate hypoxia or be due to drugs (e.g., atropine).

A suddenly dilated pupil, or unequal pupils, is a warning sign of serious problems.

The hippus response is where the pupils cannot sustain the constriction to light and redilate. Hippus response may be normal if pupils are observed under high magnification, but it is also observed at the beginning of pressure on cranial nerve III and can be associated with early transtentorial herniation.

A suddenly dilated pupil (which if fixed can be referred to as a child 'blowing' a pupil), or unequal pupils should serve as a serious warning sign, requiring immediate medical assessment and probably a computed tomography (CT) scan. See Table 6.1 for a summary of pupil changes.

THE CRANIAL NERVES

Many rhymes have been devised to help remember the cranial nerves. Here is an example (Table 6.2):

On	Finn
Old	And (acoustic – vestibulocochlear)
Olympus'	German
Towering	Viewed
Top	Some
A	Hops

Table 6.1 Summary of pupil changes

Pupil size and reactivity	Cause
Small reactive pupils	Metabolic disorders
	Medullary lesion
Pin-point pupils	Metabolic disorders
	Narcotic/organophosphate ingestion*
Fixed mid-sized pupils	Midbrain lesion
Fixed dilated pupils	Hypothermia
	Severe hypoxia
	Barbiturates (late sign)
	During and post-seizure
	Anticholinergic drugs
Unilateral dilated pupil	Rapidly expanding ipsilateral lesion
	Tentorial herniation
	Third nerve lesion
	Epileptic seizures

*Pupil constriction can also be caused by prescribed drugs, e.g., morphine/fentanyl, in addition to ingestion.
Source: with permission from Advanced Life Support Group, 2005. Advanced Paediatric Life Support: A Practical Approach, fourth ed. BMJ Publications, London.

Table 6.2 The cranial nerves

Cranial nerve	Function	Assessment
I Olfactory	Smell	Difficult to assess accurately in small children
II Optic	Vision	Assess ability to see objects near and far, object moving into visual field from periphery and identifying colours
III Oculomotor	Pupil constriction, movement of eye and eyelid	Pupils should constrict when light is applied to each; consensual constriction (constriction in response to light directed to other eye) should be observed; eye should follow moving object; eyelids should raise equally when eyes are open. Ptosis (drooping eyelid) and lateral downward deviation of eye with pupil dilatation + decreased response to light = oculomotor injury
IV Trochlear	Movement of eye (superior oblique muscle)	Assess ability of eyes to track object down through visual field; damage stops eyes moving downwards + medially. Diplopia (blurred or double vision) may be present
V Trigeminal	Sensation to most of face + movement of jaw	Cover eyes; sharp/soft to skin + assess sensation. Check clench + move jaw + chew

Continued

Table 6.2   The cranial nerves—cont'd

Cranial nerve	Function	Assessment
VI Abducens	Lateral movement of eye	Assess eye movement in socket tracking object; when object close to child, both eyes should track it + move together. Child may turn head towards weakened muscle to prevent diplopia
VII Facial	Motor innervation of face, sensation to anterior tongue + tears	Ask child to make faces (demonstrate) + assess symmetry of face. Tears should be produced when crying. Drops of sugar/salt on tongue; test taste
VIII Vestibulo-cochlear (hearing)	Hearing + equilibrium	Clap hands; startle reflex in infants; blink reflex to sudden sound. NB: Cranial nerves III and IV must be intact for normal response to following: *'Dolls eyes' manoeuvre (oculocephalic reflex):* As child's head is turned, eyes should shift in sockets in direction **opposite** to head rotation; this constitutes the normal response *Cold water calorics (oculovestibular reflex):* Normally, instillation of cold water into ear should produce lateral nystagmus (rapid involuntary movement of the eyes, up and down/side to side/rotating); not to be performed if child is conscious These tests are typically performed as part of brain stem testing
IX Glossopharyn-geal	Motor fibres to throat + voluntary muscles of swallowing + speech	Evaluate swallow, cough + gag (tests IX + X together). If possible assess clarity of speech
X Vagus	Sensory + motor impulses for pharynx	Test as above, particularly cough + gag
XI Spinal accessory	Major innervation of sternocleido-mastoid + upper trapezius	Ask child to shrug shoulders and assess contraction of trapezius muscles; child to turn head as sternocleidomastoid muscle is palpated (long muscle in neck serves to rotate head + flex neck)
XII Hypoglossal	Innervation of the tongue	Ask child to stick out tongue. Squeeze nose of infant, mouth should open + tip of tongue should rise in mouth

Source: adapted from McCance, K.L., Heuther, S. 1992. Neurologic disorders. In: Hazinski, M.F. (Ed.), Nursing Care of the Critically Ill Child, second ed. CV Mosby, St Louis, MO.

COMA IN CHILDREN

What is a coma?

This is a state where the patient is unresponsive and cannot be roused or woken by stimulation for a period of greater than 1 hour (Kirkham & Ashwal 2013).

What causes coma in childhood?

- Hypoxic–ischaemic brain injury following respiratory or circulatory failure
- Epileptic seizures
- Trauma
  - Intracranial haemorrhage, cerebral oedema
- Infections
  - Meningitis, encephalitis
- Poisoning
- Metabolic
  - Renal/hepatic failure, Reye syndrome, hypoglycaemia, ketoacidosis, hypothermia, hypercapnia
- Vascular lesions
  - Bleeding, arteriovenous malformations, arterial or venous thrombosis (adapted from Advanced Life Support Group 2005)

How does one assess coma in childhood?

A rapid measure of the level of consciousness can be recorded using the AVPU scale:

A: Alert
V: responds to Voice
P: responds to Pain (= GCS ≤8)
U: Unresponsive

Serial assessments using a more comprehensive tool (e.g., GCS) are an essential part of the ongoing monitoring of the patient and should be regularly documented on the observation chart.

IDENTIFICATION AND MANAGEMENT OF RAISED INTRACRANIAL PRESSURE

The Monro–Kellie doctrine observes that the total intracranial volume cannot expand as the skull is a rigid structure that contains a finite intracranial volume. The ICP is determined by the total intracranial volume and intracranial compliance (the change in pressure resulting from a change in volume). Skull sutures are not fixed in infancy and can expand to accommodate *gradual* increases in intracranial volume but not *acute* increases; therefore even in infancy intracranial volume is relatively constant.

Intracranial contents include:

- Brain: occupies approximately 80% of the intracranial space
- Blood – cerebral blood volume (CBV): occupies 7–10% of the total intracranial volume
- Cerebrospinal fluid (CSF): occupies 7–10% of the total intracranial volume

Intracranial volume = Brain volume + Blood volume + CSF volume.

If the volume of any of the intracranial contents increases without a commensurate and compensatory decrease in the volume of other substances in the intracranial vault, the ICP will rise.

The relationship between intracranial pressure and cerebral perfusion pressure

The normal range of ICP is:

- Infants: 1.6–6 mm Hg
- Young children: 3–7 mm Hg
- Older children/adults: 10–15 mm Hg (Chitnavis & Polkey 1998)

Transient increases can be caused by coughing or by moving from a standing to a reclining position, which causes an increase in venous pressure as a result of compensation mechanisms (below). Once the limits of these mechanisms have been reached, significant increases in ICP are seen. The optimum range of ICP for children with severe head injury is not clear; however, it is suggested that ICP should be kept below 20 mm Hg (Hazinski 1992; Shann & Henning 2003).

Cerebral perfusion pressure (CPP) is the difference between the mean systemic blood pressure (BP) and the ICP:

CCP = Mean systematic arterial pressure (MAP) – ICP

An adequate CPP is:

- Neonate >30 mm Hg
- 1 month–1 year >50 mm Hg
- 1 year–10 years >60 mm Hg
- More than 15 years >70 mm Hg (Shann & Henning 2003)

CPP will fall if the MAP falls, if the mean ICP rises, or if both occur simultaneously. The CPP can be maintained despite a rise in ICP if the MAP rises in proportion. This may or may not be associated with effective cerebral perfusion.

If there is high intracranial pressure and high cerebral perfusion pressure, there must be high blood pressure (BP). Look for the cause of the high BP (e.g., pain) and treat it. Do not give antihypertensive drugs (Shann & Henning 2003).

Causes of raised intracranial pressure

- Trauma (e.g., road traffic accident/blow to head)
- Encephalitis
- Cerebral oedema (e.g., infection/trauma/renal problems/sodium imbalance/hypoxia)
- Tumours
- CSF alteration
  - Increased production
  - Decreased absorption
  - Pathway obstruction
- Cerebrovascular alterations
  - Increased BP
  - Vein of Galen (congenital abnormality where artery joins veins in skull)
  - Sodium imbalances

Compensatory mechanisms

When CPP is altered, cerebral blood flow (CBF) is maintained by a compensation mechanism called cerebral autoregulation. When MAP decreases, cerebral vasodilatation occurs, with a large increase in CBV and ICP; when MAP increases, cerebral vasoconstriction occurs with a reduction in CBV and ICP.

- Respiratory
  - **High $P\text{CO}_2$** → vasodilation → *Raised* ICP
  - **Low $P\text{CO}_2$** → vasoconstriction → *Drop* in ICP, and cerebral perfusion
  - **Low $P\text{O}_2$** → vasodilation → *Raised* ICP
  - **Low pH** → vasodilation → *Raised* ICP
- **CSF** Can be displaced into spinal canal if the ICP is high
- **Temperature** For every 1°C rise in body temperature, cerebral metabolism may rise by up to 19%, leading to a rise in ICP (Fisher 1997)
- **Stimulation** Stress → systemic vasoconstriction → BP + CBF increased → Raised ICP.

> Once the limits of compensation have been reached, a further increase in intracranial volume will result in a rise in intracranial pressure (ICP). Progressive small rises in intracranial volume will produce progressively greater rises in ICP.

Clinical signs and symptoms

A child with raised ICP may demonstrate an alteration in the following:
- Level of consciousness: likely to deteriorate
- Pupil reaction: unequal/unreactive/dilated
- Heart rate: decreasing
- BP: increasing

- Respiratory rate/pattern: slower and irregular
- Motor activity/reflexes/development of abnormal posturing: decorticate (flexion) or decerebrate (extension)
- Reduced response to pain (demonstrating flaccidity)

The child may complain of a headache, or develop nausea and vomiting.

In severe instances, Cushings triad – hypertension/bradycardia/apnoea – may occur. This is a late and ominous sign and must be treated as an emergency.

A CT scan or a magnetic resonance imaging (MRI) scan may be taken to assist with the assessment of the child's condition.

Management

The goals of managing raised ICP are:

1. Ensure effective cerebral perfusion through the maintenance of good systemic perfusion and control of ICP
2. Preserve cerebral function
3. Prevent secondary insults to the brain

Intubation and mechanical ventilation should be undertaken for the following:

- Coma – GCS ≤8 (= AVPU scale at P)
- Loss of protective laryngeal reflexes
- Ventilatory insufficiency – hypoxaemia, hypercapnia
- Spontaneous hyperventilation causing $P\text{CO}_2$ less than 3.5 kPa
- Inappropriate respiratory pattern (e.g., apnoeas or very slow respiratory rate)

Hyperventilation and $P\text{CO}_2$: General evidence suggests that the $P\text{CO}_2$ should be kept within the lower end of the normal range (4.5–5.5 kPa). While hypocapnia produces a reduction in ICP and an increase in CPP, it also reduces CBF, to the extent of causing ischaemia (Stringer et al 1993; Skippen et al 1997). While prophylactic hyperventilation should be avoided, some suggest that mild hypercapnia—$P\text{CO}_2$ of 4–4.5 kPa—may be beneficial where raised ICP is refractory to sedation, analgesia, paralysis, and hyperosmolar therapy. Aggressive hyperventilation may be useful for brief periods where there is an acute neurologic deterioration or impending coning—usually while another management option is being instituted.

Blood pressure: Monitor closely; maintain within normal range for the child or slightly hypertensive to maintain adequate CPP and counteract raised ICP (White et al 2001). Do not reduce high BP in this setting as it is essential to maintain CBF. Studies comparing dopamine with noradrenaline (norepinephrine) in hypotensive patients have demonstrated that noradrenaline augments cerebral perfusion and increases flow velocity in a predicable manner (Johnston et al 2004) and it is therefore considered to be the vasoactive drug of choice.

Fluids and electrolytes: The importance of maintaining a good BP, central venous pressure (CVP), and CPP is balanced by the need to fluid-restrict. This may lead to high normal ranges in serum osmolality and serum sodium, which alleviates cerebral oedema and reduces ICP. Saline of 0.9% is generally the fluid of choice. Ensure blood glucose is kept within the normal range—insulin infusion may be necessary in some cases. Check and correct calcium, magnesium, potassium, and PO_4.

Hyperosmolar therapy: Traditionally osmotic agents, such as mannitol and hypertonic saline, have been used to reduce ICP by increasing the osmotic pressure of plasma, drawing fluid out of the interstitial space in the brain, into the vascular space. They may have other beneficial effects such as reducing viscosity of blood improving CBF and stimulating the release of local nitric oxide (Gwer et al 2010). Although the evidence in paediatrics is limited, systematic reviews have demonstrated that hypertonic saline appears to be superior to mannitol in achieving a sustained reduction in ICP and is therefore recommended as the osmotic agent of choice. Mannitol should be reserved for cases where hypertonic saline is not available or readily accessible (Gwer et al 2010; Wakai et al 2013).

Hypertonic (3%) saline *can be administered as a bolus dose of* 3–5 mL/kg or as a continuous infusion to achieve a specific ICP target. The osmotic effect can be monitored by measuring the serum sodium levels. If there is concern regarding ICP, levels of greater than 150 mmol/L are considered necessary and appropriate.

Mannitol (20%) should only be administered as a bolus dose of 0.5–1 g/kg; a single dose may be effective in reducing brain swelling. Repeated doses are not recommended as mannitol may pass from the blood into the injured area of the brain and aggravate the swelling (Wakai et al 2013).

Position: General evidence recommends:
- Midline – nose – sternum – umbilicus (Singh 1997)
- 30-degree head up-tilt (Feldman et al 1992)
- Support neck laterally—avoid the use of collars, which may impede venous return
- Placing central venous lines in either the subclavian or internal jugular veins should be undertaken with caution as this may obstruct venous drainage and thus increase ICP
- Avoid extreme hip flexion—increases intrathoracic pressure and thus ICP

Noise reduction: Sudden loud noises can cause a startle reflex—which can be associated with a rise in ICP
- Monitors, alarms, telephones—try to silence these promptly
- Prevent people talking negatively/airing their concerns about the child's condition/accident/prognosis near the bed space because such comments may cause anxiety and a subsequent rise in ICP (Schinner et al 1995).

Drugs: Analgesia and sedation are used to manage noxious and painful stimuli and to facilitate effective ventilatory support:
- Morphine/fentanyl as a continuous infusion with an additional bolus prior to stimulatory events (e.g., suctioning)
- Paralysis: It is suggested that neuromuscular blocking (paralysing) agents reduce ICP by a variety of mechanisms, including a reduction in airway and intrathoracic pressure with the

facilitation of cerebral venous outflow and by the prevention of shivering, posturing, or breathing against the ventilator (Hsiang et al 1994). Continuous paralysis risks the masking of seizures, which can be addressed by continuous electroencephalogram (EEG) monitoring

- Administer antacids until enterally fed

 Although propofol is still used in some centres in the UK, continuous infusion of propofol for either sedation or the management of refractory intracranial hypertension in infants and children is not recommended (Center for Drug Administration and Research 2001).

Temperature: Hyperthermia is associated with an increase in damage following brain injury by various mechanisms, including increasing cerebral metabolism, inflammation, lipid peroxidation, cell death, and acute seizures. The ideal temperature is the subject of much debate, but it is generally considered pragmatic to target a temperature of approximately 36°C.

- The prevention and aggressive treatment of fever and iatrogenic hyperthermia after head injury is emphasised (Singh 1997).
- Cooling below 35°C is no longer recommended as meta-analyses of therapeutic hypothermia trials following cardiac arrest (Bisrititz et al 2015) and traumatic brain injury (Zhang et al 2015) have not demonstrated any benefit in children. A large multi-centre trial of therapeutic hypothermia (target temperature 33°C) compared to normothermia (target temperature 36.8°C) did not confer any survival or improved functional outcome following cardiac arrest in children (Moler et al 2017).

CARE

- Staggering versus clustering—assess child and plan care accordingly
- Minimal handling
- Minimal physio/suctioning
- Avoid constipation/full bladder
- Avoid rapid changes in position
- Use log rolling to maintain alignment and prevent exacerbation of neck or spinal injury
- Consider bolus of sedation and informing child of all activities prior to carrying them out.

MONITORING

- Heart rate and rhythm
- BP and CVP
- ICP and CPP
- S_aO_2 and continuous $ETCO_2$

- Temperature
- Fluid balance
- Neuro assessment

INTRACRANIAL PRESSURE MONITORING

ICP monitoring is a valuable addition to the clinical assessment of the patient. It is extremely helpful in the evaluation of trends in the patient's condition, particularly in response to therapy. ICP measurements should always be interpreted in conjunction with the patient's clinical appearance.

Two methods of monitoring ICP are:
- **Ventricular pressure monitoring:** A catheter is inserted through a burr hole in the skull into the lateral ventricle and is attached to a fluid-filled (or fibreoptic) monitoring system.
- **Subarachnoid screw pressure monitoring:** The subarachnoid screw is inserted through a burr hole in the skull and attached to a fluid-filled (or fibreoptic) monitoring system (e.g., Camino bolt).

 NB Fibreoptic catheters are zeroed before they are placed, but fluid systems require zeroing on a daily or shift basis, with the transducer being levelled at the outer aspect of the eye.

Hourly charting of ICP on an appropriate chart should record the following:
1. The average number ICP that hour (the number used to calculate the CPP)
2. The highest peak ICP observed that hour

This method makes it possible to accurately record trends in the ICP.

Once the ICP is stable, there should be a gradual return to normal care; that is:
- Increase fluids
- Decrease ventilation
- Stop paralysis
- Decrease sedation
- Continue neurologic assessment
- Continue to normalise care until extubation is possible

Cerebrospinal fluid

CSF is mainly produced by the choroid plexuses in the lateral, third and fourth ventricles. From these production sites, the CSF fills the ventricular system and follows a pathway incorporating the subarachnoid space.

CSF flows over and around the brain and spinal cord, providing buoyancy and support, and maintaining the constant chemical composition of the extracellular fluid in which the central nervous system (CNS) metabolic activity occurs. The absorption of CSF into the venous circulation is via the arachnoid villi, which act as one-way valves and are located in the superior sagittal sinus.

CSF is produced at an approximate rate of:
- 20 mL/h in adults
- 5–10 mL/h in toddlers
- 3–5 mL/h in infants (Evans 1987)

CSF is made up of:
- White cells
- Water
- Oxygen
- Carbon dioxide
- Protein
- Glucose
- Sodium
- Potassium
- Chloride.

INDICATIONS FOR CEREBROSPINAL FLUID DRAINAGE

Extraventricular drainage diverts CSF from the ventricles in the brain when the normal physiologic mechanisms are unable to do so. It can be used:
- To monitor intraventricular pressure and output of CSF
- To divert CSF that contains bacteria or blood
- In the emergency treatment of a malfunctioning internal shunt and hydrocephalus
- To control ventricular pressure

HYDROCEPHALUS

This is the result of an increase of CSF within the cranial vault, which causes ventricular dilatation. The types are:
- Communicating hydrocephalus: occurs when the arachnoid villi are obstructed and unable to reabsorb the CSF (e.g., in subarachnoid haemorrhage)
- Noncommunicating hydrocephalus: caused by an obstruction in the flow of CSF within the ventricular system; causes include congenital malformation/tumour

TREATMENT

To treat hydrocephalus, a temporary or permanent ventricular shunt is surgically inserted to divert CSF.

A temporary shunt is a straight, silastic ventricular catheter, usually placed in the right lateral ventricle through a burr hole made in the parasagittal region of the skull, just anterior to the right coronal suture. The catheter is then attached directly to drainage tubing by an interlocking connector that has an access port. This type of setup is called a simple extraventricular drain.

A permanent shunt is usually in the form of an internal ventriculoperitoneal shunt, where the CSF is drained from the ventricles as above, but it is then tunnelled under the scalp, neck, and chest wall to the abdomen, ending in the peritoneal cavity, where the draining CSF is absorbed (Birdsall & Grief 1990).

EXTRAVENTRICULAR DRAINS

Several systems are available; generally, a measuring chamber is positioned to drain CSF at a set pressure through the attached drainage system. Refer to local policies for specific management.

COMMON DIAGNOSTIC TESTS

Electroencephalography

The electroencephalograph (EEG) is a recording of the electrical activity arising from different areas of the brain.

These areas of activity can be quantified, localised, and compared with normal EEGs for the patient's age to assist in the diagnosis of seizure activity or CNS injury or dysfunction. An isoelectric (flat) EEG in a nonsedated, nonhypothermic patient is one of the criteria used to confirm brain death.

An EEG is performed using electrodes placed on specific areas of the scalp—the number of these and their positioning depends on the specific machine used.

Computed tomography scan

Computed axial tomography (CAT) consists of a series of x-rays that are analysed and reconstructed by a computer to produce cross-sectional images. In these circumstances, the x-ray pictures of the skull will produce cross-sectional images of the intracranial contents. The images produced by the scan allow differentiation of intracranial spaces and normal grey/white matter.

The CAT scan is a reliable, painless, and noninvasive method of visualising a variety of neurologic disorders, including space-occupying lesions, haematomas, haemorrhages, hydrocephalus, and brain abscesses.

 A higher radiation dose is used for computed tomography than for conventional x-rays, but the value of this test is believed to outweigh this risk.

 If an intracranial lesion is identified (e.g., an extradural haematoma), the child will need urgent transfer to a neurosurgical centre. The referring centre should transport the child to avoid delay.

Magnetic resonance imaging scan

MRI is the application of a strong external magnetic field around the patient, which causes rotation of the cell nuclei in a predictable direction at a predictable speed. The result of the rotation of the nuclei is a resonant image that is extremely well defined and enables the visualisation of soft tissues better than any other noninvasive device (Hazinski 1992). It is particularly valuable for the visualisation of tumours, shunts, and tissue or organ thicknesses. The scan also enables detailed visualisation of areas of spinal cord compression following trauma.

Both CT and MRI scans can take up to 30 minutes to complete, depending on the area that is scanned. As the patient needs to be completely still, it is important that the child is adequately sedated, paralysed if appropriate, and monitored throughout the procedure.

A contrast medium may be administered intravenously, to assist in clarifying the areas being examined.

The cerebral function analysing monitor

The electroencephalogram, or EEG, is a recording of the electrical activity within the brain. By recording this activity and then analysing it, valuable information can be obtained to assist in diagnosing seizure activity or CNS injury/dysfunction.

Different institutions have their own methods of obtaining continuous EEG recordings of the critically ill child.

DIABETES INSIPIDUS

Central or neurogenic diabetes insipidus can be observed in children who sustain the following:

- Head injuries
- Central nervous system infections
- Intraventricular haemorrhages
- Neurosurgery

Neurogenic diabetes insipidus results from decreased production of antidiuretic hormone (ADH). When ADH is not synthesised by the hypothalamus, circulating ADH levels are negligible. Renal collecting tubules therefore remain relatively impermeable to water, resulting in insufficient reabsorption. Large amounts of water are lost in urine. Intravascular volume is quickly depleted, and haemoconcentration produces hypernatraemia. The osmotic gradient causes fluid to shift from the intracellular to the intravascular space and that fluid is quickly lost from the circulation. Intravascular hypovolaemia stimulates aldosterone secretion, leading to the reabsorption of water and sodium from the proximal renal tubule. If the child's fluid intake is limited to intravenous (IV) therapy, and he or she is not able to drink freely, unrecognised diabetes insipidus can quickly produce hypovolaemia, hypernatraemia, and serum hyperosmolality.

Signs and symptoms

- Polyuria is the excretion of large amounts of very dilute urine with low osmolality, low sodium concentration, and very low specific gravity; it is important to detect this condition early because the critically ill child can become hypovolaemic and hypernatraemic very quickly
- Irritability, tachycardia, low CVP, weak peripheral pulses and hypotension, metabolic acidosis, prolonged capillary refill time
- In the infant, the anterior fontanelle is depressed
- Reduced body weight

Management

- Rapid replacement of urinary fluid and electrolyte losses and provision of ADH in the form of the drug DDAVP (vasopressin)
- Close monitoring of fluid balance, intravascular volume, systemic perfusion, and electrolyte balance
- Positive response to vasopressin will be seen by a decrease in urine volume to approximately 1 mL/kg/h, a rise in urine specific gravity to more than 1.010, and osmolality to 280–300 mmol/L (Hazinski 1992)
- By calculating fluid replacement on hourly urine output, it is easier to taper this in response to vasopressin

SEIZURES

Seizures (fits) are sudden, abnormal discharges of cerebral neurons (BMJ 1997). They may be generalised (activity spread through the subcortical area, bilateral tonic–clonic activity possibly associated with loss of consciousness) or focal (activity localised in a small area of the cerebral cortex, unilateral tonic–clonic activity).

- **Tonic phase:** Rigidity of muscles due to spasm
- **Clonic phase:** Convulsive jerking movements, commonly of limbs and trunk

Clinical signs of fitting may include changes in the following:

- BP
- Heart rate
- Respiratory pattern
- Convulsions
- Cyanosis

Commonly, specific charts are used to document episodes of fitting, where the following details are recorded:

- Description of the abnormal movements (e.g., smacking lips followed by repeated jerking of right arm)
- Duration
- Whether self-resolving or, if medication was required, which drugs were administered and their effect

It would also be beneficial to record whether the fits were spontaneous or triggered by an intervention (e.g., someone touching or moving the child).

 As abnormal movements do not necessarily constitute fits, **write what you see** to prevent inaccurate interpretation.

When an intubated child has been paralysed and sedated, clinical signs of fitting can be masked; the use of EEG monitoring in these circumstances can be valuable.

Causes of seizures

- Structural lesions; for example:
  - Cerebral infarction
  - Tumour
  - Haematoma
  - Abscess
- Infection
  - Systemic
  - CNS
  - Encephalitis/meningitis
  - High-grade pyrexia
- Toxic ingestion
- Metabolic disorders
- Head trauma
- Seizure disorders (e.g., epilepsy)
- Hypoxic–ischaemic encephalopathy

Status epilepticus

This occurs either when a fit lasts for longer than 30 minutes, or when successive seizures occur so frequently that the patient does not recover fully between them.

Status epilepticus can be fatal; death may be due to:
- Complications of the convulsion (e.g., obstruction of the airway or aspiration of vomit)
- Overmedication
- Underlying disease process

Injury to the brain during status epilepticus occurs as a result of one or more of the following:
- Direct injury from repetitive neuronal discharge
- Systemic complications of the convulsions, especially hypoxia from airway obstruction and later acidosis when systemic hypotension occurs

- The underlying disease process

The most common causes of status epilepticus in children are:
- Febrile status epilepticus
- Sudden reduction in antiepileptic medication
- Acute cerebral trauma
- Idiopathic epilepsy (i.e., cause unknown)
- Bacterial meningitis
- Encephalopathy (including Reye syndrome)
- Poisoning (BMJ 1997)

Aims of treatment:
- Maintain ABCD
- Stop fit
- Reduce risk of further fitting
- Treat cause
- Reduce risks associated with treatment

Urgent investigations required:
- Glucose
- Sodium
- CAT scan if suspect:
  - Focal seizures
  - Trauma
  - Space-occupying lesion

The treatment protocol for status epilepticus is set out in Fig. 6.2 (ALSG 2016). Thiopental is a general anaesthetic. It is particularly valuable in patients with neurologic involvement because of its ability to acutely reduce ICP; therefore it has a cerebroprotective effect (Singer & Webb 1997).

It is an alkaline solution, which will cause irritation if it leaks into subcutaneous tissues; watch for signs of cannula extravasation.

By reassessing the child after each step of the treatment protocol in Fig. 6.2, or guidelines similar to it, the effects of treatment can be evaluated and the need for further intervention can be decided.

DYSTONIA

Dystonia is defined as 'a movement disorder in which involuntary sustained or intermittent muscle contractions cause twisting and repetitive movements and abnormal postures' (Sanger et al 2003). Dystonia is often more prominent when voluntary movement is attempted, or in certain postures. It is the most common movement disorder in children and impairs quality of life with pain and progressive deformity (Lumsden et al 2013). Infants and children with dystonic conditions may require PICU admission during acute periods of deterioration known as 'status dystonicus' or 'dystonic storm' with intense, generalised, and painful muscle contractions, or as a consequence of their treatment, which may lead to respiratory depression and increased drooling.

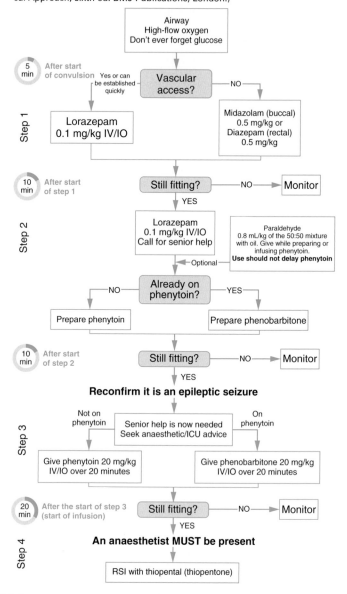

Fig. 6.2 Emergency treatment status epilepticus. *ICU*, Intensive care unit; *IO*, intraosseous; *IV*, intravenous; *RSI*, rapid sequence induction. (From Advanced Life Support Group, 2016. Advanced Paediatric Life Support: A Practical Approach, sixth ed. BMJ Publications, London.)

Aetiology of dystonia in childhood

The causes of dystonia in childhood can be considered as acquired or genetic (Van Egmond et al 2015).

- **Acquired** causes include drug reaction, encephalitis (including NMDA receptor), structural brain lesions (e.g., stroke), and cerebral palsy (nonprogressive injury to the developing brain often occurs during the perinatal period).
- **Genetic** causes include inherited errors of metabolism (organic acidaemia, GLU-1 deficiency, lysosomal storage disorders, dopa-responsive dystonia, and metal storage) and specific genetic conditions, which are either monogenic (assigned single gene locus) or genetic conditions in which dystonia is an important feature alongside other associated neurologic (e.g., ataxia, hypotonia, epilepsy) and systemic features (hepatosplenomegaly, dysmorphism).

It is important to identify the specific conditions as early treatment and intervention may prevent progress of the disorders.

Treatment

The treatment for dystonia must involve the whole multidisciplinary team from the early stages. The natural history of these conditions is that they often progress for the first 5 years, which requires regular reassessment of the patient's response and clinical condition. The cornerstones of treatment include medication, botulinum toxin injections, and deep brain stimulation.

ORAL MEDICATIONS

- Trial of levodopa for all patients to treat/exclude dopa-responsive dystonia
- Trihexyphenidyl
- Oral baclofen or diazepam with progressive drowsiness, drooling, and droopiness (poor trunk and neck control) with escalating doses; the risk of aspiration and respiratory depression warrant careful observation and monitoring of patients
- Clonidine is a useful oral adjunct with less respiratory depression in severe cases
- Gabapentin can help to manage pain and mood disorders

Botulinum toxin is licensed for treatment lower limb spasticity and cerebral palsy but can also be effective for treating other localised dystonia such as neck, hands, and elbows.

Deep brain stimulation (DBS) consists of a neurostimulator, which is usually placed under the collarbone with leads attached to electrodes that are placed in the basal ganglia. The electrodes are used to reduce the abnormal signalling from these areas of the brain. The device is turned on and adjusted using a handheld wireless device.

Numerous scoring systems are available to assess children with dystonia, but these systems are complex and require specialist training. Two specialist teams (Children's Neuroscience Centre at the Evelina London Children's Hospital, and the Paediatric Neurology & Neurodisability Department at Royal Belfast Hospital for Sick Children) have developed a simple scoring system to meet this need, called the Dystonia Severity Action Plan (Table 6.3).

Status dystonicus or dystonic storm

Acute potentially fatal episodes of severe generalised dystonia can cause complications, such as hyperpyrexia, respiratory failure, and rhabdomyolysis, leading to renal failure. These episodes may be exacerbated by underlying problems, such as constipation, gastro-oesophageal reflux, dislocated hips or other orthopaedic problems, and infection; these factors should be treated to alleviate symptoms. Supportive care, which may include invasive ventilation and haemofiltration for rhabdomyolysis, initially should be aggressive followed by a slow weaning process. Treatment options include clonidine, benzodiazepine, and propofol infusions. Up to one-third of cases may require DBS insertion (McCrae 2013).

DEMYELINATING CONDITIONS

Myelin is the fatty white substance that surrounds nerve fibres (axons) acting as an insulator to increase the speed of conduction of the nerve impulses (Fig. 6.3).

There are some inflammatory conditions that specifically target and damage the myelin sheath, known as demyelinating conditions. These conditions include:

- Guillain-Barré syndrome (GBS)
- Acute disseminated encephalitis (ADEM)
- Transverse myelitis

GUILLAIN-BARRÉ SYNDROME

GBS is an autoimmune disorder where the patient's immune system attacks part of the peripheral nervous system, usually following a respiratory or gastrointestinal infection (*Campylobacter jejuni* and cytomegalovirus most commonly) and classically presents as a demyelinating neuropathy with ascending weakness (Yuki & Hartung 2012). Muscles begin to lose the ability to respond to the brain; the brain receives fewer sensory signals, thus affecting the ability to feel heat, pain, or other sensations, and tingling and muscle weakness generally begin in hands and feet.

Typical signs and symptoms

- Numbness, tingling, and pain
- Bilateral and ascending weakness in arms and legs, which progressively worsens over time; maximum severity may be reached in hours or up to 3 weeks and then may plateau for 2 days to 6 months before the improvement phase occurs

Table 6.3 Dystonia severity score and action plan

Severity	Assessment	Plan
Grade 1: The child sits comfortably and has regular periods of uninterrupted sleep. Child stable on medication	No assessment needed	Continue at home or going to school as usual Discharge home if recovering from acute decompensation
Grade 2: The child is irritable and cannot settle Dystonic posturing interferes with sitting activities The child can only tolerate lying despite usual baseline medication	Seek advice from local team including fresh assessment within next few days	Adjust medication as preplanned or initiate new plan.
Grade 3: Not able to tolerate lying and/or unable to get to sleep or sleep disturbed No evidence of metabolic decompensation, with creatinine kinase <1000 IU/L	No response to adjusted medication? Urgent assessment/review required	Further adjustments to medication Metabolic screen required to look for signs of decompensation; observe in hospital if indicated; be prepared to escalate management
Grade 4: Early multiorgan failure: Clinically as above with: Pyrexia (in absence of infection) Evidence of metabolic compromise (e.g., acidosis, elevated potassium, low calcium, evidence of rising creatinine, and/or urea) Evidence of myoglobinuria, creatinine kinase >1000 IU/L	This is an emergency, urgent hospital admission required for multisystem support and attempt to prevent frank renal failure and disseminated intravascular coagulation.	Measure creatinine kinase levels monitored regularly along with urea and electrolytes, renal and liver function Nasogastric or gastrostomy or rectal medication if tolerated and working IV Medication

Continued

Table 6.3 Dystonia severity score and action plan—cont'd

Severity	Assessment	Plan
Grade 5: Immediate life-threatening: As above with: Full metabolic decompensation Respiratory, cardiovascular, or renal compromise Requires intensive care	Child needs HDU/PICU	Consider need for: IV infusion of clonidine* and/or midazolam Dialysis/haemofiltration ventilation – specifically if spasms causing airway compromise, bulbar dysfunction with secretions compromising airway, evidence of respiratory failure or impending exhaustion Liver support Intrathecal baclofen infusion Deep brain stimulation

*Non-respiratory depressant.
HDU, high dependency unit; *IV,* Intravenous; *PICU,* paediatric intensive care unit.
From Lumsden, D., Lundy, C., Fairhurst, C., Lin, J.P., 2013. Dystonia severity action plan: a simple grading for medical severity of status dystonicus and life-threatening dystonia. Dev. Med. Child. Neurol. 55, 671–672.

Fig. 6.3 Diagram of a neuron showing the myelin sheath. (http://ehumanbiofield.wikispaces.com/neurons+jo)

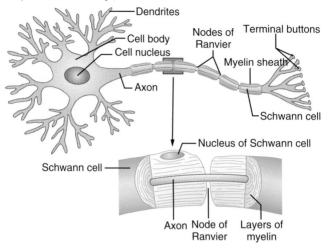

- 45–75% of patients with GBS experience cranial nerve involvement, which may include facial palsy, diplopia, dysarthria, dysphagia, opthalmoplegia, pupillary disturbances
- Sensory changes – paresthesia, loss of vibration, proprioception, touch
- Pain – the mechanism of this is uncertain but may be from direct nerve injury, paralysis, or immobilisation
- Autonomic changes – dysfunction in sympathetic and parasympathetic nervous systems, which can lead to tachycardia, bradycardia, facial flushing, paroxysmal hypertension, orthostatic hypotension, anhidrosis, or diaphoresis
- Respiratory disturbances – approximately 40% of GBS patients present with some respiratory weakness, which may include slurred speech, difficulty in swallowing, shortness of breath or dyspnoea on exertion, and approximately one-third of GBS patients may require ventilator support for respiratory weakness
- Reflexes may be reduced or absent on presentation

Diagnosis – signs and symptoms can be varied, but specific findings, such as rapid development and ascending weakness, absent reflexes and absence of fever, may indicate GBS but other tests may be used to aid diagnosis:

- Lumbar puncture (LP) and analysis of CSF (in GBS there may be elevated CSF protein [>0.55 g/L]) with normal or low white cell count (van den Berg et al 2014)

- Electromyography and nerve conduction studies but in the first 2 weeks of illness with GBS they may not show any abnormality (Rinaldi 2013)
- MRI and CAT scan of the spine may show enhancement of the spinal nerve roots on MRI in Guillain Barré Syndrome and can also be useful to exclude alternative diagnosis such as a tumour causing spinal cord compression
- Blood tests – to exclude other possible causes of weakness (e.g., low potassium). Low serum sodium has been found in patients with GBS due to the inappropriate secretion of an ADH, leading to water retention (Spasovski et al 2014)

Treatment

There are two main treatment options in GBS: plasmapheresis or IV immunoglobulin. These two treatments are equally effective and a combination of the two is not significantly better than a single option (Hughes et al 2014). Plasmapheresis filters antibodies and other immune cell-derived factors that could contribute to nerve damage from the bloodstream, and it has been shown to speed recovery when used within 4 weeks of the onset of symptoms (Hughes et al 2003). High-dose IV immunoglobulins (derived from a pool of thousands of donors) appears to reduce the immune attack on the nervous system. This therapy should be started within 2 weeks of the onset of symptoms; it is easily administered but can cause liver inflammation and kidney failure (Dantal 2013).

Other therapy includes:
- Respiratory support including ventilation
- Pain relief
- Deep vein thrombosis prophylaxis
- Physiotherapy, occupational therapy, psychologic support, speech and language assessment, rehabilitation, and a dietician

Despite optimum care, a 5% mortality has been reported in GBS as a result of complications, infections, blood clots, cardiac arrest due to autonomic neuropathy, and up to 20% of adult patients remain severely disabled but this is less common in children (Yuki & Hartung 2012). The Guillain-Barré Syndrome Support Group provides information and support for families:
www.gaincharity.org.uk

ACUTE DISSEMINATED ENCEPHALITIS

ADEM is a rare condition that can occur at any age, but it is more common in children than adults, with a peak age of 5–8 years. In some (but not all) cases there is a preceding trigger such as a vaccination or infection (Koelman & Mateen 2015). The hallmark of this condition is widespread inflammation of the brain and spinal cord with loss of myelin (white matter). There are usually multiple lesions in the cerebral hemispheres, brainstem, and spinal cord (Alper 2012). It can present with a wide variety of clinical signs depending on the location and the severity of the brain lesions:

- Encephalopathy (altered level of consciousness, lethargy, and even coma)
- Altered behaviour (irritability and confusion)
- Weakness in the upper and/or lower limbs
- Ataxia (loss of balance)
- Seizures
- Cranial nerve palsies
- Headache and vomiting.

Diagnosis

- MRI scans demonstrate multiple T2-enhancing (bright) lesions in the brain and often include the spinal cord
- A LP may be necessary to exclude meningitis once it is evident that it is safe to perform the LP. The CSF usually shows inflammation with an increased cell count and protein.

Treatment

- Supportive care with ventilation and seizure control may be required in severe cases.
- There are no randomised controlled studies comparing treatment. The first line of treatment usually includes pulsed doses of IV methylprednisolone (20–30 mg/kg, maximum 1 g/day) for 3–5 days. The IV steroids are followed by a tapering dose of oral steroids.
- If steroid therapy is not effective, the second-line treatment consists of IV immunoglobulin (2 g/kg) divided over 2 days. Plasmapheresis is considered as a last resort treatment for patients who fail to respond to steroids and immunoglobulins.

Prognosis

- The majority of patients (75%) recover after treatment and only experience a single episode.
- A small group may develop a relapse or recurrence; this may occur at the time of tapering oral steroids. Recommencing steroid therapy can reduce symptoms.
- The recovery period may take days to months. Very occasionally children with ADEM may go on to develop multiple sclerosis.
- Very severe cases can be fatal with a 5% mortality described in the literature (Scolding 2014).

TRANSVERSE MYELITIS

Transverse myelitis is an immune-mediated demyelination that affects the spinal cord and presents with sudden onset of motor, sensory, and autonomic symptoms. The name 'transverse' is not used to describe the spinal cord pathology but rather the bandlike sensory disturbance that is often associated with this condition (Wolf et al 2012). It is a rare condition only affecting one to eight people per million; approximately 20% of cases occur in children.

Diagnosis (Wolf et al 2012):

- The diagnosis can only be confirmed when other important conditions, such as a spinal cord tumour, spinal cord compression, and ischaemic lesion, have been excluded.

The American Academy of Neurology has proposed specific diagnostic criteria (2002):

- Evidence of spinal cord inflammation typically spanning multiple vertebral segments
  - Enhancing spinal cord lesion (on MRI)
  - CSF increased cell count (>10 cells/mm^3) or increased immunoglobulin type G index
- Time to maximum disability 4 hours to 21 days

Presentation

- Children often present with a prodromal mild illness weeks before the onset of symptoms; less commonly, transverse myelitis may follow a vaccine or trauma. There is no specific vaccine type or viral illness that is clearly linked to transverse myelitis.
- Pain, sensory, motor, and autonomic deficits begin over hours and progress over a few days (range 2–30 days). The symptoms usually plateau within a week.
- Autonomic instability is common and includes fluctuating temperature, heart rate and rhythm, breathing rate, and bladder and bowel function.
- If the lesion is in the lower back there is usually pain and loss of power in the legs. Higher spinal cord lesions affect the legs, arms, and respiratory muscles. The motor problems begin as flaccid paresis with loss of deep tendon reflexes in the affected area (e.g., arms), but upper motor neuron signs of brisk reflexes and increased tone may develop below the lesion (e.g., legs) over time.

Treatment

- As with all serious conditions in childhood, it is important to assess the adequacy of the patient's airway, breathing, and circulation. A high spinal cord lesion may affect the respiratory muscles, in which case intubation and ventilation may be essential.
- Autonomic symptoms may lead to urinary retention, which should be managed by catheterisation.
- There are no randomised controlled studies supporting any specific treatment regimen; however, corticosteroids have been shown to reduce the length of disability and to improve the overall outcome. High-dose methylprednisolone (10–30 mg/kg/day max 1g/day) for 5–7 days should be followed by a tapering course of oral steroids.

- Limited evidence exists for additional therapies but plasmapheresis is recommended for fulminant demyelinating conditions, such as transverse myelitis and GBS. Occasionally, IV immunoglobulin (2 g/kg over 2 days) and in rare cases IV cyclophosphamide may be administered.
- Spasticity may be relieved with baclofen or benzodiazepines.
- Pain is a significant feature of this condition and can be relieved by regular muscle stretching but may require specific treatments, such as gabapentin or carbamazepine.
- Paresis requires early initiation of rehabilitation to preserve muscle strength and prevent deformity. Involvement of the occupational and physiotherapy team early with a programme and splinting is highly recommended.
- Flaccid paresis increases the risk of deep vein thrombosis; age-appropriate prophylaxis should be initiated following local guidance.
- Early attention to bladder and bowel symptoms with involvement of specialist teams (e.g., urology) may help to limit long-term consequences.
- There is a high risk of depression and anxiety, particularly among the teenagers and adolescents affected. The most effective interventions are aimed at improving parent–child communication.

Prognosis

- The time to be able to walk is, on average, 1 month (range: 2–365 days).
- Rehabilitation should begin as soon as possible to maintain the range of motion and to preserve strength.
- Complete recovery occurs in 33–50% of all affected patients.
- There is a small group who have a poor recovery, remain nonambulatory, and have ongoing sphincter problems (10–20%). The poorer prognosis is associated with the rapid onset of symptoms and the need for ventilation.
- The other group of patients recover but have mild residual symptoms, such as paresthesia.

MYASTHENIA GRAVIS

Myasthenia gravis is a chronic disease (unless it occurs in the neonatal period) marked by abnormal fatigability and weakness of selected muscles. The degree of fatigue is so extreme that these muscles are temporarily paralysed. The muscles initially affected are those around the eyes, mouth, and throat, resulting in drooping of the upper eyelids (ptosis), double vision, and dysarthria (unclear speech). In extreme cases it can lead to respiratory failure. It is an autoimmune disease in which autoantibodies bind to cholinergic receptors on muscle cells, which impairs the ability of the transmitter acetylcholine to induce muscular contractions (adapted from Williams & Asquith 2000).

There are three types of myasthenia gravis seen in children:

- **Neonatal:** This occurs in infants born to myasthenic mothers. It involves muscles associated with the distal cranial nerves, causing dysphonia and dysphagia. It resolves spontaneously within the first 5 days of life.
- **Congenital:** The onset occurs within the first few days of life. Mothers of these infants rarely have myasthenia gravis but it may present in siblings. Respiratory failure is very unusual, but the infants will be poor feeders, and extraocular muscles will be affected.
- **Juvenile:** This may be present after the age of 2 years, but it is most commonly present during adolescence. It first presents in the muscles supplied by the lower cranial nerves. This is the form of myasthenia gravis seen in adults (Williams & Asquith 2000).

Management

- Diagnosis is made by titres for acetylcholine receptor antibodies, electromyogram, and a Tensilon test; Tensilon (edrophonium) is a short-acting anticholinergic drug given intravenously. The child will almost immediately show a dramatic, temporary increase in muscle strength.
- Anticholinesterase drug therapy is commonly in the form of neostigmine or pyridostigmine.
- Immunosuppression may reduce the production of acetylcholine receptor antibodies so corticosteroids may be used.
- Plasmapheresis may give temporary remission as acetylcholine receptor antibodies are protein-bound.
- Thymectomy may increase muscle strength as the thymus gland may increase the development of acetylcholine receptor antibodies; this may have long-term implications for the development of the immune system in children.

MENINGITIS

Meningitis is an acute inflammation of the meninges and CSF, which occurs more commonly in children than adults, particularly in children between 1 month and 5 years of age. It is most commonly caused by bacteria, although it can also be viral. In addition to *Neisseria meningitidis* and tuberculous meningitis, there is an age-related association with different causative organisms (see Table 6.4).

Immunisation against *Haemophilus influenzae* type B (Hib vaccine), meningitis C, and pneumococcus is now incorporated into the childhood immunisation schedule.

Signs and symptoms

- Difficult to assess in infants: extreme irritability, with high-pitched 'cerebral cry' or lethargy with vomiting and fever
- If ICP is high, anterior fontanelle may be full and tense

Table 6.4 Causes of bacterial meningitis with age	
0–2 months	Group B streptococci
	Enteric *(Escherichia coli, Klebsiella, Proteus, Listeria)*
2–4 months	Group B streptococci
	Streptococcus pneumoniae
	Haemophilus influenzae type B
	Meningococcus
More than 4 months	*Streptococcus pneumoniae*
	Meningococcus
	Haemophilus influenzae type B (in under 5-year-olds)

Source: with permission from Stack, C., Dobbs, P., 2004. Essentials of Paediatric Intensive Care. Greenwich Medical, London.

- Child may complain of headache and photophobia (extreme sensitivity to light)
- Neck stiffness
- Kernig sign (pain associated with extension of the knee when the thighs are flexed)
- Brudzinski sign (flexion of neck stimulates flexion at knees and hips)

The importance of early recognition of symptoms so that effective treatment can be commenced as soon as possible cannot be overemphasised.

Management

Intubation and ventilation may be necessary to maintain a patent airway and to treat raised ICP.

- If meningitis is suspected, while awaiting confirmation of diagnosis the administration of IV antibiotics should commence; centres have their own protocols, but ceftriaxone and cefotaxime are the antibiotics of choice.
- Full blood screen for analysis will be performed, including blood cultures.
- Full neurologic assessment with careful attention to any focal signs or cranial nerve involvement.
- Fluid restriction according to local policy.
- LP to obtain CSF specimen may be performed **unless** the child is believed to have raised ICP or an altered level of consciousness, when it would be omitted.
- Management of raised ICP if indicated, as previously discussed.
- It is now common practice in many PICUs for children with meningitis to be nursed on an open unit, rather than in a cubicle, once the first dose of IV antibiotics has been given (refer to local infection control policy).
- Once the causative agent has been identified, the appropriate antibiotics will be prescribed.

- If the child shows signs of meningococcal sepsis; for example, poor capillary refill time and toe–core gap, purpuric skin rash (small dark red spots [petechiae] caused by capillaries bleeding into the skin), deranged clotting and hypotension (late sign), that do not respond to boluses of fluid, multiorgan support including high-frequency oscillation, inotropes and renal replacement therapy may be required. For evidence-based guidelines to manage sepsis see Chapter 12.

> NB Provision of prophylactic oral antibiotics to family members and others who have had recent, prolonged, close contact with the child, is common. Examples of these are ciprofloxacin or rifampicin. When rifampicin is administered, to avoid alarm, those taking it need to be informed that it turns bodily secretions (e.g., urine) red. If rifampicin is administered to women of child-bearing age, it is important to inform them that this drug obliterates the action of the contraceptive pill.

Meningitis is a notifiable disease; therefore the medical staff will have to notify the public health inspector of the occurrence.

Viral meningitis may require only supportive care, as this form is usually much milder than bacterial meningitis.

POSTERIOR REVERSIBLE LEUKOENCEPHALOPATHY SYNDROME

Posterior reversible leukoencephalopathy syndrome (PRES) is a clinical and radiologic diagnosis, which presents with headache, seizure, altered level of consciousness, and visual disturbances accompanied by radiologic changes. The MRI findings may be typical involving the posterior cortex/occipoparietal lobes, but also may be more extensive including diffuse changes and can even extend to the brainstem (Fig. 6.4).

The MRI changes are not always reversible, and the CT scan may be normal in these cases. The EEG can show slowing of background activity in keeping with encephalopathy.

The most common identified trigger was a hypertensive crisis, but PRES has also been described following treatment with calicineurin inhibitors (e.g., tacrolimus) and cyclosporin-A. PRES is well described in children with cancer, particularly haematologic malignancies, often in association with hypertension (97%) and corticosteroid therapy (78%).

The majority of children recover following treatment of hypertension (see Chapter 4, Hypertensive Crisis Management) or following withdrawal of the medication that has triggered the event. However, there is a small risk of mortality and long-term morbidity, including persistent imaging abnormalities and epilepsy, in a small number of cases.

SPINAL MUSCULAR ATROPHY

Spinal muscular atrophy (SMA) is caused by a defect in the SMN1 gene, which leads to insufficient levels of the SMN protein. Motor neurons rely on this protein for survival, so an inadequate amount leads

Fig. 6.4 Scans demonstrating typical changes associated with posterior reversible leukoencephalopathy syndrome (PRES). (A) Computed tomography (CT) scan: bilateral low density changes in parietal and occipital lobes. (B) Magnetic resonance imaging (MRI) scan: hyperintensity in parietal and occipital lobes signalling reduced diffusion. (From Barber, C., Leclerc, R., Gladman, D., Urowitz, M.B., Fortin, P.R., 2011. Posterior reversible encephalopathy syndrome: an emerging disease manifestation in systemic lupus erythematosus. Semin. Arthritis. Rheum. 41 (3), 353–363.)

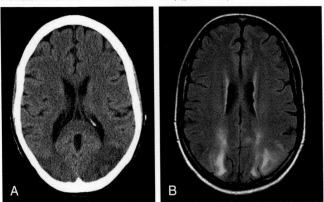

to degeneration of the lower motor neurons. This is a genetic autosomal recessive disease characterised by a slowly progressive muscle weakness and atrophy of limb muscles due to the destruction of lower motor neurons in the brainstem and spinal cord.

There are four main types of SMA; the first two types are described and are based on the age of onset, severity, and progression of symptoms:

SMA type 1: This is the most severe and the baby will have symptoms of hypotonia, reduced limb movements, feeding difficulties, and impaired breathing before 6 months of age. Most of these children will develop respiratory failure before the age of 2 years. There is significant worldwide variation on the management of children with SMA type 1 (Geevasinga & Ryan 2007; Dybwik et al 2010). The benefits and ethics of ventilation have been assessed. The British Thoracic Society (2012) issued guidelines for the respiratory management of children with neuromuscular weakness and this recommends that doctors engage patients and their parents in a mutual participation in decision making, with full disclosure of all information in a sensitive and timely manner.

SMA type 2: Symptoms usually emerge between 6 and 18 months of age. Children may sit but not stand or walk without assistance;

around 40% will develop respiratory failure in childhood (British Thoracic Society 2012). Progression of the disease is variable and life expectancy is reduced but some children will live into young adulthood.

Diagnosis

This may be made by physical examination looking for signs, such as muscle wasting and weakness, reduced or absent tendon reflexes and twitching of individual muscle fibres, by genetic testing, electromyography, and muscle biopsy.

Treatment

There is no cure for SMA. Treatments focus on managing symptoms:
- Use of benzodiazepines and baclofen may reduce spasticity
- Glycopyrolate or atropine (or botulinum toxin injected into salivary glands) may be used for excessive saliva
- Dietetic advice to optimise nutrition and often a feeding tube may be required
- Physiotherapy
- Noninvasive ventilation and other types of ventilation may be considered with quality of life discussions (Spinal Muscular Atrophy Support UK – www.smasupportuk.org.uk).

REFERENCES

Advanced Life Support Group, 2005. Advanced Paediatric Life Support: A Practical Approach, fourth ed. BMJ Publications, London.

Advanced Life Support Group, 2016. Advanced Paediatric Life Support: A Practical Approach, sixth ed. BMJ Publications, London.

Alper, G., 2012. Acute disseminated encephalomyelitis. J. Child. Neurol 27 (11), 1408–1425.

American Academy of Neurology, 2002. Transverse Myelitis Consortium Working Group. Proposed diagnostic criteria and nosology of acute transverse myelitis. Neurology 59, 499–505.

Birdsall, C., Grief, L., 1990. How do you manage extraventricular drainage? Am. J. Nurs 90 (11), 47–49.

Bisrititz, J.F., Horton, L.M., Smaldrone, A., 2015. Therapeutic hypothermia in children after cardiac arrest: asystematic review and meta-analysis. Pediatr. Emerg. Care 31 (4), 296–303.

BMJ, 1997. Advanced Paediatric Life Support – The Practical Approach, second ed. British Medical Journal, London.

British Thoracic Society Respiratory Management of Children with Neuromuscular Weakness Guideline Group, 2012. Guidelines for respiratory management of children with neuromuscular weakness. Thorax 67 (Supp1), i1–i40.

Center for Drug Administration and Research 2001 Pediatric Exclusivity Labeling Changes. US Food and Drug Administration, Washington, DC.

Available online at: http://www.fda.gov/cder/pediatric/labelchange.htm. Accessed 5 September 2006.

Chitnavis, B.P., Polkey, C.E., 1998. ICP monitoring. Care Crit. Ill 14 (3), 80–84.

Dantal, J., 2013. Intravenous immunoglobulins: in-depth review of excipients and acute kidney injury risk. Am. J. Nephrol 38 (4), 275–284.

Dybwik, K., Tollali, T., Nielsen, E.W., et al., 2010. Why does the provision of home mechanical ventilation vary so widely? Chron Respir Dis 7, 67–73.

Evans, O.B., 1987. Manual of Child Neurology. Churchill Livingstone, New York.

Feldman, Z., Kanter, M., Robertson, C., et al., 1992. Effect of head elevation on intracranial pressure and cerebral blood flow in head injured patients. J. Neurosurg 76, 207–211.

Fisher, M.D., 1997. Pediatric traumatic brain injury. Crit. Care Nurs. Q 20 (1), 36–51.

Geevasinga, N., Ryan, M.M., 2007. Physician attitudes towards ventilator support for spinal muscular atrophy type 1 in Australasia. J. Paediatrics. Child. Health 43, 790–794.

Gwer, S., Gatakaa, H., Mwai, L., et al., 2010. The role for osmotic agents in children with acute encephalopathies: a systemic review. BMC Peditr 10, 23.

Hazinski, M.F. (Ed.), 1992. Nursing Care of the Critically Ill Child, second ed. CV Mosby, St Louis, MO.

Hsiang, J.K., Chesnut, R.M., Crisp, C.B., et al., 1994. Early, routine paralysis for intracranial pressure control in severe head injury: is it necessary? Crit. Care Med 22, 1471–1476.

Hughes, R.A., Swan, A.V., van Doorn, P.A., 2014. Intravenous immunoglobulin for Guillain Barré syndrome. Cochrane Database Syst. Rev 9, CD002063.

Hughes, R.A., Wijdicks, E.F., Barohn, R., et al., 2003. Practice parameter: immune-therapy for Guillain Barré syndrome: report of the Quality Standards Subcommittee of the American Academy of Neurology. Neurology 61 (6), 736–740.

Johnston, A.J., Steiner, L.A., Chatfield, D.A., et al., 2004. Effect of cerebral perfusion pressure augmentation with dopamine and norepinephrine on global and focal brain oxygenation after traumatic brain injury. Intensive Care Med 30, 791–797.

Kirkham, F.J., Ashwal, S., 2013. Coma and brain death. Hand Clin Neurol 111, 43–61.

Koelman, D.L., Mateen, F.J., 2015. Acute disseminated encephalomyelitis: current controversies in diagnosis and outcome. J. Neurol 262 (9), 2013–2024.

Lower, J., 2002. Facing neuro assessment fearlessly. Nursing 32 (2), 58.

Lumsden, D., Lundy, C., Fairhurst, C., et al., 2013. Dystonia Severity Action Plan: a simple grading for medical severity of ststus dystonicus and life-threatening dystonia. Dev. Med. Child Neurol 55, 671–672.

McCrae, N., 2013. Childhood dystonia. ACNR 13 (5), 18–20.

Moler, F.W., Silverstein, F.S., Holubkov, R., et al., 2017. Therapeutic hypothermia after in-hospital cardiac arrest in children. N Engl J Med 376, 318–329.

Rinaldi, S., 2013. Update on Guillain Barré syndrome. J Peripher Nerv Syst 18 (2), 99–112.

Sanger, T.D., Delgado, M.R., Gaebler-Spira, D., et al., Task force on childhood motor disorders, 2003. classification and definition of disorders causing hypertonia in childhood. Pediatrics 111 (1), 89–97.

Schinner, K., Chisholm, A., Grap, M., et al., 1995. The effects of auditory stimuli on intracranial pressure and cerebral perfusion pressure in traumatic brain injury. J Neurosci Nurs 27, 348–354.

Scolding, N., 2014. Acute disseminated encephalomyelitis and other inflammtory demyelinating variants. Hand Clin Neurol 122, 601–611.

Shann, F., Henning, R., 2003. Paediatric Intensive Care Guidelines. Collective, Parkville, Victoria.

Simpson, D., Reilly, P., 1982. Paediatric coma scale. Lancet 2, 450.

Singer, M., Webb, A., 1997. Oxford Handbook of Critical Care. Oxford University Press, Oxford.

Singh, N.C. (Ed.), 1997. Manual of Pediatric Critical Care. WB Saunders, Philadelphia, PA.

Skippen, P., Seear, M., Poskitt, K., et al., 1997. Effect of hyperventilation on regional cerebral blood flow in head-injured children. Crit Care Med 25, 1402–1409.

Spasovski, G., Vanholder, R., Allolio, B., et al., on behalf of the Hyponatraemia Guideline Development Group, 2014. Clinical practice guideline on diagnosis and treatment of hyponatraemia. Eur J Endocrinol 17 (3), 1–47.

Stringer, T., Hasso, A.N., Thompson, J.R., et al., 1993. Hyperventilation-induced cerebral ischemia in patients with acute brain lesions: demonstration by xenon-enhanced CT. Am J Neuroradiol 14, 475–484.

Teasdale, G., Jennett, B., 1974. Assessment of coma and impaired consciousness, a practical scale. Lancet 2, 81–84.

van den Berg, B., Walgaard, C., Drenthen, J., et al., 2014. Guillain Barré syndrome: pathogenesis, diagnosis, treatment and prognosis. Nat Rev Neurol 10 (8), 469–482.

Van Egmond, M.E., Kuiper, A., Eggink, Sinke R., et al., 2015. Dystonia in children and adolescents: a systematic review and a new diagnostic algorithm. J Neurol Neurosurg Psychiatry 86, 774–781.

Wakai, A., McCabe, A., Roberts, I., et al., 2013. Mannitol for traumatic brain injury. Cochrane Database Syst Rev 8, CD001049.

White, J.R., Farukhi, Z., Bull, C., et al., 2001. Predictors of outcome in severely head-injured children. Crit Care Med 29, 534–540.

Williams, C., Asquith, J. (Eds.), 2000. Paediatric Intensive Care Nursing. Churchill Livingstone, London.

Wolf, V., Lupo, P.J., Lotze, T.E., 2012. Pediatric acute transverse myelitis overview and differential diagnosis. J Child Neurol 11, 1426–1436.

Yuki, N., Hartung, H.P., 2012. Guillain Barré syndrome. N Engl J Med 366 (24), 2294–2304.

Zhang, B.F., Wang, J., Lui, Z.W., et al., 2015. Meta-analysis of the efficacy and safety of therapeutic hypothermia in children with acute traumatic brain injury. World Neurosurg 83 (4), 567–573.

FURTHER READING

Foster, C., Nadel, S., 2002. New therapies and vaccines for bacterial meningitis. Expert Opin. Investig. Drugs 11, 1051–1060.

Society of Critical Care Medicine, 2003. Guidelines for the acute medical management of severe traumatic brain injury in infants, children and adolescents. Crit. Care. Med. Suppl 31, S417–S491.

ONCOLOGY EMERGENCY

7

Whilst the admission of children with a malignancy to a paediatric intensive care unit (PICU) is relatively rare at around 3% (PICANeT 2016), these children may be extremely sick and require specialist and urgent care. Admissions to the PICU may result from growth of a malignant tumour that causes pressure or obstruction and perhaps requires immediate surgery or, more commonly, from complications of treatment leading to severe electrolyte derangement and/or infection. This chapter will cover common conditions requiring PICU admission and snippets of valuable information when caring for a child receiving treatment for cancer. It is essential, of course, to seek expert advice and specialist guidance, but the following information will provide general principles and links to further specialist information available online.

CARING FOR AN ONCOLOGY PATIENT IN PAEDIATRIC INTENSIVE CARE UNIT – GENERAL PRINCIPLES

- Oncology patients have a significantly increased susceptibility to infection (if neutropenic).
- Nurse in a side room (and if neutropenic use positive pressure air flow).
- Chemotherapy may be excreted in body fluids for 7 days postadministration and therefore all waste should be considered cytotoxic and must be disposed of appropriately according to hospital protocol and while wearing personal protective equipment.
- Any cytotoxic spillage must be cleaned using a specific cytotoxic spillage kit.
- Intravenous (IV) line care must be fastidious (see below).
- Chemotherapy must be prescribed only by an experienced oncologist (usually on a specific chemotherapy drug chart) and administered by a specifically trained nurse.
- Blood transfusions: careful consideration must be taken regarding specific requirements; for example, leucocyte depleted, irradiated and cytomegalovirus (CMV)-negative. Check requirements with the oncology team.

CENTRAL VENOUS ACCESS

Children undergoing treatment for a malignancy will usually have some type of long-term central venous catheter (CVC) in situ. There are advantages and disadvantages to each, but the most common types include peripherally inserted central catheter (PICC), skin tunnelled cuffed CVCs (e.g., Hickman, Broviac, and implanted port, such as PORT-A-CATHs). The catheter tip usually sits in the superior vena cava just at the entrance to the right atrium.

GENERAL PRINCIPLES OF CARE OF LONG–TERM CENTRAL VENOUS CATHETERS

- Aseptic nontouch technique.
- Daily assessment of all IV lines for signs of infection.
- Change dressing at insertion site every 7 days, or more frequently if wet, soiled; use own hospital protocol (some centres change bungs on end of lines also).
- Clean access port/needle free hub with 70% alcohol, 2% chlorhexidine wipe for 30 seconds using vigorous friction rub and allow to dry naturally.
- Assess patency prior to giving drugs. Use 10-mL syringe of normal saline and flush in 2 mL and then withdraw to ensure blood can easily flow back and that the line is patent. Then flush more normal saline to clear the line of blood.
- 10-mL syringes should be used when first accessing any CVC as smaller syringes can exert high pressures, which can damage the catheter. Using a 10-mL syringe it is easier to feel back pressure from an occlusion (Conn 1993), but if a flush is easily given and blood is able to be withdrawn, then smaller syringes may be used to give drugs (Hadaway 1998).
- Turbulent flushes (a push–pause pulsing flush) may be used, which causes turbulent flow and will clear medication or blood components from the internal wall of the CVC (Dougherty & Lister 2008).
- The use of positive pressure flushing off helps to maintain CVC patency (RCN 2010).
- Heparin versus normal saline: the evidence for heparin flushes is inconclusive (UK Medicines Information 2012). Various centres have different practices regarding the use of normal saline or heparin and local policy should be adhered to.
- Consider the use of urokinase as thrombolytic if CVC is blocked; this may be left in the line or given as a very slow infusion (check local oncology protocol).

(For guidance about accessing a Port-A-Cath and care of a PICC line, see end of chapter – a reminder for trained staff only.)

CHEMOTHERAPY – COMMON SIDE EFFECTS

It is not within this guide's remit to describe chemotherapy regimes; refer to specialist information:
www.medicines.org.uk
However, it is useful to be aware of common side effects of chemotherapy agents. Many patients are treated according to established protocols and these should be made available to the PICU team.

Mucositis – this is characterised by pain, inflammation, and ulceration of the gastrointestinal (GI) tract from mouth to anus. It usually starts 5–10 days after the administration of chemotherapy (some patients who have had radiotherapy can develop mucositis). It can cause severe pain, reduced fluid and oral intake, altered taste perception and weight loss, and is particularly associated with increased risk of infection as mucosal barriers are breached. Treatment is largely supportive (analgesia and total parenteral nutrition if needed) along with meticulous and regular oral hygiene, mouthwash.

Do not use rectal probes or give drugs per rectum if the child has mucositis or is neutropenic.

Myelosuppression – This is a reduction in the bone marrow's ability to produce blood cells, which can lead to anaemia, neutropenia, and thrombocytopenia, which is usually a side effect of chemotherapy or radiotherapy (usually 7–10 days after). This can be life threatening due to the risks of bleeding and infection. A daily full blood count should be taken and if required blood and platelet transfusions may be given. Colony stimulating factor (CSF) may be used to accelerate neutrophil recovery (discuss with the oncology team). Erythropoietin is occasionally considered as an alternative to blood transfusion. Granulocyte (buffy coat) infusions may occasionally be considered for severe sepsis (must be discussed with the oncology team).

Nausea and vomiting – This may be caused by the cancer itself; for example, abdominal mass/bowel obstruction, a cancer-related cause (e.g., pain, blood in stomach), or a treatment-related cause (e.g., chemotherapy, opioids, or radiotherapy). It is important to elicit the cause so the appropriate antiemetic agent or combination of drugs can be prescribed. Assess the patient regularly and provide timely administration of antiemetic therapy.

Anaphylaxis and infusion-related reactions – Some chemotherapy drugs and many of the monoclonal antibodies have a relatively high risk of hypersensitivity reactions, which may range from mild to anaphylaxis (Table 7.1). Some chemotherapy regimens administer steroids and other drugs to minimise the risk of hypersensitivity reactions.

Table 7.1 Chemotherapy drugs with reports of immediate hypersensitivity reactions		
High Risk	**Common**	**Less Common**
Asparaginase	Docetaxel	Amsacrine
Paclitaxel	Carboplatin	Anthracyclines
Cetuximab	Oxaliplatin	Bleomycin
Rituximab	Pegylated liposomal doxorubicin	Cisplatin
Trastuzumab	Gemcitabine	Etoposide
		Melphalan
		Methotrexate
		Mitomycin C
		Bevacizumab

London Cancer. North and East, 2013. Guidelines for management of intravenous systemic anti-cancer therapy related hypersensitivity reactions including anaphylaxis. www.londoncancer.org/media/79795/London-C.

Signs and symptoms of hypersensitivity reaction/anaphylaxis:
- Skin reactions – urticarial, facial flushing, angioedema
- Rigors
- Pyrexia
- Tachycardia
- Rhinitis
- GI – nausea, vomiting, diarrhoea, abdominal pain
- Airway – tongue/throat swelling, stridor, hoarseness
- Breathing – increased respiratory rate, wheeze, hypoxia, cyanosis, decreased oxygen saturations less than 92%
- Circulation – hypotension, dizziness, reduced consciousness
  (See weblink for U.S. Department of Health and Human Services, National Institutes of Health and National Cancer Institute Table for Criteria for Common Toxicity, www.ctep.cancer.gov.)
  Paediatric Anaphylaxis Algorithm – in Resuscitation chapter

Extravasation – This is inadvertent leakage of a drug from the vascular pathway into the surrounding tissue with the potential for a mild skin reaction to severe necrosis possibly requiring amputation. Many drugs used in PICU can cause extravasation injury, including inotropes, antibiotics, concentrated electrolytes, hyperosmolar agents, and cytotoxic agents. As with all IV administration, the appropriately trained personnel should administer the medication, using the right patient, drug, prescription, route, at the right time, first ensuring the access device is clean, dry, well secured and in the vein, and all the correct checks should be carried out while the drug is infusing:
- Pressure setting set on pump
- Infusion site checked hourly or more frequently according to local protocols
- Pump pressures should be recorded
- A rise in pump pressure must be investigated
- The site of insertion of the IV device must be visible
- The child should be observed or asked about soreness or pain at the site; family concerns must be answered.

The following signs of infiltration/extravasation must be recognised by the team caring for the child and immediate action taken:
- Swelling
- Tenderness/discomfort/pain
- Taut skin
- Blanching at the cannula site
- Leakage of fluid at the insertion site
- Numbness or tingling/pins and needles
- Inability to withdraw blood where prior to infusion this had been possible
- Redness/blistering/tissue necrosis/ulceration (Dougherty & Lister 2008)

Immediate action is required:
- Stop the infusion/administration of the drug
- Aspirate as much of the residual drug as possible
- Disconnect drug and administration set, but keep it to ascertain how much drug has been administered

- DO NOT FLUSH THE CANNULA/PORT
- Explain your actions to the child/family
- Leave the IV device in situ (the plastic surgeon may use this to administer antidote)
- Draw around red/extravasated area with a felt-tip pen
- Inform senior doctor (and plastic surgeons if cytotoxic drug involved)
- Closely monitor site for colour, sensitivity, and swelling, and elevate if a limb is involved
- Administer analgesia if required
- Document in patient's notes
- Locate 'extravasation kit' if required
- If extravasation site deteriorates, re-refer to plastics team
- Specific management may depend on the nature of the extravasated drug; discuss with the oncology team urgently if a chemotherapy agent involved (Paediatric Haematology and Oncology: Supportive Care Protocols 2014).

Specific side effects

Nephrotoxicity – not all patients who are given nephrotoxic chemotherapeutic agents develop kidney injury, but risk factors for chemotherapy-induced nephrotoxicity include:

- Tumour lysis syndrome (TLS) – rapid destruction of tumour cells (usually lymphoma or leukaemia) and urate nephropathy
- Innate drug toxicity
- Tumour-related kidney effects; for example, obstruction
- Indirect renal involvement; for example, volume depletion (secondary to nausea, vomiting, and diarrhoea), effective volume depletion (cardiomyopathy, ascites), metabolic effects
- Patient factors; for example, age, underlying kidney injury, immune response
- Renal drug handling (Perazella 2012)

Drugs noted to have adverse renal effects include methotrexate, cisplatin, and ifosfamide.

Preventative measures and supportive care include monitoring electrolytes, IV fluids/hyperhydration, 2-mercaptoethane sulfonate Na (MESNA), electrolyte supplementation, forced diuresis, and in some cases dialysis.

Cardiotoxicity – Direct cardiotoxicity may result from anthracyclines chemotherapy agents (e.g., doxorubicin, daunorubicin) or from radiotherapy to the chest. This may result in cardiomyopathy, arrhythmias, myocardial ischaemia, hypertension, or thromboembolism. Different factors influence the incidence of cardiotoxicity and these include:

- Type of drug, dose, cumulative dose, administration schedule, route of administration, concomitant drug therapy, association with radiotherapy (but can occasionally occur, unpredictably, at low doses).
- Patient age, presence of cardiovascular disease, prior mediastinal radiotherapy (Bovelli et al 2010).

Table 7.2 Chemotherapy-induced cardiotoxic effects	
Drugs associated with congestive heart failure	Anthracyclines, anthraquinolones
	Cyclophosphamide
	Trastuzumab and other monoclonal antibody-based tyrosine kinase inhibitors
Drugs associated with ischaemia or thromboembolism	Antimetabolites (fluorouracil, capecitabine)
	Antimicrotubule agents (paclitaxel, docetaxel)
	Cisplatin
	Thalidomide
Drugs associated with hypertension	Bevacizumab
	Cisplatin
	Sunitinib, sorafenib
Drugs associated with other toxic effects	
Tamponade and endomyocardial fibrosis	Busulfan
Haemorrhagic myocarditis (rare)	Cyclophosphamide (high-dose therapy)
Bradyarrhythmias	Paclitaxel
Raynaud phenomenon	Vinblastine, bleomycin
Autonomic neuropathy	Vincristine
QT prolongation or torsades de pointes	Arsenic trioxide
Pulmonary fibrosis	Bleomycin, methotrexate, busulfan, high-dose cyclophosphamide

Bovelli, D., Plataniotis, G., Roila, F., 2010. Cardiotoxicity of chemotherapeutic agents and radiotherapy-related heart disease: ESMO Clinical Practice Guidelines. Ann. Oncol. 21(suppl 5), 277–282.

Onset may be acute after transfusion, within 1 year of therapy or up to 30 years after treatment (e.g., in anthracycline-induced cardiotoxicity the patient may present with dilated cardiomyopathy a year after treatment). Refer to Table 7.2 for reported chemotherapy induced cardiotoxic effects.

Neurotoxicity – Chemotherapy can damage the nervous system and this may be either the direct or indirect effect of the neurotoxic agents. The neurotoxicity effect is usually only temporary and resolves on cessation of treatment, but some effects may be permanent and therefore could have a significant effect on quality of life. Table 7.3 identifies chemotherapy agents associated with neurotoxicity (Nielsen and Brant 2002). Specific neurotoxicities that may require intensive care include:

- Methotrexate encephalopathy – occurring up to 3 weeks after IV or intrathecal methotrexate resulting in seizures, encephalopathy, or focal neurology – usually resolves with supportive management.
- Ifosfamide encephalopathy – acute encephalopathy occurring during or shortly after ifosfamide infusion. Treatment is with methylene blue.
- Posterior reversible encephalopathy syndrome (PRES) – may present with seizures, hypertension, encephalopathy, and visual disturbance – can occur after a number of different chemotherapy agents or steroids.

Table 7.3	Chemotherapy agents associated with neurotoxicity	
Drug	Neurotoxicity	Incidence, severity, dose dependence
Paclitaxel	Demyelination of nerve fibres	Dose level affects incidence and severity of neuropathic signs
Vincristine	Degeneration and atrophy of axons-peripheral nerve damage – numbness in extremities, paraparesis, urinary retention, constipation, myalgia, loss of pain and temperature sensation	Risk factors include doses exceeding 2 mg/m²
Cisplatin	Demyelination of nerve cells – burning sensations, loss of Achilles tendon and deep tendon reflexes, sensory ataxia	Neurotoxicities most often seen with a cumulative dose of 300–500 mg/m²
Cytarabine	Cerebellar dysfunction, encephalopathy, peripheral neuropathy, seizures	Doses exceeding 1 g/m² – usually there is recovery from neurologic sequelae within a few days after cessation of treatment
Ifosfamide	CNS toxicity – confusion, dizziness, cranial nerve dysfunction, seizures, coma	Incidence of CNS toxicity 12%, children more susceptible, recovery usually within few days of stopping treatment
Methotrexate	Demyelination of nerve fibres and CNS toxicities – headache, lethargy, nausea and vomiting, cranial nerve dysfunction	CNS toxicity seen when administered intrathecally. (Rarely, repeated intrathecal doses may result in progressive necrotising leucoencephalopathy)

CNS, Central nervous system.
Nielsen, E., Brant, J., 2002. Chemotherapy-induced neurotoxicity: assessment and interventions for patients at risk. Am. J. Nurs. 102, 16–19.

 In any oncology patient presenting with new neurology, it is also important to consider haemorrhage and infection in the differential diagnosis.

Hepatotoxicity – This is a liver injury associated with impaired function due to exposure to a drug. Patients receiving chemotherapy require careful assessment of their liver function prior to and during treatment as all patients are at risk of either:
• Direct chemotherapy-induced hepatotoxicity
• Altered hepatic drug metabolism
• Potentiation of preexisting liver disease
Hepatotoxic drug reactions are unpredictable due to immunologic mechanism or metabolic response. Preexisting health issues (e.g., immunosuppression, tumour, hepatitis, nutritional deficiencies, or total

parenteral nutrition) all can affect the liver's susceptibility to injury. Hepatotoxicity may manifest initially with vague clinical symptoms of fatigue, anorexia, nausea, dark urine, right upper quadrant pain, and jaundice. Other symptoms include steatosis, hepatic fibrosis, cirrhosis, and venoocclusion. Elevation in serum enzymes alanine aminotransferase (ALT) and alkaline phosphatase (ALP) indicate a liver injury, whereas an increase in prothrombin time, albumin concentration, and bilirubin levels measure overall liver function.

Many chemotherapy agents can induce hepatotoxicity, which may have transient and dose-related effects; these include methotrexate, cytarabine, L-asparaginase, cyclophosphamide, vincristine, etoposide, and antibiotics (e.g., doxorubicin, daunorubicin).

ONCOLOGY EMERGENCIES

Febrile neutropenia

Febrile neutropenia or neutropenic sepsis are terms often used interchangeably, but both lack a standard definition. Neutropenic sepsis is common, and potentially causes the deaths of over 1 in 500 people of all ages diagnosed with cancer, with the highest rate of increase of neutropenic sepsis deaths in the 15- to 24-year-old age group (Office of National Statistics 2001–2010). Patients at highest risk are those with:

- Prolonged and/or severe neutropenia ($<0.2 \times 10^9$/L)
- Co-existent mucositis
- Acute haematologic malignancies
- Chronic immunosuppression
- Indwelling CVC

Neutrophils are found in the blood and bone marrow and are an innate part of the immune system as they not only kill bacteria by phagocytosis, but also activate T cells (Nathan 2006). Neutrophils circulate in the blood for some time between 8 hours and 5 days (Pillay et al 2010). Bone marrow can be affected by chemotherapy, and the neutrophil count falls to its lowest level most commonly 5–7 days after the administration of chemotherapy (Holmes 2002).

The National Institute for Health Clinical Excellence (NICE 2012) identified a lack of consensus regarding its definition, prevention, diagnosis, and treatment, but summarised that it is often identified by:

- Neutropenia with a neutrophil count $\leq 0.5 \times 10^9$/L
- Fever 38°C (range of 37.5°C–39°C at some centres) (NICE 2012)

Presentation – neutropenia, fever, and typically warm shock; hypotension. Bounding pulses with a wide pulse pressure.

(NB: Consider chemotherapy induced cardiotoxicity; for example, anthracyclines such as doxorubicin.)

 NB RESPOND QUICKLY TO SIGNS OF INFECTION IN THE NEUTROPENIC PATIENT WITH BROAD-SPECTRUM ANTIBIOTICS. THIS IS LIFE SAVING.

Goals of management include early administration of broad-spectrum IV antibiotics and management of shock. Other recommendations include:

- A 'door to needle' time of 30–60 minutes for antibiotics to be given in neutropenic sepsis and shock (NCEPOD 2008; NCAG 2009)
- Early investigations – for example, blood cultures, serum lactate, and goal-directed resuscitation (Dellinger et al 2012)
- Meticulous examination of the child for infection (including line sites and perineum), infection screen, chest x-ray if clinically indicated, full blood count, C-reactive protein, coagulation, liver and renal function, and urinalysis in all children under 5 years
- Resuscitation – usually fluid responsive (60–100 mL/kg)
- Early inotrope support (first-line peripheral dopamine at 5–10 μg/kg/min, then noradrenaline at 0.1–1.0 μg/kg/min; may need new central venous line if the use of the indwelling vascular line causes instability)
- Early non-invasive ventilation for cardio-respiratory support
- Intubation if fluid- or inotrope resistant shock is evident
- After first-line antibiotics (piperacillin/tazobactam in 2- to 16-year-olds ± an aminoglycoside), consider liposomal amphotericin for suspected fungal infection (NICE 2012); however, local guidelines should be utilised, and previous positive microbiology considered (has there been any resistant organisms?)

The safety and efficacy of piperacillin/tazobactam has not been established in children 0–2 years.

- Consider removal of indwelling vascular device if there is refractory shock, bacterial showering, falling platelets
- Consult the oncology centre about the use of granulocyte-colony stimulating factor (G-CSF) (to stimulate bone marrow to produce white blood cells)
- Rectal temperature contraindicated due to a risk of bacterial translocation when the thermometer is inserted into the anus
- Protective isolation (positive air flow cubicle)

Tumour lysis syndrome

This is an acute metabolic derangement usually as a result of a rapid reduction in tumour mass with resultant rapid release of intracellular contents into the bloodstream following chemotherapy. TLS occurs most often in children with Burkitt lymphoma, acute lymphoblastic leukaemia, and non-Hodgkin lymphoma. It is characterised by:

- Hyperuricaemia (≥8 mg/dL)
- Hyperkalaemia (≥6 mmol/L)
- Hyperphosphataemia (≥6.65 mg/dL)
- Hypocalcaemia (≤7 mg/dL)

The Cairo-Bishop definition of TLS is the development of two or more of the above criteria within 3 days before or 7 days after the initiation of chemotherapy (Cairo & Bishop 2004). A consensus panel of experts subsequently identified a model of low-, medium- and high-risk TLS classifications and recommendations (Cairo et al 2010).

Children with TLS may present with life-threatening cardiac arrhythmias (hyperkalaemia), acute renal failure with a rise in creatinine to 1.5, the upper limit of normal, (hyperphosphataemia), muscle cramps, cardiac arrhythmias, seizures, and tetany (hypocalcaemia).

Preventative therapy is the goal with identification of the patients at risk prior to the administration of chemotherapy. Intravenous hydration is given to improve renal perfusion and glomerular filtration and to increase urine output, minimising the likelihood of uric acid or calcium phosphate precipitation in renal tubules. The use of rasburicase (rapidly breaks down serum uric acid) or allopurinol (decreases formation of new uric acid) is well documented in the Cochrane review (Cheuk 2010). However, if the child requires admission to the PICU, the mainstays of treatment will include:

- Close monitoring of electrolytes and careful correction – check serum electrolytes, phosphate, uric acid, calcium, and creatinine 4-hourly.
- If hyperkalaemia or hypocalcaemia is present – do 12-lead electrocardiogram and if cardiac arrhythmias or K+ ≥5.5, treat hyperkalaemia using the hyperkalaemia protocol (see below). Hypocalcaemia may be treated using IV calcium gluconate if symptomatic
- Rasburicase 0.05–0.2 mg/kg IV over 30 minutes for hyperuricaemia
- Aluminium hydroxide 50–150 mg/kg/24 h PO for phosphate ≥2.1 mmol
- Isotonic saline hydration (≤10 kg 200 mL/kg/day or >10 kg 3 L/m²/day) Reduce in acute renal failure and monitor Na+
- A diuretic may be used to maintain urine output (loop diuretic; e.g., frusemide may be preferable as this increases not only diuresis but also potassium secretion)
- Worsening renal function must be closely observed and the patient should be considered for early initiation of dialysis to control rapidly rising serum electrolytes
- Consider the need to modify drug dosages in the presence of renal insufficiency
- Intubation for cardiorespiratory compromise

Management of Hyperkalaemia (APLS 2016)

Principles of hyperkalaemia management (ALSG 2016) – algorithm in Resuscitation chapter

If K+ high plus arrhythmia – give calcium gluconate 0.1 mmol/kg IV

If no arrhythmia, give nebulised salbutamol (2.5–10 mg)

If repeat serum K+ high, assess pH and if pH <7.34 give sodium bicarbonate 1–2 mmol/kg IV or if pH >7.35 give 5 mL/kg glucose 10% and insulin 0.05 units/kg/hour IV

Calcium resonium 1 g/kg PO or PR may be used to remove K+ from the body (or dialysis)

Superior vena cava obstruction/syndrome

The superior vena cava (SVC) returns all blood from the head, neck, and upper limbs into the right atrium. SVC obstruction is mostly associated with advanced malignancy that causes gradual and increasing compression of the SVC. It can also be recognised with a more abrupt presentation in thrombotic events or secondary to defibrillator or pacemaker leads (Aryana et al 2007) and dialysis catheters (Greenwell et al 2007).

The high-risk tumours in paediatrics are lymphoblastic lymphoma and Hodgkin disease.

Presentation – the extent of obstruction and speed of development will dictate the presentation, since obstruction is better tolerated when the onset has been slow and the collateral veins have developed; however, this process usually takes several weeks. It is characterised by:

- Dilated veins in head, neck, and sometimes chest wall
- Facial plethora
- Dyspnoea
- Cough
- Chest pain
- Dysphagia (oedema around digestive tracts)
- Periorbital oedema
- Headaches (due to distension of cerebral vessels against dura)
- Cardiovascular compromise and raised intracranial pressure (ICP) (impeded venous return)
- Stridor (an alarming sign that there is narrowing of pharynx and larynx due to oedema)
  These symptoms may be worse if the patient is supine.

Diagnosis is made clinically and caution should be taken in undertaking computed tomography (CT) or magnetic resonance imaging (MRI) scans, which necessitate the patient lying flat.

Management requires prompt recognition of the syndrome but includes:

- Sitting the child up with face-mask oxygen
- Minimal handling and no sedation to avoid worsening obstruction
- Immediate consultant/senior anaesthetic review
- Upright chest x-ray (may need chest drain for large symptomatic effusions)
- IV access and diagnostic bloods
- General anaesthesia should be avoided where at all possible as the patient may decompensate with the induction of anaesthesia; intubate if absolutely necessary, for example, with decreased level of consciousness due to raised ICP, but be aware that intubation and ventilation may prove difficult.
- Treat intracranial hypertension with 3% saline (3 mL/kg)
- Neuroprotection if intubated (normal P_{co_2})

Malignant airway obstruction

Upper or lower airway obstruction can be caused by various paediatric malignancies including lymphomas, neuroblastoma, and germ cell tumours.

The obstruction may be due to external compression or infiltration of the tumour within the trachea and bronchi causing severe narrowing.

Presentation – symptoms may be nonspecific but include:
- Dyspnoea (most common symptom)
- Cough
- Wheeze
- Stridor
- Haemoptysis (reported in up to 45% of patients with obstructing tumours [Mathisen & Grillo 1989])

Symptoms may appear minimal until the airway is critically narrow – so clinical presentation does not reflect the degree of obstruction. This is a life-threatening situation (Chen et al 1998).

Symptoms are often worse at night, particularly when the patient is supine.

Diagnosis is made with chest x-ray and CT scans but airway obstruction should always be considered in patients with a history of malignancy and new respiratory symptoms (Lewis et al 2011). The priority, however, is careful and appropriate management with the most senior personnel:
- Sit the patient upright with face-mask oxygen
- Senior anaesthetic review
- HIGH-RISK INTUBATION – anaesthetic team and paediatric intensive care consultant to confer on timing, location, and induction required and 'difficult airway team/ENT (ear/nose and throat specialists)' to be involved; use reinforced tracheal tubes
- Bronchoscopy may be utilised as stents may be the treatment of choice in patients with acute airway compression secondary to extrinsic tumour compression (Wood 2003)
- Discuss the use of steroids before histology in severe cases (may interfere with histology so consider risk/benefit)

Spinal cord compression
This is a medical emergency that requires rapid diagnosis and treatment if permanent paralysis is to be avoided.

Spinal cord compression

When a primary cancer metastasises to the spine or epidural space, it can cause compression of the thecal sac and spinal cord. It is a common complication that can cause pain and potential irreversible loss of neurologic function and can affect almost 5% of cancer patients (Vachani 2006; Cole & Patchell 2008; Simon et al 2012).

Symptoms of spinal cord compression usually have an insidious progression and include:
- Back pain (most common symptom)
- Motor symptoms – fatigue, disturbance of gait, difficulty in walking

- Sensory – sensory loss and paraesthesia
- Autonomic dysfunction – neurogenic shock, paralytic ileus, loss of thermoregulation, drop in peripheral resistance causing hypotension
- Sphincter disturbances
- Cervical spine lesions can cause quadriplegia – with paralysis of the diaphragm requiring ventilation
- Thoracic spine lesions can cause paraplegia
- Lumbar spine; lesions can affect L4, L5 and sacral nerve roots
- Neurologic signs:
  - Lhermitte sign – flexion of the neck causes an electric shock type sensation, which radiates down the spine and into the limbs
  - Upper motor neurone signs in the lower limbs (Babinski sign – upgoing plantar reflex, hyperreflexia, clonus, spasticity)
  - Lower motor neurone signs in the upper limbs (atrophy, hyporeflexia)
  - Tendon reflexes may be absent at the level of the compression: increased below the level of compression and normal above the level of compression

Clinical features of spinal cord compression depend upon the extent and rate of development.

The gold standard for diagnosis is an MRI scan of the whole spine, unless there is a specific contraindication, within 24 hours in the case of spinal pain and any symptoms suggestive of spinal cord compression (NICE 2008).

Management and treatment include:

- Nurse supine with neutral spine alignment (log roll to turn) until bony and neurologic stability are ensured
- High-dose dexamethasone – can be started prior to imaging if there is a high level of clinical suspicion/neurologic signs.
- Urgent paediatric neurosurgical/oncology multidisciplinary team discussion should be held as whether to start urgent empirical chemotherapy or to surgically decompress. Chemotherapy may be started prior to the histologic confirmation of diagnosis if there is progressing neurology.
- Radiotherapy is rarely used at initial diagnosis but may be used in patients with relapsed disease.
- Analgesia
- Catheterise for bladder dysfunction
- Prophylaxis of venous thrombus
- Management of hypotension

Graft-versus-host disease

Graft-versus-host disease (GvHD) can be a major complication in allogenic stem cell transplant. It is an immune reaction where the donor's immune system attacks the recipients, and depending on the risk factors present, the incidence is 10–80% (Sullivan 2004). The Haemato-oncology subgroup of The British Committee for Standards in Haematology (BCSH) and The British Society of Blood and Marrow Transplantation (BSBMT) (2012) have made recommendations for the diagnosis and management of acute and chronic GvHD and organ-specific management of GvHD in both children and adults (Dignan et al 2012). At diagnosis, the grade of acute GvHD should be documented, detailing the extent of individual organ involvement as this has prognostic significance. Grading is 1–4.

Signs, symptoms, and diagnosis:

- Skin – the most common organ involved at the outset of acute GvHD with typically a maculopapular rash on the palms and soles, which can then spread over all the body. (In severe forms, it can appear like toxic epidermal necrolysis.)
- GI tract – diarrhoea, nausea, vomiting, anorexia, weight loss, abdominal pain
- Liver – jaundice, painful hepatomegaly, dark urine, pale stools, fluid retention, raised conjugated bilirubin, ALP and gamma-glutamyl-transpeptidase, bile acids, cholesterol – and in severe cases a coagulopathy, hyperammonaemia, and pruritis

Management of Grade 1 acute GvHD

- Skin GvHD is usually responsive to a topical steroid
- Optimise levels of calcineurin inhibitors
- Systemic therapy is not usually required
- Antihistamines are used for pruritis and topical tacrolimus (0.03%) may be used (not a licensed indication) in 2–15 year-olds (Dignan et al 2012)

Management of a GvHD Grade II–IV

- Seek specialist help
- These patients are likely to require systemic corticosteroids
- Second-line therapy includes the consideration of the cell-based immune modulatory approach and monoclonal antibodies, but falls outside the remit of this guide.

Venoocclusive disease (sinusoidal obstruction syndrome)

Venoocclusive liver disease (VOD), also known as sinusoidal obstruction syndrome due to associated characteristic histopathologic findings (De Leve et al 1999), occurs as a result of conditioning treatment administered prior to a stem cell transplant. Diagnosis is made based on clinical criteria shown in Table 7.4 including modified Seattle and Baltimore criteria (McDonald et al 1984; McDonald et al 1993; Jones et al 1987).

Table 7.4 Clinical criteria for venoocclusive disease	
Modified Seattle Criteria – within 20 days of transplant, two of the following must be present	Baltimore Criteria Bilirubin must be >34.2 µmol/L (2 mg/dL) within 21 days of transplant AND two of the following must be present
Bilirubin >34.2 µmol/L (2 mg/dL)	Hepatomegaly
Hepatomegaly or right upper quadrant pain	Ascites
Weight gain (>2% of pretransplant weight)	Weight gain (>5% of pretransplant weight)

VOD can be graded according to severity but these criteria can be assigned retrospectively. Paediatric patients are particularly at risk of VOD and those less than 6.7 years old were found to be at significant risk for VOD (Cesaro et al 2005).

Patients with severe VOD were found to have increased weight gain and jaundice early after transplant, and frequently developed respiratory, cardiac, or renal failure (McDonald et al 1993).

Treatment (Joint Working Group – recommendations of Haemato-oncology Subgroup of the BCSH and the BSBMT [Dignan et al 2012]).

- Defibrotide (has antithrombotic, antiinflammatory, and antiischaemic properties, protects against endothelial cell injury, but has not been associated with an increased risk of bleeding) is recommended in the treatment of VOD in children. This drug is unlicensed but is recommended in prophylaxis and treatment in VOD.
- Careful management of fluid balance and diuretic therapy in severe fluid overload.
- Early consultation with specialist hepatology and critical care is recommended. Tissue plasminogen activator (TPA) is not recommended due to the risk of haemorrhage. N-acetylcysteine is not routinely recommended due to lack of efficacy.

Oncology terminology

Autologous bone marrow transplant – the patient's own stem cells are collected and frozen and then infused back into the patient after they have received high-dose chemotherapy to eliminate cancer cells.

Allogenic bone marrow transplant – stem cells from a matched donor are harvested, stored, then infused into the patient. The patient will first receive high-dose chemotherapy to eliminate cancer cells and impair or destroy bone marrow function so that the donor cells are not rejected.

Specialist oncology drugs

Allopurinol is a xanthine oxidase inhibitor that prevents the development of uric acid in renal tubules, but it cannot break down existing uric acid, which is already deposited.

Defibrotide is a polydeoxyribonucleotide derived from porcine tissue and has antithrombotic, antiinflammatory, thrombolytic, and antiischaemic properties (Corbacioglu et al 2006).

G-CSF is a glycoprotein that stimulates the bone marrow to produce, mature, and activate neutrophils and then release them into the blood stream. It is used to help prevent infection and neutropenic fever caused by chemotherapy. The generic name is filgrastim.

MESNA is an organosulfur compound used as an adjuvant in chemotherapy involving cyclophosphamide and ifosfamide to protect the lining of the bladder.

Rasburicase is a recombinant urate oxidase which can reduce urate levels by metabolising urate to the more soluble compound, allantoin (Moreau 2005) (avoid in G6PD deficiency and known allergy to rasburicase).

Care of peripherally inserted central catheter line

Position – PICC lines may be in the scalp, external jugular, antecubital fossa, or long saphenous vein.

- The line tip should be OUTSIDE the heart on chest x-ray to avoid tamponade (at T2 if the PICC is in the upper limb, or below the diaphragm if the PICC is in the lower limb).
- BCSH determined that a chest x-ray must be performed to check the correct position before use (Bishop et al 2007).

Record – in notes, the date of insertion, length, insertion site, catheter tip position, and name of operator who inserted PICC.

Nursing Care – observe the site for signs of infection or line dislodgement and document findings:

- A transparent dressing should be used to cover the site, and this should be changed weekly after cleaning the site, using an aseptic nontouch technique if there are no signs of infection or oozing from the site
- Follow the manufacturer's guidance about catheter flushing protocol – some PICC lines may be used for blood taking, but some may not be used (follow manufacturers' guidance).
- Always use a 10-mL syringe (no smaller) and discuss the use of heparin or saline as evidence is ambiguous, but always use a pulsatile flush method (Vigier et al 2005).
- Neonatal and paediatric PICC lines may require continuous infusions to maintain patency.

Removal of a PICC line – the line should be pulled out slowly and gently to avoid line breakage; apply pressure to site for 5 minutes to stop bleeding:

- Check line length once removed to ensure the whole line has been removed
- Send line tip for microscopy and culture if required
- Inform doctor immediately if the line breaks or it has not been entirely removed
- Document in the patient's notes the date, time, and length of PICC line removed

Accessing a PORT-A-CATH (Smiths Medical)

PORT-A-CATHs may be placed in the arm or chest, but either way, the tip of the catheter should be properly positioned in the superior vena cava, and this must be confirmed by chest x-ray or fluoroscopy. If the portal is sited in an arm, avoid using this arm to withdraw blood unless using the portal, and avoid taking manual blood pressures to avoid potential damage. Only trained personnel should access a PORT-A-CATH (Fig. 7.1).

Access Needles – do not use standard hypodermic needles as they may cause damage to the septum; use only noncoring needles when accessing the portal. Use GRIPPER needles, which are either a safety Huber tip (a Huber needle is a hollow needle with an angle tip to prevent coring), or a noncoring safety needle with an extension set for infusions (Fig. 7.2).

Fig. 7.1 Injectable port.

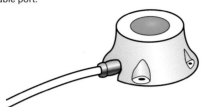

Fig. 7.2 Preferred GRIPPER needles (based on an image from Smiths Medical). (A) GRIPPER needle with injection cap Y-site. (B) GRIPPER PLUS needle with Luer-activated neddleless Y-site. (C) PORT-A-CATH 90° needle. (D) PORT-A-CATH straight needle. (E) GRIPPER PLUS POWER P.A.C. needle.

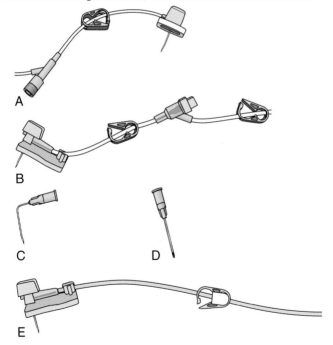

Accessing the portal

Equipment required: PORT-A-CATH GRIPPER noncoring needle set (with or without an extension set), mask, sterile gloves, antiseptic solution, 5-mL heparin solution (10–100 IU/mL), 10-mL syringes, 10-mL flush of normal saline, and transparent dressing.

It is essential to confirm portal and catheter integrity before any injection or infusion therapy, so follow these guidelines:

- Inquire and/or observe whether the patient has experienced any symptoms that might warn of catheter fragmentation and/or catheter embolisation since the system was last accessed; for example, shortness of breath, chest pain, or palpitations. If any of these are observed or reported, an x-ray is recommended to determine whether there are any problems with the catheter.
- Examine and palpate the portal pocket and catheter tract for erythema, swelling, or tenderness, which might indicate system leakage, and if this is suspected an x-ray is recommended.
- Set up the sterile field and supplies.
- Prepare the site by cleaning the skin with antiseptic solution per institutional policy.
- Anaesthetise the skin if required for needle puncture.
- Using a 10-mL or larger syringe, prime the noncoring PORT-A-CATH access needle and extension set to remove all air.
- Locate the portal by palpation. Immobilise the portal using thumb and fingers of the nondominant hand.
- Always access the portal at a 90° angle to the septum.
- Insert the needle steadily through the skin and portal septum until you feel the bottom of the portal. Do not tilt or rock the needle once the septum is punctured as this may cause fluid leakage or damage to the septum.
- Aspirate for blood return. Difficulty in withdrawing blood may indicate catheter blockage or improper needle position.
- Using a 10-mL or larger syringe, flush the system with 10 mL of normal saline, taking care not to exert excessive force to the syringe. Difficulty in injecting or infusing fluid may indicate catheter blockage. Observe the portal pocket and catheter tract whilst flushing to observe for swelling or pain; these symptoms could indicate fluid extravasation into the portal pocket or catheter tract.
- If the portal is not going to be used immediately, use either a heparin or saline lock, but follow local policies and procedures. (See Fig. 7.3.)

Fig. 7.3 GRIPPER needle inserted into septum at 90° angle (based on an image from Smiths Medical).

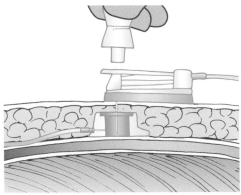

REFERENCES

Aryana, A., Sobota, K.D., Esterbrooks, D.J., et al., 2007. Superior vena cava syndrome induced by endocardial defibrillator and pacemaker leads. Am. J. Cardol. 99, 1765–1767.

Bishop, L., Dougherty, L., Bodenham, A., et al., 2007. Guidelines on the insertion and management of central venous access devices in adults. British Committee for Standards in Haematology. Int. J. Lab. Hematol. 29, 261–262.

Bovelli, D., Plataniotis, G., Roila, F., 2010. Cardiotoxicity of chemotherapeutic agents and radiotherapy-related heart disease: ESMO Clinical Practice Guidelines. Ann. Oncol. 21 (suppl. 5), 277–282.

Cairo, M.S., Bishop, M., 2004. Tumour lysis syndrome: new therapeutic strategies and classification. Br. J. Haematol. 127 (1), 3–11.

Cairo, M.S., Coiffer, B., Reiter, A., et al., 2010. Recommendations for the evaluation of risk and prophylaxis of tumour lysis syndrome (TLS) in adults and children with malignant diseases: an expert TLS panel consensus. Br. J. Haematol. 149, 578–586.

Cesaro, S., Pillon, M., Talenti, E., et al., 2005. A prospective survey on incidence, risk factors and therapy of hepatic veno-occlusive disease in children after hematopoietic stem cell transplantation. Haematologica. 90, 1396–1404.

Chen, K., Varon, J., Wenker, O.C., 1998. Malignant airway obstruction: recognition and management. J. Emerg. Med. 16 (1), 83–92.

Cheuk, D.K.L., Chiang, A.K.S., Chan, G.C.F., et al., 2010. Urate oxidase for the prevention and treatment of tumour lysis syndrome in children with cancer. Cochrane. Database. Syst. Rev. 6, CD006945.

Cole, J.S., Patchell, R.A., 2008. Metastatic epidural spinal cord compression. Lancet. Neurol 7 (5), 459–466.

Conn, C., 1993. The importance of syringe size when using an implanted vascular access device. J. Vasc. Access Networks. 3, 11–18.

Corbacioglu, S., Honig, M., Lahr, G., et al., 2006. Stem cell transplantation in children with infantile osteopetrosis is associated with a high incidence of VOD, which could be prevented with defibrotide. Bone. Marrow. Transplant. 38, 547–553.

De Leve, L.D., McCuskey, R.S., Wang, X., et al., 1999. Characterisation of a reproducible rat model of hepatic veno-occlusive disease. Hepatology 29, 1779–1791.

Dellinger, R.P., Mitchell, M., Levy, M.D., et al., 2012. Surviving Sepsis Campaign; international guidelines for the management of severe sepsis and septic shock. Crit. Care. Med. 41 (2), 580–637.

Dignan, F.L., Clark, A., Amrolia, P., et al., 2012. Diagnosis and management of acute graft-versus-host disease. Haemato-oncology Task Force of the British Committee for Standards in Haematology and the British Society for Blood and Marrow Transplatation. Br. J. Haematol. 1–16.

Dougherty, L., Lister, S., 2008. Drug administration cytotoxic drugs. In: The Royal Marsden Hospital Manual of Clinical Nursing Procedures, seventh ed. Wiley Blackwell, Oxford.

Greenwell, M.W., Basye, S.L., Dhawan, S.S., et al., 2007. Dialysis catheter induved superior vena cava syndrome and downhill esophageal varices. Clin. Nephrol. 67, 325–330.

Hadaway, L., 1998. Major thrombotic and nonthrombotic complications: loss of patency. J. Intraven. Nurs. 21, 5.

Holmes, F.A., Jones, S.E., O'Shaughnessy, J., et al., 2002. Comparable efficacy and safety profiles of once-per-cycle pegfilgrastim and daily injection filgrastim in chemotherapy-induced neutropenia: a multicentre dose-finding study in women with breast cancer. Ann. Oncol. 13 (6), 903–909.

Jones, R.J., Lee, K.S., Beschomer, W.E., et al., 1987. Venoocclusive disease of the liver following bone marrow transplantation. Transplantation 44 (6), 778–783.

Lewis, M.A., Hendrickson, A.W., Moynihan, T.J., 2011. Oncologic emergencies: pathophysiology, presentation, diagnosis and treatment. CA. Cancer. J. Clin. 61, 287–314.

London Cancer. North and East, 2013. Guidelines for management of intravenous systemic anti-cancer therapy related hypersensitivity reactions including anaphylaxis. www.londoncancer.org/media/79795/London-C.

Mathisen, D.J., Grillo, H.C., 1989. Endoscopic relief of malignant airway obstruction. Ann. Thorac. Surg. 48, 469–475.

McDonald, G.B., Hinds, M.S., Fisher, L.D., et al., 1993. Veno-occlusive disease of the liver and multi-organ failure after bone marrow transplantation: a cohort study of 355 patients. Ann. Int. Med. 118, 255–267.

McDonald, G.B., Sharma, P., Matthews, D.E., et al., 1984. Veno-occlusive disease of the liver after bone marrow transplantation: diagnosis, incidence, and predisposing factors. Hepatology 4, 116–122.

Moreau, D., 2005. Pharmacological treatment of acute renal failure in intensive care patients. Contrib. Nephrol. 147, 161–173.

Nathan, C., 2006. Neutrophils and immunity: challenges and opportunities. Nat. Rev. Immunol. 6 (3), 173–182.

National Chemotherapy Advisory Group, 2009. Chemotherapy Services in England: Ensuring quality and safety a report from the National Chemotherapy Advisory Group. http://www.theacp.org.uk/news/22-aug-2009-ncag-report-published.asp?term=Chemotherapy+services+in+England%3A+Ensuri.

National Institute for Health and Clinical Excellence, 2008. Metastatic spinal cord compression: diagnosis and management of adults at risk of and with metastatic spinal cord compression. NICE guideline CG75. www.nice.org.uk.

National Institute for Health and Clinical Excellence, 2012. Neutropenic sepsis: prevention and management of neutropenic sepsis in cancer patients. NICE clinical guideline 151. www.nice.org.uk.

NCEPOD, 2008. For better or worse: a review of the care of patients who died within 30 days of receiving systemic anti-cancer therapy. http://www.ncepod.org.uk/2008sact.html.

Nielsen, E., Brant, J., 2002. Chemotherapy-induced neurotoxicity: assessment and interventions for patients at risk. Am. J. Nurs. 102, 16–19.

Office of National Statistics 2001–2010. http://www.statistics.gov.uk/hub/index.html.

Paediatric Haematology and Oncology: Supportive Care Protocols, 2014. A collaborative publication from Great Ormond Street Hospital for Children NHS Foundation Trust, The Royal Marsden NHS Foundation Trust, fourth ed. University College Hospital NHS Foundation Trust. www.londoncancer.org/media81610/Supportive-Care-Protocol-4th-Edition.

Perazella, M.A., 2012. Onco-nephrology: renal toxicities of chemotherapeutic agents. Clin. J. Am. Soc. Nephrol. 7, 1713–1721.

PICANeT, 2016. Annual Report. Paediatric Intensive Care Audit Network. www.picanet.org.

Pillay, J., den Braber, I., Vrisekoop, N., et al., 2010. In vivo labelling with $2H_2O$ reveals a human neutrophil lifespan of 5.4 days. Blood 116 (4), 625–627.

Royal College of Nursing (RCN), 2010. Standards for Infusion Therapy. www.rcn.org.uk/_data/assets/pdf_file/0005/78593/002179.pdf.

Simon, T., Niemann, C.A., Hero, B., et al., 2012. Short and longterm outcome of patients with symptoms of spinal cord compression by neuroblastoma. Dev. Med. Child. Neurol. 54 (4), 347–352.

Smiths Medical. www.smiths-medical.com

Sullivan, K.M., 2004. Graft-vs-host disease. In: Blume, K.G., Forman, S.J., Appelbaum, F.R. (Eds.), Thomas' Haematopoietic Cell Transplantation. Blackwell Publishing Ltd, Oxford, pp. 635–664.

United Kingdom Medicines Information, 2012. Should heparin based flushing solutions be used in preference to saline to maintain the patency of indwelling intravascular catheters and cannulae?.Available at: www.evidence.nhs.uk/search?q=%22Should+heparin+based+flushing+solutions+be+used+in+preference+to+saline%22.

United States Department of Health and Human Services, National Institutes of Health, National Cancer Institute, 2010. Common Terminology Criteria for Adverse Events (CTCAE) Version 4.03. www.ctep.cancer.gov.

Vachani, C., 2006. Spinal cord compression. OncoLink. www.oncolink.org.

Vigier, J.P., Merckx, J., Coquin, J.Y., et al., 2005. The use of hydrodynamic bench for experimental simulation of flushing venous catheters: impact on the technique. Rev. Eur. de. Techn. Biomed. 26 (2), 147–149.

Wood, D., 2003. Airway stenting. Chest. Surg. Clin. North. Am. 13, 211–229.

FLUIDS AND NUTRITION

8

It is important to weigh children or appropriately calculate their weight on admission to hospital as this provides the base for fluid administration and drug doses. Table 8.1 therefore gives mean weights of babies and children on the 50th centile, which can be used as a guide, or can be calculated using the following guideline for estimated weight. Special care is required when prescribing for neonates because there is an increased risk of toxicity due to reduced drug clearance. Also note that for most drugs, the adult maximum drug dose should not be exceeded when prescribing for children. If children are overweight, ideal weight related to height and age should be used to calculate drug doses (BNF for Children 2015–2016).

GUIDELINES TO CALCULATE ESTIMATED WEIGHT

Estimated body weight in a child aged younger than 12 years (APLS 2016)
Weight 0–1 year old = (Age in months / 2) + 4
Weight 1–5 years = (Age in years × 2) + 8
Weight 6–12 years = (Age in years × 3) + 7

Table 8.2 shows recommended daily energy requirements for healthy infants and children. Table 8.3 is a guide to fluid requirements per 24 hours according to the weight of the infant or child and includes average (standard) fluid requirement and ½ average. This chart serves as a guide for fluid administration, which should be adjusted to suit the patient's clinical condition. It is important to note that if children are given intravenous (IV) maintenance fluids in hospital, serum sodium should be measured daily to identify and treat hyponatremia before the patient develops symptoms (e.g., seizures) (Holliday et al 2004).

- Increased fluids may be required in patients with a pyrexia, with burns, undergoing phototherapy, or to replace lost volume
- Decreased fluids may be necessary in patients following cardiac surgery or patients in renal or heart failure.
  - ½ average recommended for children at risk of syndrome of inappropriate antidiuretic hormone (SIADH), including patients with bronchiolitis and other respiratory infections, postoperative patients and children on opiates and ventilation. SIADH is explained in detail in the Handy Hints chapter.

Table 8.1   Guide to weight: mean weight of babies and children on 50th centile

Age	Mean weight (kg)
Newborn term	3.5
3 months	6.1
6 months	7.6
1 year	9.0
3 years	14
5 years	18
7 years	23
10 years	32
12 years	39
14 years	49–50

Source: BNFC 2015–2016 – derived from UK WHO growth charts 2009 and UK 1990 standard centile charts by extrapolating 50th centile.

Table 8.2   Estimated average daily energy requirement by age

Age	Kilocalories/24 h
1–2 months	502–574
3–4 months	550–598
5–6 months	574–622
7–12 months	646–718
3 years	1076–1171
6 years	1482–1577
9 years	1721–1840
12 years	2103–2247
15 years	2390–2820

The lower end of the range refers to females and the upper end refers to males.
Source: Scientific Advisory Committee on Nutrition (SACN), 2011. Dietary reference values for energy. London <www.sacn.gov.uk accessed> (accessed 09.05.17.)

Table 8.3   Fluid requirements: maintenance recommendations

Weight	Average/day (mL/kg/day)	½ Average/day (mL/kg/day)	Average (mL/kg/hour)	½ Average (mL/kg/hour)
2–10 kg	100	50	4	2
10–20	80	40	3	1.5
20–50	50	25	2	1
>50 kg*	2500 mL/day *NOT per kg	1250 mL/day *NOT per kg	100 mL/h *NOT per kg	50 mL/h *NOT per kg

* = NOT per kg (For children > 50 kg a total daily fluid allowance recommended which is not based on their weight)
Modified from Holliday, M.A., Friedman, A.L., Segar, W.E., Chesney, R., Finbery, L., 2004. Acute hospital-induced hyponatremia in children: a physiologic approach. J. Paediatr. 145, 584–587.

ENTERAL FEEDING

The benefits of early enteral feeding in the critical care setting are well known (Kreymann et al 2006; Nguyen et al 2008; Marik 2014; Mehta 2014; Mikhailov 2014). The gut has an important immunomodulatory role in critical illness, which is aided by enteral feeding. Beneficial effects include stimulation of mucosal blood flow, regulating gut permeability by maintaining normal intercellular channel function, and limiting pathogenic bacterial overgrowth via promoting (1) release of bile salts, (2) secretory immunoglobulin A (IgA) production from gut-associated lymphoid tissue, and (3) stimulation of peristalsis. When infants or children are admitted to paediatric intensive care, enteral feeding is commenced whenever possible and usually within the first 24–48 hours. Many units have developed practice guidelines to facilitate establishment of full enteral feeding and encourage teams to consider feeding within the first 2 hours of admission or at the start of each shift. A novel guideline introduced in Evelina London Children's Hospital (ELCH) following three prospective audits (one preintroduction and two post guideline) used individual gastric emptying time (GET) and showed by enterally feeding patients in accordance to their individual GETs pursuant to the ELCH Guideline, they were:

 (a) **fed more**
 (b) **fed earlier**
 (c) **fed primarily by 2–6-hourly bolus feeds or continuous nasojejunal feeding**, instead of hourly bolus feeds or continuous nasogastric (NG) feeding (Knight et al 2015)

Rationale for this guideline is twofold. First, it seeks to minimise gastric distension. Gastric distension increases the release of amylin, an amino acid cosecreted with insulin, which potently inhibits gastric motility (Mayer et al 2002; Kairamkonda et al 2008). This guideline seeks to minimise gastric distension and so minimise the release of amylin by BOLUS feeding each patient by reference to and NO FASTER than their individual GET. Secondly, feeding by reference to gastric residual volumes is justified. If feed is being tolerated, gastric aspirates will be 0–6% of the original feed; if not being tolerated, gastric aspirates may be 261–494% (Mayer et al 2002; Kairamkonda et al 2008). If tolerated, provided you feed NO FASTER than the individual's GET, the feed should have all been absorbed by the end of that GET. Therefore if an individual's GET is 4 hours, it does not matter whether you give 30 mL or 90 mL, by the end of the 4 hours, it should have been absorbed.

The ELCH Pediatric Intensive Care Unit (PICU) Guideline, in Fig. 8.1, entails two steps. First, define the individual's GET by (1) aspirating the patient's stomach, discarding this aspirate, and then giving a test feed of 2 mL/kg, additional to his or her fluid allowance for that hour; and (2) aspirating the stomach (returning the aspirate each time) every 2 hours, for up to 6 hours, to see how quickly the test feed is absorbed. The individual's GET is defined as when more than 50% of the test feed has been absorbed.

Secondly, commence bolus feeding immediately the GET is defined, at the frequency equal to the individual's GET, 2, 4, or 6 hourly. The

Fig. 8.1 Enteral feeding guideline based upon individual gastric emptying times. (From references Knight et al 2015; Mayer et al 2002; Jabbar et al 2003; McClave 2006; Skillman & Mehta 2012; Marik 2014.)

PICU: Enteral Feeding using Gastric Emptying Times (GET)

The aim is to initiate enteral feeding as soon as possible, UNLESS CONTRAINDICATED, by reference to each individual's GET Feeding NO faster than the individual's GET minimises gastric distension and production of amylin, an amino acid which potently inhibits gastric motility.

Contra-indications: bowel obstruction; surgical plan specifically excludes enteral feeding; severe vomiting; pre-surgery or pre extubation (6 hours before for solid food, fizzy drink or milk feed; 4 hours before for EBM; 2 hours before for clear fluid); and first 48 hours post aortic arch surgery. NB Feeding should be recommended post extubation as soon as clinically appropriate following a doctor's review.

STEP. 1: Define the individual's GET

(a) Aspirate the stomach and DISCARD the aspirate. Chart this discard.

(b) Give a test bolus feed of 2 mL/kg (up to a maximum of 80 mL) via an NG. DO NOT count this as part of the fluid allowance for that hour; it is extra; but DO chart this test feed, adding it into the input for that hour.

(c) Aspirate the stomach every 2 hours (for up to 6 hours) and return the aspirate. The individual's GET is the time when > 50% of the test feed has been absorbed.

(d) If the GET is > 6 hours, assume gastroparesis; do NOT feed gastrically; pass a naso-jejunal tube and feed jejunally (see NJ guideline)

STEP. 2: Establish a feeding regime.

(a) Follow this unless a specific alternative regime has been set by the metabolic team.

(b) Immediately start bolus feeding at the frequency of the individual's GET (2, 4 or 6 hourly). If a baby of < 5 kg and the GET is 6 hours, please discuss with the doctors continuing some IV fluid to maintain an appropriate blood glucose.

(c) Prior to every bolus feed (other than the test feed in Step.1) aspirate the NG and REPLACE the aspirate.

Fig. 8.1, cont'd

(d) Each bolus should be the maximum allowed within the individual's
   fluid allowance.

(e) Once the feeding regime is well established, the aim is to normalise
   feeding frequency relative to:

- (a) age (<1 month: 2 hourly; 1–12 months: 2–4 hourly; >12 months:
   4–6 hourly)

- (b) the individual's norm (e.g. bolus feeding in the day and
   continuous at night). So, as appropriate, check aspirates
   between feeds to see if the GET has decreased or try feeding
   less often. Also, promptly patient is extubated or chronic patient
   is stabalised discuss liberating feed allowance with the doctors.

(f) If on aspirating the NG > 50% of the last bolus feed remains, return
   the aspirate, wait 2 hours and then re-aspirate. If the next
   aspirate is minimal, consider it a one-off change and continue
   bolus feeding as before. If the aspirate is still > 50% of the last
   bolus feed go back to STEP.1 and re-define the GET and
   consider re-commencing IV maintenance while doing this.

Miscellaneous:

• If a gastrostomy is in situ, still consider passing an NG so aspirates
   can be measured more accurately.

• Infection control: ALWAYS use non-touch clean technique; limit total
   hang-time to 24 hours for sterile feeds (i.e. spiked bags) and
   4 hours for decanted/non-sterile feeds; change giving set every
   24 hours; see local guidelines: storage and identification of
   expressed breast milk.

amount of each bolus is the individual's feed allowance multiplied by
the individual's GET. For example, an individual permitted 10 mL an
hour of enteral feed within his hourly fluid allowance will be given 20
mL 2-hourly if his GET is 2 hours, 40 mL 4-hourly if his GET is 4
hours, or 60 mL 6-hourly if his GET is 6 hours.

If 50% or more of the test feed remains unabsorbed within 6 hours,
gastroparesis is presumed and jejunal feeding, which is always continuous, is commenced as soon as practicable. Jejunal feeds may be absorbed
whether there are bowel sounds or the stomach is working (Jabbar et al
2003; McClave 2006; Marik 2014).

GET may be influenced by feed composition – aqueous, breast milk,
formula, semisolid, and solid feed were found to have increasing mean

gastric residence times (Bonner et al 2015) – method of feeding (tube feed versus oral) (Chen et al 2013) and also drugs affecting motility.

Nasogastric tube placement and use

Because many children in PICU are sedated and ventilated, NG tubes are usually inserted to enable enteral feeding and the administration of oral medication and to reduce gastric distention. There is a small risk that the NG tube may be misplaced into the lungs on insertion or that the tube may become displaced out of the stomach at any stage. Between 2011 and 2016 there were a reported 95 'Never Events' where a misplaced NG tube was not detected before use (The National Patient Safety Agency 2016). It is therefore vital that staff consider the following before feeding via the NG tube.

CORRECT METHODS

- Measuring the pH of aspirate using pH indicator strips is recommended (feeding can commence if pH is 5.5 or less).
- Radiography is recommended but should not be used routinely.

 None of the existing methods for testing the position of NG tubes is totally reliable.

- Carry out an individual risk assessment prior to administering anything via the NG tube, at least once daily and following episodes of vomiting, retching, or coughing.
- Note and document length of NG tube and mark correctly placed NG tube at nares.
- Review and agree local action required.
- Report misplaced incidents via local risk management reporting systems (National Patient Safety Agency 2005).

Fig. 8.2 represents the correct procedure for commencing NG feeds.

Gastrostomy use and care

Gastrostomies may be placed percutaneously via endoscopy (percutaneous endoscopic gastrostomy [PEG]), via laparoscopic (LAP) techniques including LAP-assisted PEG, and standard open gastrostomy methods (Akay 2010). The reasons for gastrostomy insertion include feeding problems in children with neurodisabilities, special feeding requirements for children with metabolic conditions, and continuous feeding to improve growth (e.g., in children with short gut or chronic renal failure).

The following information represents general care of a gastrostomy and is not specific postoperative care. Any gastrostomy requires a good

Fig. 8.2 Confirming the correct position of nasogastric feeding tubes in infants and children. Published by the National Patient Safety Agency in *Patient Safety Alert 05,* February 2005 (see www.npsa.nhs.uk/advice). The flowchart was developed to provide staff with a guide to minimise risk in placing nasogastric feeding tubes; however, staff should continue to make decisions based on individualised risk assessment appropriate to local circumstances, and to seek clinical and/or professional advice where necessary.

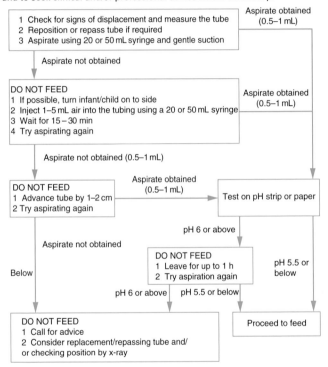

transabdominal and intragastric seal. When the stoma site is completely healed, then most gastrostomy tube manufacturers recommend that the tube should be rotated 360° once a week by holding the tube vertically to ensure the skin does not adhere to the gastrostomy unless fitted with a jejunal extension, because rotation could displace it. Use local policies and specific manufacturer's instructions to guide care, but here are a few pointers:

• At least 6 weeks after insertion, once a week, the tube should be moved gently in and out by 2–3 cm to prevent buried bumper syndrome. The bumper can become buried as soon as 3 weeks after surgery. Buried bumper presents as feeding problems, leak at the site or pain. If the bumper does become buried, it should be removed immediately to prevent perforation of the stomach and peritonitis (Rahnemai-Azar 2014).

- For balloon gastrostomies, a weekly balloon check is required. Deflate the balloon using a 10-mL syringe and record the volume of aspirate. If the volume is correct, reinflate using the correct volume of sterile water or cooled boiled water. If aspirate is less than the expected volume according to the product guide, reinflate using cooled boiled or sterile water, wait 10 minutes and reaspirate to see if any fluid has leaked. If still leaking, this may indicate that a new balloon gastrostomy is required.
- Keep gastrostomy sites clean and dry – clean and inspect site daily for signs of infection or leakage.
- Access balloon port only for weekly check.
- Use a 10-mL or larger syringe for flushing pre and post medications.
- Rinse any equipment to be reused (e.g., connectors) in sterile water and leave out to air dry.
- In case of tube blockage, NEVER force a flush. Try to draw back any free fluid. Turbulent flush gently with warm water and leave for 30 minutes. If still blocked, try using carbonated water or specific solutions recommended by the local surgical team.
- If the tube falls out, act immediately so that the stoma does not close. Reinsert balloon gastrostomy and tape to abdomen until it can be replaced, or in the case of a PEG, replace with an NG tube inserted 2–3 cm into the stoma and taped to abdomen; in either case, ask for relevant help.
- Site granulomas – seek guidance because topical prescriptions may be indicated.

Insertion and care of a nasojejunal tube

If gastric motility is impaired, enteral feeds may be optimised by feeding jejunally because the small intestine's motility and absorption can remain satisfactory with or without bowel sounds (Marik 2014).

How to insert a nasojejunal (NJ) tube (adapted from Meyer et al 2007):

1. Ensure an NG tube is in situ.
2. Explain procedure to child and family.
3. Collect equipment – polyurethane silk NG tube, radiopaque without a weighted tip and ideally chilled, 2 × 50 mL oral syringes, a 10-mL syringe, pH paper, measuring tape, sterile water, DuoDERM and Tegaderm or other such securing tape
4. Measure insertion length (Ellet & Beckstrand 2001):
   (a) Gastric length – tip of nose to edge of ear by cheek to halfway between xiphisternum and umbilicus
   (b) Jejunal length – tip of nose to edge of ear by cheek to xiphisternum to iliac crest plus 5 cm (Fig. 8.3)

Fig. 8.3 Measuring nasojejunal tube length. (From Knight, D., Durward, A., Tibby, S., Stanley, I., 2015. Evaluation of novel feeding guideline based on individual gastric emptying times shown by 3 prospective audits. PICS Conference, UK Paediatric Intensive Care Society, Birmingham 2015.)

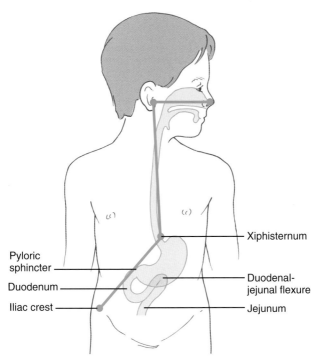

Pyloric sphincter

Duodenum

Iliac crest

Xiphisternum

Duodenal-jejunal flexure

Jejunum

5. Use clean technique throughout.
6. Position the patient: elevate bed head to 30°, clinical condition permitting, put patient left side up and with head midline, slightly anteroflex neck (i.e., chin toward chest).
7. BEFORE inserting, lubricate NJ tip with sterile water and push guidewire right in.
8. Insert NJ into the stomach initially through either nostril, and confirm gastric placement as per your unit guideline (to provide something to aspirate, 10–20 mL of sterile water may be put down the original NG tube). ONLY AFTER gastric placement has been confirmed, flush NJ with 10 mL of water to lubricate guidewire and leave in situ. NEVER lubricate guidewire before gastric placement is confirmed, because lubricant alters the pH (NPSA 2012).

9. Insert NJ into jejunum only after gastric placement is confirmed:
   (a) Empty and decompress the stomach by aspirating the old NG and gently pressing down on the stomach.
   (b) Advance the NJ tube slowly, 1 cm at a time, rotating it close to the nostril. Having a 50-mL syringe on the NJ may help rotation. Continuous low-grade resistance should be felt on advancing through the pylorus and small intestine.
   (c) On reaching the jejunal length, with or without the guidewire in, do the NJ air-test (see later). If the NJ air-test fails, pull the NJ back to the gastric length and try repassing – it often takes several attempts. If the NJ air-test is passed, x-ray before use. (See Fig 8.4 for x-ray showing correct placement of NJ.) Only after x-ray confirmation that NJ is in the correct position should the guidewire be removed. You can NEVER REINSERT the guidewire when the tube is in the patient (per manufacturer's instructions).

Nasojejunal tubes: checking position

WHEN to check:
- On initial placement
- Before commencing any continuous feed

Fig. 8.4 X-ray showing correct placement of a nasojejunal tube (post pyloric if it crosses across the spine twice; jejunal if it then goes through 360° as it passes the duodenal flexure).

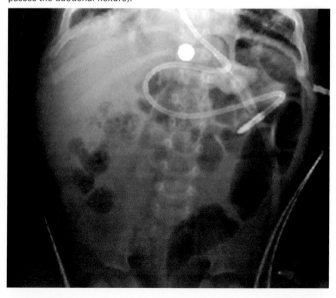

- If clinical judgment indicates that the NJ may have migrated upward (e.g., post coughing or vomiting), or new unexplained respiratory symptoms

If you have any concerns about position, do not commence or continue feeds until you are confident it is in the correct position.

HOW to check:

- NJ air-test. Insert 8–10 mL of air slowly down NJ and immediately aspirate it. If <2 mL is aspirated, this indicates it is post pyloric (Harrison et al., 1997). For new insertions, position must be confirmed by x-ray before use. If air cannot be inserted, the NJ is probably kinked or coiled.
- X-ray for all new insertions before use and in exceptional cases to clarify NJ position. Routine x-rays should include the abdomen for any patient with an NJ in situ.
- Other indicators of NJ placement should be used with caution, NOT as primary clarification:
  - External length
  - NJ aspirates – difficult to obtain, usually pH of ≥6, yellow or greenish brown due to bile staining, but once feed has started, aspirates look like feed.

Extra Considerations:

- Always feed continuously; never bolus feed, because the small intestine responds poorly to distension. There is no need for a break, so feed continuously 24 hours/day.
- If feeding via NJ route, aspirate the NG every 4 hours to check whether there is any feed in stomach, which would indicate that the NJ has migrated into the stomach.
- Always have an NG in situ for giving most oral medications, aspirating the stomach as required.
- Document the date of NJ insertion, length at nose, size.

TYPES OF FEEDING AND PRODUCTS AVAILABLE

Breastfeeding is the best form of nutrition for infants. Exclusive breastfeeding is recommended for the first 26 weeks of life, then from 6 months, breastfeeding alongside complementary foods (WHO 2003). However, there are many suitable formulas available to give a baby who for whatever reason cannot be breastfed. Suitable products appropriate to age and weight for children in hospital who are unable to eat normally are discussed as follows.

Infant milks and children's feed
USE OF MILK PRODUCTS AND CHILDREN'S FEEDS

All infant formula milk feeds contain protein, fats, carbohydrates, vitamins, and minerals.

- Younger than 6 months, breastfeed or use first baby milk formula, as preferred.
- 6–12 months use first milk formula as previous plus varied complementary foods

PREMATURE BABIES

Premature babies have higher energy requirements (110–135 kcal/kg/day) compared with term infants (96–120 kcal/kg/day) (Agostoni et al 2010). Breast milk is the feed of choice, but added minerals and vitamins will also be required. If formula feed is required, the following are available in the United Kingdom.

Preterm babies with birthweight less than 2 kg

- SMA Pro Gold Prem 1, Nutriprem 1, Hydrolysed Nutriprem

Preterm babies greater than 2 kg until 6 months corrected gestational age

- SMA Pro Gold Prem 2, Nutriprem 2.

FULL-TERM BABIES

High energy for infants

These should be used only under dietetic supervision:
- Infatrini, SMA high energy formula, Similac High Energy

Whey-based milks

These are the closest in composition to breast milk and are recommended for the first year if formula feeding is preferred. These may have either cow's milk or goat's milk protein as the main protein source, and they have been found to be equivalent in terms of safety and allergenicity. These include cow milk based:
- SMA Pro First Infant milk, Cow & Gate 1 First Infant milk, Similac First Infant Milk, Milupa Aptamil First, Kendamil First Infant milk, Babynat 1 Infant milk

And goat milk based:
- Holle Organic Infant Goat milk formula, Nannycare First Infant milk, Kabrita Gold 1 First Infant milk

Casein-based milks

These milks have a larger proportion of casein content, which is intended to make the baby feel full for longer and thus are often marketed as suitable for hungry babies, but there is no evidence that babies sleep or settle for longer if given these feeds (Thorkelsson 1994).
- SMA Extra Hungry, Cow & Gate Infant milk for Hungrier babies, Hipp Organic Combiotic Hungry Infant milk, Aptamil Hungry milk.

Soya milk

Soya-based formula is not recommended in infants unless recommended by a health professional and may not be the first choice in

cow's milk sensitivity or lactose intolerance because the safety of soya-based infant feed is still debated.
- Infants (up to 60%) are as likely to be allergic to soya beans as to cow's milk protein (Whitington & Gibson 1997)
- Concern has been raised over the use of soya formula in infants younger than 6 months because of its phyto-oestrogen content, which can mimic sex hormones. Although there is a potential risk that phyto-oestrogens could cause dysmenorrhoea in females and decreased fertility in males in later life, a systematic review found no strong evidence of negative effects on reproductive and endocrine function (Vandenplas et al 2014).

FULL-TERM BABIES' MILK SUITABLE FOR INFANTS FROM 1 YEAR OF AGE

From the age of 1 year, infants and children may be given:
- Any milk from cows, goats, or sheep as long as it has been pasteurised
- Unsweetened, calcium-fortified soya milk, oat milk, or almond milk

 NB Rice milk is not recommended for children younger than 4.5 years due to its inorganic arsenic content (Food standards agency 2009).

Follow-on formulas

There is no evidence that follow-on formulas offer any nutritional or health advantage over whey-based infant formula in babies who are artificially fed (SACN 2007). They also may contain higher levels of iron, sucrose, glucose, and other nonmilk sugars. They are NOT suitable for babies younger than 6 months:
- SMA Pro Follow-On Milk, Cow & Gate 2 Follow-On Milk, Aptamil 2 Follow-On Milk, Holle Organic Infant Follow-On Formula, Nanny Care Follow-On Milk

CHILDREN'S FEEDS
Standard whole protein feeds (1–6-year-olds/8–20 kg)

1 kcal/mL standard feeds:
- Nutrini, Frebini Original, PediaSure

1 kcal/mL standard feeds with fibre:
- Nutrini multifibre, Frebini Original Fibre, PediaSure Fibre.

High energy whole protein feeds (1–6-year-olds/8–20 kg)

1.5 kcal/mL high energy feeds:
- Nutrini Energy, Frebini Energy, PediaSure Plus

1.5 kcal/mL high energy feeds with fibre:
- Nutrini Energy Multifibre, Frebini Energy Fibre, PediaSure Plus Fibre

Peptide-based feeds

Peptide-based feeds may be recommended in some instances where feed intolerance is poor.

1 kcal/mL feeds:
- Nutrini Peptisorb, Peptamen Junior, Pediasure Peptide

1.5 kcal/mL feeds:
- Nutrini Energy Peptisorb, Peptamen Junior Advanced

Additional energy/protein supplements may be added to feeds under dietetic supervision. Supplements include:
- *Calories* – Duocal, Calogen, Maxijul
- *Protein* – Maxipro, Vitapro

All formula milks in the United Kingdom are gluten free (Shaw 2014).

Other Specialist Formulas

If your child is admitted to hospital, requiring a special diet for cultural or medical reasons, it is advised that you contact your dietician for guidance on the appropriate formula to use.

Manufacturers change the composition of formulas, so suitability may change.

Vegetarian Milk

The only vegetarian milk powders suitable for babies younger than 6 months that are available on the UK market currently are:
- Similac First Infant Milk, Kendamil Mehadrin First Infant Milk, and Holle Organic Goat's Milk Formula

Vegan Milk

Currently there is no infant milk formula available in the United Kingdom suitable for vegans.

Halal Milk Formula

Some of the infant milk powder formula are Halal approved, but always check the label.

For example, Aptamil, Cow and Gate, and SMA powdered milks are Halal approved BUT the ready-made formulas of these brands are NOT.

Cow's Milk Protein Allergy

Cow's milk protein allergy (CMPA) is estimated to affect 2–3% of the population (Luyt et al., 2014). Clinical manifestation can vary because CMPA can be IgE or non-IgE mediated (Table 8.4). IgE-mediated CMPA tends to result in immediate onset of allergic symptoms occurring within 1 hour of ingestion of dairy products, whereas non–IgE-mediated

Table 8.4   Typical presentation of cow's milk protein allergy – IgE mediated versus non-IgE mediated

System	IgE-mediated CMPA	Non–IgE-mediated CMPA
Cutaneous	Pruritus without skin lesions Urticaria Angiooedema Atopic eczema exacerbation	Atopic eczema exacerbation
Gastrointestinal	Vomiting Diarrhoea Bloody stools Gastrooesophageal reflux Abdominal pain	Vomiting/posseting Dysphagia Diarrhoea Constipation Blood in stools
Respiratory	Rhinitis Nasal congestion Wheeze Cough Stridor Difficulty breathing	
Cardiovascular	Anaphylaxis Hypotonia Hypotension/shock Prostration	
General	Anaphylaxis Irritability Failure to thrive	Irritability (colic) Failure to thrive

CMPA, Cow's milk protein allergy.
Adapted from Luyt, D., Ball, N., Makwana, M., 2014. BSACI guideline for the diagnosis and management of cow's milk allergy. Clin. Exp. Allergy 44, 642–672.

symptoms tend to occur 2 or more hours after ingestion. Symptoms are immune mediated and reproducible on milk exposure.

Diagnosis, treatment, and prognosis of cow's milk protein allergy

The cornerstone of allergy diagnosis is allergy-focused history. This is usually combined with skin prick testing or serum assay testing (IgE) to confirm diagnosis in IgE-mediated CMPA. National Institute of Clinical Excellence (NICE) guideline CC116 provides guidance on taking an allergy-focused history (2011). Treatment of CMPA involves complete avoidance of dairy, including all milk and milk products. Prognosis is favourable, with most children outgrowing their CMPA. Reintroduction methods used depend on the allergic presentation (NICE guidance, 2011).

Feeding an infant with cow's milk protein allergy

Breastfeeding. The majority of breast-fed infants with CMPA will tolerate milk protein exposure via breast milk. If symptoms persist, then a 2-week trial of maternal dairy avoidance should be tried. Maternal education on dairy avoidance and appropriate alternatives should be provided by a dietitian, and additional calcium and vitamin D supplementation may be required. The reference nutrient intake for calcium for a lactating woman is 1250 mg calcium.

Mixed feeding or formula feeding. Standard cow's milk–containing formula (e.g., Aptamil, Cow and Gate, HIPP, or SMA) should be replaced with an extensively hydrolysed formula (EHF) in most circumstances (see indications for amino acid formula [AAF]). These are formulas with proven hypoallergencity, in which the milk protein has been hydrolysed (broken down) using enzymes, resulting in a change in the chemical structure. Consequently, the IgE antibody no longer recognises the milk protein and, as a result, does not bind to it and does not cause the allergic symptoms. EHF will be tolerated by 90% of the cow's milk–allergic population.

EHFs are recommended as a first line treatment in cow's milk protein intolerance.

EHFs currently available in the United Kingdom are listed in Table 8.5.

Elemental amino acid formula

Amino acid formulas. Amino acid–based formulas are hypoallergenic formulas made from individual amino acids. These have greater cost implication and, although suitable for the treatment of CMPA, are usually reserved for the following presentations: multiple food allergies, severe cow's milk allergy (history of previous anaphylaxis to milk), allergic symptoms or severe atopic eczema when exclusively breastfed, severe forms of non–IgE-mediated cow's milk allergy such as eosinophilic oesophagitis, enteropathies and food protein–induced

Table 8.5 Types of extensively hydrolysed formula			
Extensively hydrolysed formula (EHF)	**Suitable age range**	**Protein source**	**Lactose present (Y/N)**
Althera (450 g)	From birth	Whey	Y
Aptamil Pepti 1 (400/800 g)	Birth to 6 months	Whey	Y
Aptamil Pepti 2 (400/800 g)	From 6 months	Whey	Y
Nutramigen 1 with LGG (400 g)	Birth to 6 months	Casein	N
Nutramigen 2 with LGG (400 g)	From 6 months	Casein	N
Cow & Gate Pepti Junior (450 g)	From birth	Whey	N
Pregestimil LIPIL (400 g)	From birth	Casein	N
Similac Alimentum (400 g)	From birth	Casein	N
Peptamen Junior (400 g)	From 1 year	Whey	N

NB: Guidance on how to prepare different EHF varies please see manufactures guidance on tin.

enterocolitis syndrome (FPIES), faltering growth, and those who have reacted to or refusing to take an EHF who are at nutritional risk.

Amino acid formulas currently available in the United Kingdom are listed in Table 8.6.

Infant low-lactose formula

Lactose intolerance is caused by a lactase enzymatic deficiency. As a result, lactose, the sugar present in cow's milk and milk products, cannot be broken down in the large colon. Consequently, water is pulled back into the large colon, causing diarrhoea. Primary lactose intolerance is rare in infants. Secondary lactose intolerance is often seen post gastroenteritis due to the brush border being damaged. In these situations, lactose should typically be avoided for 4–6 weeks before being reintroduced. There are a number of lactose-free formulas on the market that can be purchased (Table 8.7).

Current recommendation for the use of soya formula in cow's milk protein allergy. Soya formula can be used for the treatment of CMPA. However, it is not recommended and if parents wish to use soya formula, advice should be provided by a competent health care professional.

Current recommendation for the use of goat milk formula in cow's milk protein allergy. Due to the protein homology between cow's milk and other mammalian milks (e.g., goat or sheep's milk), these are not recommended for the treatment of CPMA (Luyt et al 2014). Therefore goat's milk formula or over-the-counter mammalian milks are not recommended in the treatment of CMPA.

Table 8.6 Amino acid formulas	
Amino acid formula (AAF)	**Suitable age range**
Alfamino (400 g)	From birth
Neocate Junior (400 g)	From 1 year of age
Neocate LCP (400 g)	From birth
Nutramigen Puramino (400 g)	From birth

LCP, Long-chain polyunsaturated fatty acids.

Table 8.7 Lactose-free formulas	
Lactose-free formula	**Suitable age range**
Aptamil LF	From birth
Enfamil O-Lac	From birth
SMA LF	From birth

LF, Lactose free.

Current recommendations for children with CMPA older than 1 year:

Specialist EHF and AAF can be used to manage CMPA until 2 years. However, from 1 year of age, if a child is thriving and the diet is assessed by a dietitian as nutritionally adequate, an over-the-counter calcium-enriched milk alternative will usually replace the specialist formula. Calcium-enriched milk alternatives can be made from hemp, oat, rice, soya, or tree nuts (almond, cashew, and hazelnut).

Fructose-based and low-calcium infant formula

- Galactomin 19, Locasol

Other products

- Monogen, Medium chain triglycerides (MCT) Pepdite, Heparon Junior (for use in patients with chylothorax or liver disease)
- Kindergen (renal patients)

VITAMIN SUPPLEMENTS

It is recommended that:

- breast-fed babies are given a daily vitamin D supplement from birth (NICE 2014)
- all children (except babies who receive more than 500 mL of infant formula/day) aged 6 months to 5 years are given vitamin supplements containing vitamin A, C, and D every day (NICE 2008; Imdad et al 2010)

SPECIAL DIETS FOR SPECIAL KIDS

Infants and children with certain inborn errors of metabolism often have specific dietary requirements. General principles of dietary needs are highlighted; they are only intended as a guide to give nurses some ideas of general requirements and will not replace specialist advice from dietetic services.

Ketogenic diet

The ketogenic diet is a prescribed low-carbohydrate, high-fat diet, and the aim of the diet is to change the energy source to produce ketones.

Children whose seizures have not responded to antiepileptic medication should be referred to a specialist tertiary paediatric epilepsy centre for consideration of the use of a ketogenic diet (NICE 2012). The ketogenic diet is also prescribed for children with GLUT 1 deficiency and may also be used in some patients with pyruvate dehydrogenase deficiency.

If a child on a ketogenic diet requires intravenous fluids, where possible give normal saline 0.9%, but if fasting or blood sugar level is less than 3 mmol/L, use a dextrose-containing solution (2.5% or 5%) to maintain blood glucose between 3 and 4 mmol/L.

The following should be considered (depending on clinical condition) for a child on a ketogenic diet who is unwell and admitted to a PICU:

pH and blood gases
Blood ketones
Blood sugars – laboratory and bedside
Urea and electrolytes

Care and consideration must be used when prescribing medication for children on a ketogenic diet so that where possible the carbohydrate is as low as possible. Avoid sucrose, fructose, dextrose, sorbitol, glucose, mannitol, glycerol, starch, maize starch, lactose, and maltodextrin.

Recommended to have the medications checked by the pharmacy team so that they are 'keto friendly'.

COELIAC DISEASE

- Coeliac disease is a malabsorption syndrome in which the proximal intestinal mucosa loses its villous structure and the absorptive function becomes impaired.
- It is precipitated by the ingestion of gluten in foods. Coeliac disease can result in severe symptoms such as steatorrhoea, abdominal discomfort, and weight loss. However, this presentation is quite rare and symptoms are usually less specific (e.g., iron-deficiency anaemia, fatigue, or calcium deficiency).
- A strict, lifelong gluten-free diet is required.

CYSTIC FIBROSIS

- Cystic fibrosis is a hereditary disorder with widespread dysfunction of exocrine glands, characterised by chronic pulmonary disease, pancreatic deficiency, abnormally high levels of electrolytes in the sweat, and occasionally biliary cirrhosis.
- Most patients will require pancreatic enzyme replacement therapy.
- A high-protein, high-energy diet is required with added fat-soluble vitamins.

DIABETES MELLITUS

- Diabetes mellitus is a metabolic disorder in which the pancreas becomes unable to maintain normal insulin production, causing hyperglycaemia, glycosuria, and polyuria.
- In children, this is frequently controlled by a combination of diet and insulin.
- A well-balanced diet is required with minimal refined sugars, free fructose, and an even distribution of carbohydrate throughout the day.

Inborn errors of metabolism

Inborn errors of metabolism comprise a group of disorders in which a single gene defect causes a clinically significant block in a metabolic pathway, resulting in either an accumulation of substrate behind the block or deficiency of the product. Disorders can be classified into nutrient groups and are listed later. Early discussion with a senior doctor and dietician who specialise in metabolic disorders is essential.

ILLNESS MANAGEMENT OF INBORN ERRORS OF METABOLISM

During illness, disorders of intermediary metabolism result in catabolism and increased toxic metabolites resulting in metabolic decompensation which can include metabolic acidosis, encephalopathy, hyperammonaemia, and hypoglycaemia. The aim of illness management is to minimise catabolism and reduce toxic metabolites. All patients are encouraged to carry their emergency regimen with them at all times.

If the enteral route is viable, an emergency regimen (Dixon & Leonard 1992) containing a prescribed amount of glucose polymer every 2 hours or continuously is given. The concentration of glucose polymer is age dependent (Table 8.8).

If the enteral route is not viable, intravenous dextrose (at least 10%) should be prescribed (neonate 6–10 mg carbohydrate/kg/min and children 6–8 mg carbohydrate/kg/min). Intravenous lipid may be required to optimise energy intake. For some inborn errors of metabolism, a specialised regimen containing glucose polymer and a specific metabolic feed is required.

DISORDERS OF PROTEIN METABOLISM

These include phenylketonuria (PKU), maple syrup urine disease (MSUD), homocystinuria (HCU), and tyrosinaemia type 1 (TYR). In the United Kingdom, PKU, MSUD, and HCU are included in the newborn blood spot screening program. The aim of treatment is to restrict protein and provide a supplement containing specific amino acids, vitamins, and trace elements. If the child with PKU, HCU, or TYR becomes unwell, he or she is not at risk of decompensation and does not require an emergency regimen. Intake of the amino acid

Table 8.8 Concentration of glucose polymer according to age		
Age (years)	Glucose polymer concentration (% carbohydrate)	Daily volume
Up to 1	10	150–200 mL/kg
1–2	15	95 mL/kg
2–6	20	1200–1500 mL
6–10	20	1500–2000 mL
≥10	25	2000 mL

supplement should continue. If the child with MSUD becomes unwell, he or she is at risk of metabolic decompensation (see later for details).

PHENYLKETONURIA

- PKU is a disorder of amino acid metabolism characterised by a deficiency of the liver enzyme phenylalanine hydroxylase, which is needed to break down the amino acid phenylalanine to tyrosine.
- Phenylalanine is essential for growth, so once the initially high level of phenylalanine has been reduced by a phenylalanine-free diet, it is gradually reintroduced at a low level.
- A diet low in phenylalanine with a phenylalanine-free supplement of amino acids, vitamins, and trace elements will be required for life.

MAPLE SYRUP URINE DISEASE

MSUD is caused by a deficiency of branched chain 2-ketoacid dehydrogenase enzyme complex, which results in the accumulation of three branch chain amino acids – leucine, isoleucine, and valine.

- The infant presents in the first few days of life with encephalopathy, which may be mistaken for sepsis, and the characteristic urine that smells of maple syrup.
- A low leucine diet is required with a branch chain–free amino acid supplement, with vitamins and minerals.
- If the child becomes unwell, all protein intake is stopped and an emergency regimen comprising the branch chain–free supplement and additional calories is required. When these children become very sick, they may require haemofiltration to reduce the level of leucine.

ORGANIC ACIDAEMIAS

These disorders are characterised by a specific organic aciduria and often present with vomiting, encephalopathy, neutropenia, and thrombocytopenia. Metabolic decompensation can cause acidosis, ketosis, lactic acidosis, and mild to moderate hyperammonemia. There are several organic acidaemias, all due to different malfunctioning or absent enzymes resulting in a block of the breakdown of different amino acids. Two of the organic acidaemias are included in the UK newborn blood spot screening (glutaric aciduria type 1 and isovaleric aciduria).

The basic principles of dietary management include a low protein diet and supplements of vitamins, minerals, and trace elements; energy supplements are also required.

- During periods of illness, the patient is at risk of developing metabolic acidosis due to accumulation of organic acids, so protein intake is usually withdrawn for a few days and an emergency diet, predominantly of a glucose polymer is given. In acute decompensation, these children may have a rising level of lactate and may require haemofiltration.

- Supplements of carnitine or other amino acid derivatives may be required. These patients may be on a low dose of metronidazole to reduce their gut flora, as propionic acid is formed in the gut.

UREA CYCLE DEFECTS

Urea cycle defects result from an inability to detoxify nitrogen and are characterised by severe hyperammonaemia and respiratory alkalosis with a typical onset in the first few days of life.

- The infant or child may present with neurologic abnormalities (e.g., encephalopathy) due to toxic levels of ammonia and acidosis and may require haemofiltration.
- A low protein diet is required to try to keep ammonia levels as low as possible, plus supplements of vitamins, minerals, and trace elements.
- In illness, children are at risk of hyperammonaemia and so protein intake is stopped and a standard emergency regimen is required.

DISORDERS OF FAT METABOLISM

These include fatty acid oxidation defects (e.g., medium- and very-long-chain acyl-CoA dehydrogenase [MCAD and VLCAD, respectively] deficiencies). They are characterised by hypoketotic hypoglycaemia, mild-moderate hyperammonaemia, rhabdomyolysis, cardiomyopathy, and liver dysfunction. MCAD is included in the UK newborn blood spot screening. Dietary management of long-chain defects includes a minimal fat diet, feeds containing medium-chain triglycerides, regular feeds, and standard emergency regimen in illness.

DISORDERS OF CARBOHYDRATE METABOLISM

Glycogen storage diseases

GLUCOSE-6-PHOSPHATASE DEFICIENCY

- This is an enzyme deficiency of glucose-6-phosphatase, which disrupts normal maintenance of plasma glucose levels.
- It usually presents in infancy with hepatomegaly, hypoglycaemia, and metabolic acidosis.
- The aim of management is to avoid hypoglycaemia and correct other biochemical abnormalities. Frequent glucose/carbohydrate feeds are required, and, in older children, corn starch boluses can be used.
- In illness, children are at risk of hypoglycaemia, so an emergency regimen of glucose polymer, Maxijul solution, is required to provide sufficient carbohydrate.
- Individuals with glucose-6-phosphate dehydrogenase (G6PD) deficiency are susceptible to developing acute haemolytic anaemia when they take common drugs, so when prescribing for these patients, consult British National Formulary for Children or other trusted source for advice.

GALACTOSAEMIA

- Galactosaemia is an inborn error of galactose metabolism as a result of enzyme deficiency.
- Most infants present in first week of life with jaundice, failure to thrive, vomiting, hepatomegaly, and cataracts because breast milk and most infant formulas contain galactose.
- Treatment is a lifelong lactose-free diet. Soya-based formula or feeds are used.

TOTAL PARENTERAL NUTRITION

Total parenteral nutrition consists of sterile solutions that are made up in pharmacy and are administered directly into the blood stream via a vein. The solutions:

- are made up of amino acids, carbohydrates, and lipids
- should be protected from light to prevent the formation of free radicals
- should be stored in a fridge until used
- should be administered via a central line, especially if the glucose concentration is greater than 12.5%, and on a unique line saved for the sole use of total parenteral nutrition (TPN)
- should be double-checked against the prescription before administration
- should be changed using aseptic precautions.

Patients on TPN should:

- have daily urea and electrolytes until their regime is established, after which – two to three times a week is sufficient
- check glucose levels at least 12-hourly initially until stable
- if patient has hyperbilirubinaemia, send daily bilirubins and confirm conjugated bilirubin status weekly
- check triglyceride levels when initiating TPN or if levels are high or in severe sepsis
- after a fortnight, measure plasma chemistry for selenium and zinc and then measure monthly. (Adapted from Guy's, St Thomas', Kings College and Lewisham Hospitals 2010.)

On occasion, it is necessary to make up solutions of dextrose that are not available as standard commercially prepared products (Table 8.9).

How to prepare 0.9% sodium chloride in 10% glucose

Remove 15 mL from a 500-mL bag of 10% glucose and discard. Draw up 15 mL of 30% sodium chloride and add to bag of 10% glucose and mix well.

Table 8.9 How to prepare 12.5% and 15% glucose solutions

Concentration required (%)	Quantity of 50% glucose (mL)	
12.5	31.25	Add to 468.75 mL of 10% glucose
15	62.5	Add to 437.5 mL of 10% glucose

How to prepare 3% solutions of sodium chloride

Remove 36 mL from a 500-mL bag of 0.9% sodium chloride and discard. Draw up 36 mL of 30% sodium chloride and add to the 0.9% sodium chloride bag.

Dextrose solutions

- 4% dextrose and 0.18% saline solution contains 4 g of dextrose and 30 mmol of sodium and chloride per 100 mL
- 5% dextrose contains 5 g dextrose/100 mL
- 10% dextrose contains 10 g dextrose/100 mL
- 50% dextrose contains 50 g dextrose/100 mL.

INSENSIBLE LOSS

This occurs mostly through the skin and the respiratory tract and accounts for approximately 30 mL/kg/24 h. However, fever will increase insensible loss by 12% per 1°C rise in temperature above 37.2°C (Shann 2003).

BURNS

See Chapter 12 for estimation of percentage burns and fluid replacement regimes.

REFERENCES

Advanced Life Support Group, 2016. Advanced Paediatric Life Support: A Practical approach to Emergencies (APLS), 6th ed. Wiley Blackwell.

Agostoni, C., Buonocore, G., Carnielli, V.P., et al., 2010. Enteral nutrition supply for preterm infants: commentary from the European Society for Paediatric Gastroenterology, Hepatology and Nutrition Committee (ESPGHAN). JPGN. 50, 1–9.

Akay, B., Capizzani, T.R., Drongowski, R.A., et al., 2010. Gastrostomy tube placement in infant and children: is there a preferred technique? J. Pediatr. Surg. 46 (6), 1147–1152.

BNF British National Formulary for Children. 2015–2016 Prescribing for Children: Weight, Height and Gender. BMJ. Group. London

Bonner, J.J., Vajjah, P., Abduljalil, K., et al., 2015. Does age affect gastric emptying time? A model-based meta-analysis of data from premature neonates through to adults. Biopharm. Drug. Dispos. 36, 245–257.

Chen, W., Codreanu, I., Yang, J., et al., 2013. Tube feeding increases the gastric emptying rate determined by gastroesophageal scintigraphy. Clin. Nuclear Med. 38, 962–965.

Dixon, M.A., Leonard, J.V., 1992. Intercurrent illness in inborn errors of intermediary metabolism. Arch. Dis. Child 67, 1387–1391.

Ellet, M.L., Beckstrand, J., 2001. Predicting the distance for nasojejunal tube insertion in children. J. Soc. Pediatr. Nurs. 6 (3), 123–132.

Food Standards Agency, 02/09, 2009. Survey of total and inorganic arsenic in rice drinks. Food Survey Information Sheet. www.food.gov.uk.

Guy's, St Thomas', King's College and University Lewisham Hospitals, 2010. Paediatric Formulary, eighth ed. Guy's, St Thomas', King's College and Lewisham Hospitals, London.

Holliday, M.A., Friedman, A.L., Segar, W.E., et al., 2004. Acute hospital-induced hyponatremia in children: a physiologic approach. J. Paediatrics. 145, 584–587.

Imdad, A., Herzer, K., Mayo-Wilson, E., et al., 2010. Vitamin A supplementation for preventing morbidity and mortality in children from 6 months to 5 years of age. Cochrane Database Syst. Rev. (Issue 12), CD008524.

Jabbar, A., Chang, W.-K., Dryden, G.W., et al., 2003. Gut immunology and the differential response to feeding and starvation. Nutr. Clin. Pract. 18, 461–482.

Kairamkonda, V., Deorukhkar, A., Bruce, C., et al., 2008. Amylin peptide is increased in preterm neonates with feed intolerance. Arch. Dis. Child. Fetal Neonatal Edn. 93, 265–270.

Knight, D., Durward, A., Tibby, S., et al., 2015. Evaluation of novel feeding guideline based on individual gastric emptying times shown by 3 prospective audits. PICS Conference, UK Paediatric Intensive Care Society, Birmingham 2015.

Kreymann, K.G., Berger, M.M., Deutz, N.E., et al., DGEM (German Society for Nutritional Medicine), 2006. ESPEN Guidelines in enteral nutrition: intensive care. Clin. Nutr. 25, 210–223.

Luyt, D., Ball, H., Makwana, N., et al., 2014. BSACI guideline for the diagnosis and management of cow's milk allergy. Clin. Exp. Allergy 44, 642–672.

Marik, P.E., 2014. Enteral nutrition in the critically ill: myths and misconceptions. Crit. Care Med. 42 (4), 962–969.

Mayer, A.P.T., Durward, A., Turner, C., et al., 2002. Amylin is associated with delayed gastric emptying in critically ill children. Intensive Care Med. 28 (3), 336–340.

McClave, S.A., 2006. Critical care nutrition: getting involved as a gastrointestinal endoscopist. J. Clin. Gastroenterol. 40 (10), 870–890.

Mehta, N.M., 2014. Feeding the gut during critical illness – It is about time. JPEN. 38 (4), 410–414.

Meyer, R., Harrison, S., Cooper, M., et al., 2007. Successful blind placement of nasojejeunal tube in Paedaitric Intensive Care; Impact of training and audit. J. Adv. Nurs. 60 (4), 402–408.

Mikhailov, T.A., Kuhn, E.M., Manzi, J., et al., 2014. Early enteral nutrition is associated with lower mortality in critically ill children. JPEN. 38 (4), 459–466.

National Patient Safety Agency (NPSA), 2005. Reducing the harm caused by misplaced nasogastric feeding tubes. National Patient Safety Agency, London.

National Patient Safety Agency (NPSA), 2012. Harm from flushing nasogastric tubes before confirmation of placement. National Patient Safety Agency, London. NPSA/2012/RRR001. www.nrls.npsa.nhs.uk.

National Patient Safety Agency (NPSA) 2016 Patient Safety Alert. Nasogastric tube misplacement: continuing risk of death and severe harm. NHS/PSA/RE/2016/006. www.improvement.nhs.uk. accessed 13/06/2017. Nasogastric Feeding Tubes Alert. National Patient Safety Agency, London

Nguyen, N.Q., Fraser, R.J., Bryant, L.K., et al., 2008. The impact of delaying enteral feeding on gastric emptying, plasma cholecystokinin, and peptide YY concentrations in critically ill patients. Crit. Care Med. 36 (5), 1469–1474.

NICE Guidance, 2008. updated 2014 Maternal and Child Nutrition. Public Health guideline (PH11). National Institute for Health and Care excellence. www.nice.org.uk.

NICE Guidance, 2011. Food allergy in children and young people. NICE Clinical Guideline (CG116). National Institute for Health and Care excellence. www.nice.org.uk/guidance/CG116.

NICE Guidance, 2012. Epilepsies: diagnosis and management. Clinical Guideline (CG137) 1.12.1. National Institute for Health and Care excellence. www.nice.org.uk.

NICE Guidance, 2014. Vitamin D: increasing supplement use among at risk groups. Public Health Guideline (PH56). National Institute for Health and Care excellence. www.nice.org.uk.

Rahnemai-Azar, A., Rahnemaiazar, A., Naghshizadian, R., et al., 2014. Percutaneous endoscopic gastrostomy: indications, technique, complications and management. World J. Gastroenterol. 20 (24), 7739–7751.

SACN, 2007. Subgroup on Maternal and ChildNutrition's (SMCN) response to the Infant Formula and Follow on Formula Draft Regulations. London. www.sacn.gov.uk/pdfs/position statement 2007 09 24.pdf.

Scientific Advisory Committee on Nutrition (SACN), 2011. Dietary Reference Values for Energy. London. www.sacn.gov.uk.

Shann, F., 2003. Drug doses, twelfth ed. Collective. Parkville, Victoria.

Shaw, V., 2014. Clinical paediatric dietetics, fourth ed. Oxford, Blackwell.

Skillman, H., Mehta, M., 2012. Nutrition in the critically ill child. Curr. Opin. Crit. Care (18), 192–198.

Thorkelsson, T., 1994. Similar gastric emptying rates for casein and whey predominant formulasin preterm infants. Pediatr. Res. 36 (3), 329–333.

Vandenplas, Y., Castrellon, P.G., Rivas, R., et al., 2014. Safety of soya-based infant formulas in children. Systematic review with Meta-Analysis. Br. J. Nutr. 111, 1340–1360.

Whitington, P.F., Gibson, R., 1997. Soy protein intolerance: four patients with concomitant cow's milk intolerance. Pediatrics 59, 730–732.

World Health Organisation (WHO), 2003. Global strategy for infant and child feeding. WHO, Geneva.

USEFUL WEBSITES

www.npsa.nhs.uk
www.nhsdirect.nhs.uk
www.breastfeeding.nhs.uk
www.matthewsfriends.org
www.bimdg.org.uk

BLOOD AND ELECTROLYTES

9

This chapter highlights normal blood values, specialised blood tests, general information about blood products, storage and administration, and guidance about electrolyte emergencies. Always consult and follow local policies. The normal ranges of blood values given are intended as a guide and may vary in different hospitals.

NORMAL BLOOD VOLUMES

- Preterm babies – approximately 100 mL/kg
- Infants – 80 mL/kg
- Children – 70 mL/kg

NORMAL VALUES: FULL BLOOD COUNT

Whole blood consists of plasma (water and solutes), white blood cells, red blood cells, and platelets.

White blood cells consist of:

- Neutrophils, which fight infection. Neutrophilia (↑ neutrophils) may indicate bacterial infection. Neutropenia (↓ neutrophils) may result from viral infection, overwhelming infection, an inherited immune problem, drug treatment including antibiotics, or cancer drugs
- Monocytes, which also fight infection. Monocytosis (↑ monocytes) may indicate viral infection, leukaemia, glandular fever. Monopenia (↓ monocytes) may indicate leukaemia or bone marrow failure
- Lymphocytes, which are immune cells that produce antibodies (B cells) and recognise and target the antigen and regulate immune responses (T cells). Lymphocytosis (↑ lymphocytes) implies a viral infection most commonly, whereas lymphopenia (↓ lymphocytes) may result from viral infection, inherited immune disorders, corticosteroid therapy, adrenocortical hyperfunction, or stress.
- Eosinophils, which can indicate parasitic infection or allergy. Eosinophilia (↑ eosinophils) often with asthma, eosinopenia (↓ eosinophils) after corticosteroid therapy
- Basophils, which are responsible for histamine release in systemic allergic reactions. Basophilia (↑ basophils) may be due to chronic inflammatory responses, whereas basopenia (↓ basophils) can result from corticosteroid therapy.

Red blood cells (erythrocytes) develop in bone marrow, last for 120 days, and contain haemoglobin (Hb), a protein that carries oxygen

Table 9.1   Full blood count for normal infants and children

Age	Units	Newborn (full term)	Up to 6 months	2–6 years	6–12 years
Red blood cells (RBCs)	×10^{12}/L	6.0 ± 1.0	3.8 ± 0.8	4.6 ± 0.7	4.6 ± 0.6
Haemoglobin (Hb)	g/dL	16.5 ± 3.0	11.5 ± 2.0	12.5 ± 1.5	13.5 ± 2.0
Packed cell volume (PCV)	L/L	0.54 ± 0.10	0.35 ± 0.07	0.37 ± 0.03	0.40 ± 0.05
Mean corpuscular volume (MCV)	fL	110 ± 10	91 ± 17	81 ± 6	86 ± 8
Mean corpuscular haemoglobin (MCH)	pg	34 ± 3	30 ± 5	27 ± 3	29 ± 4
Platelets	×10^9/L	150–400	150–400	150–400	150–400
White blood count (WBC)	×10^9/L	18 ± 8	12 ± 6	10 ± 5	9 ± 4
Neutrophils	×10^9/L	5.0–13.0	1.5–9.0	1.5–8.0	2.0–8.0
Lymphocytes	×10^9/L	3.0–10.0	4.0–10.0	6.0–9.0	1.0–5.0
Monocytes	×10^9/L	0.7–1.5	0.1–1.0	0.1–1.0	0.1–1.0
Eosinophils	×10^9/L	0.2–1.0	0.2–1.0	0.2–1.0	0.1–1.0
Reticulocytes	×10^9/L	200–500	40–100	20–200	20–200

Source: From Dacie, J.V., Lewis, S.M., 1997. Practical Haematology, eighth ed. Churchill Livingstone, Edinburgh.

around the body and carbon dioxide to the lungs. Polycythemia (↑ Hb) occurs at high altitude, in congenital heart disease, and with chronic hypoxia; decreased Hb may be caused by haemorrhage, iron deficiency, renal disease, or vitamin B12 deficiency.

Platelets (thrombocytes) are produced in megakaryocytes in bone marrow and have a life span of approximately 9–10 days. They form a platelet clot as part of the clotting cascade. Thrombocytopenia (↓ platelets) may result from decreased platelet production, increased destruction, or sequestration.

See Tables 9.1–9.3.

ADDITIONAL BLOOD TESTS

Anti-Xa

The plasma anti–Xa assay is a laboratory test which measures, indirectly, the activity of heparin. It is used to monitor patients who are being treated with low-molecular-weight heparin (LMWH). Monitoring is controversial because there is a poorly defined therapeutic range in different clinical settings (Barras 2013).

LMWHs bind with antithrombin (a naturally occurring anticoagulant protein), changing the molecule and increasing its anticoagulant activity. Proteins such as thrombin and clotting factor Xa are inactivated, thus disrupting the clotting cascade. Intravenous LMWH has a half-life of 2 hours, whereas subcutaneous LMWH has a half-life of approximately 4 hours, measured as anti–Xa activity (Colvin & Barrowcliffe 1993).

Table 9.2	Normal ranges for urea and electrolytes	
	Value	**Standard units**
Sodium	135–145	mmol/L
Potassium	3.5–5.0	mmol/L
Chloride	98–107	mmol/L
Bicarbonate	22–32	mmol/L
Anion gap	7–17	mmol/L
Urea	2.5–7.5	mmol/L
Creatinine	40–90	µmol/L
Calcium	2.19–2.51	mmol/L
Albumin-corrected calcium	2.19–2.51	mmol/L
Magnesium	0.65–0.95	mmol/L
Phosphate	1.2–1.8	mmol/L
Total protein	62–81	g/L
Albumin	37–56	g/L
Alkaline phosphatase	145–320	U/L
Total bilirubin	0–22	µmol/L
Alanine transaminase	0–55	U/L
Aspartate transaminase	0–35	U/L
Gamma glutamyl transpeptidase	8–78	U/L
C-reactive protein	<7	mg/L

Table 9.3	Clotting values for children		
	Abbreviation	**Value**	**Standard unit**
Prothrombin time	PT	11–16	Seconds
International normalised ratio	INR	0.8–1.1	Ratio
Activated prothrombin time	APTT	0.8–1.2	Ratio
Fibrinogen		2.02–4.24	g/L

Therapeutic anti-Xa range:

- 0.5–1 unit/mL for management of thromboembolic disease (Hirsh et al 2008; Ignjatovic et al 2010)
- 0.3–0.5 units/mL for prevention of thromboembolic disease (Hirsh et al 2008; Ignjatovic et al 2010).

LMWHs are 80% renally eliminated, so patients with renal impairment could accumulate the drug on standard doses, thus increasing the risk of bleeding (Hirsh et al 2008; Lim et al 2006). Children with renal impairment will need to be monitored closely.

NB Protamine sulphate will only partially reverse LMWH activity.

Creatinine phosphokinase

Creatinine phosphokinase (CPK or CK) is an enzyme found predominantly in skeletal muscle but also in the heart and brain. Elevated serum

CK in children usually reflects skeletal muscle damage but could indicate injury to the heart or brain. Reference values have not yet been established for those younger than 6 years, and it is important to note that strenuous exercise may cause a transient elevation.

Normal ranges (Mayo Clinic 2016):

Male 6–11 years, 150–499 U/L; 12–17 years, 94–499 U/L

Female 6–7 years, 134–391 U/L; 8–14 years, 91–391 U/L; 15–17 years, 53–269 U/L

Causes of mildly elevated CK (≥500 U/L) include:

- Spinal muscular atrophy
- Neuropathies (e.g., Charcot–Marie–Tooth disease)
- Recent immunisation
- Muscle trauma
- Viral infection
- Seizures
- Burns
- Electric shock
- Myocarditis

Causes of grossly elevated CK (3000–30 000 U/L) include:

- Muscular dystrophy (e.g., Duchenne)

Causes of extreme elevation of CK (50 000–200 000 U/L) include:

- Rhabdomyolysis (may be after extreme exercise)

Procalcitonin

Procalcitonin is an inactive protein composed of 116 amino acids, usually made in the process of producing the hormone calcitonin by C cells of the thyroid gland. It is a useful biomarker for the early diagnosis of sepsis in critically ill patients (Wackner et al 2013).

Normal values are age related (Van Rossum et al 2004; Chiesa et al 2011):

At birth – ≤2 ng/mL then rises to ≤20 ng/mL at 18–30 hours of age By 72 hours of age and until adulthood – ≤0.15 ng/mL

Raised procalcitonin levels 0.15–2.0 ng/mL may indicate a localised bacterial infection without systemic sepsis.

Procalcitonin level of ≥2.0 ng/mL are suggestive of systemic sepsis.

Procalcitonin level ≥10 ng/mL indicates severe sepsis, organ dysfunction, and high risk of death (O'Grady et al 2008).

Elevated procalcitonin becomes detectable within 2–4 hours of a triggering event, and this will peak at approximately 12–24 hours (Becker et al 2008). The level of procalcitonin secretion mirrors the severity of the inflammatory response. It is eliminated with a half-life of 24–35 hours.

Troponin

Troponins are proteins in muscle fibres that help to regulate muscle contractions. There are three different troponins: a skeletal muscle troponin and two cardiac muscle troponins. Cardiac troponin levels in healthy individuals are usually undetectable, but when there is myocardial injury, cardiac troponins are released into the bloodstream several hours after injury. Acute heart muscle damage will result in increasing troponin levels over time. In neonatal and paediatric populations, the range of normal values of troponin is still being determined, but some studies have shown seemingly healthy infants with a higher baseline of cardiac troponin concentration than in adults (Bennett et al 2011; Lipshultz et al 2008).

Normal cardiac troponin I in infants younger than 1 year is less than 0.1 ng/mL (Souto & de Carvalho 2008).

Causes of elevated cardiac troponins include:

- Myocardial infarction (with ischaemia) and cardiac troponin will increase over time but may remain high for several weeks

Rising troponins without ischaemia may be caused by:

- Tachyarrhythmia
- Pulmonary hypertension
- Pulmonary embolus
- Coronary artery spasm
- Acute cardiac failure
- Myocarditis
- Cardiomyopathy
- Trauma that injures heart
- Prolonged exercise (e.g., marathon)
- Cardioversion
- Cardiac stenting, angioplasty, radiofrequency ablation, or surgery

Elevated but unchanging troponins may be caused by:

- Congestive heart failure
- Hypertension
- Long-term renal disease
- Chronic inflammatory muscle conditions

TRANSFUSION COMPONENTS

The Joint United Kingdom Blood Transfusion and Tissue Transplantation Services Professional Advisory Committee (2014) advises:

- Potential risks and benefits must be considered when deciding whether to transfuse children
- There is potential to develop late adverse effects of transfusion in children who have received foetal or neonatal transfusions
- Enhanced donor screening provides extra safety measures for neonatal and infant transfusion
- Transfusion volumes and rates should be calculated and prescribed in millilitres, not units, to minimise circulatory overload and dosing errors
- A restrictive red cell transfusion policy (threshold 70 g/L) is safe for clinically stable children in PICU
- Many transfusions of fresh frozen plasma (FFP) in NICU and PICU should be given to nonbleeding patients with minor abnormalities in coagulation parameters of uncertain significance

- Age-specific blood components should be used as long as this does not delay urgent provision of blood
- Tranexamic acid is recommended for children with major traumatic haemorrhage (JPAC 2014)

Blood products for neonates (up to 28 days) (JPAC 2014)

A restrictive transfusion policy is primarily adopted, but the Cochrane Review (2011) highlights an undefined safe lower limit for Hb transfusion threshold (Whyte & Kirplani 2011). The British Committee for Standards in Haematology (BCSH) Transfusion Guidelines for Neonates and Older Children (2004) suggest transfusion thresholds and can be found at www.bcshguidelines.com.

Red cell transfusion in neonates (JPAC 2014)

- For exchange, transfusion should be: plasma reduced, in citrate phosphate dextrose (CPD) anticoagulant, less than 5 days old, irradiated (essential if previous intrauterine transfusion [IUT]), cytomegalovirus (CMV) negative, sickle screen negative, usually produced as group O (low-titre haemolysins), RhD negative (or RhD identical with neonate) and Kell negative, red cell antigen negative for maternal alloantibodies and indirect antiglobulin test crossmatch compatible with maternal plasma

Large-volume transfusion in cardiac surgery (JPAC 2014)

Approximately 80 mL/kg
- In saline, adenine, glucose, and mannitol (SAG-M) anticoagulant, haematocrit 0.5–0.7, transfused less than 5 days from donation (to reduce risk of hyperkalaemia), group O (or ABO compatible with baby and mother) and RhD negative (or RhD compatible with neonate), CMV negative (in neonates)
- Consider need for irradiated blood in babies with known or suspected T-cell immunodeficiency, such as DiGeorge syndrome, or if they have previously received an intrauterine blood transfusion

Top-up transfusion in neonates (JPAC 2014)

Up to 20 mL/kg
- In SAG-M anticoagulant, haematocrit 0.5–0.7, transfused up to 35 days from donation, group O (or ABO compatible with baby and mother) and RhD negative (or RhD compatible with neonate), CMV negative, consider need for irradiated blood

Neonatal platelet transfusion (JPAC 2014)

Often 10–20 mL/kg
- Single donor apheresis platelets manufactured to neonatal specifications, CMV negative, ABO RhD identical or compatible with recipient

Neonatal fresh frozen plasma and cryoprecipitate transfusion (JPAC 2014)

FFP carries a significant risk of serious acute transfusion reactions. Dose is usually 12–15 mL/kg.

- For neonates, plasma is imported from countries with low risk of variant Creutzfeldt-Jakob disease (vCJD) and is pathogen inactivated. Methylene blue (MB) is used for inactivation and often human plasma pooled and treated is used in the same way FFP is used (e.g., octaplasLG). It should be ABO identical with recipient or group AB (group O FFP should only be given to neonates of group O)

Cryoprecipitate is used as a more concentrated source of fibrinogen than FFP and is indicated when fibrinogen level is less than 0.8–1.0 g/L with bleeding from acquired hypofibrinogenaemia. Dose is usually 5–10 mL/kg.

Transfusion practice in paediatrics

All hospitals will have their own policies that must be adhered to regarding the transfusion of blood products. It is good practice to document:

- The reason for transfusion with relevant blood results in the patient notes
- If the patient/family has been given an information leaflet outlining the risks and benefits and if consent has been obtained
- Any special requirements (e.g., irradiated, CMV-negative or hepatitis–negative products)
- Name, status, and Nursing Midwifery Council or General Medical Council (NMC or GMC) number of the prescriber

Local policies will detail appropriate and accurate blood sampling, correct ordering, identification of the right patient, maintenance of the blood product in the correct environment, documentation, appropriate observation and monitoring of the patient prior to, during and after transfusion, safe transfusion, and following correct procedures returning labels or untransfused units to the labs. It is essential to report any transfusion reactions.

 If a blood transfusion is necessary, ensure it is the RIGHT blood to the RIGHT patient at the RIGHT time and in the RIGHT place.

MAJOR HAEMORRHAGE

Crash blood/emergency release blood

This is O-negative (universal donor) blood, which can be given to anyone in an emergency situation where a patient's blood group is unknown, to save a life. Hospitals will have local policy around the supply of 'crash' blood.

The Royal College of Paediatrics and Child Health recommends the use of tranexamic acid in children after major trauma 15 mg/kg (maximum of 1 g) diluted to a convenient volume in N/saline or 5% glucose,

Patients ABO group	Red cells	Platelets*	Fresh frozen plasma[†]	Cryoprecipitate
Group 0				
First choice	0	0	0	0
Second choice		A	A or B	A or B
Third choice			AB	
Group A				
First choice	A	A	A	A
Second choice	0[‡]	0[§]	AB	0 or B
Third choice			B[§]	
Group B				
First choice	B	A[§]	B	B
Second choice	0[‡]	0[§]	AB	0 or A
Third choice			A[§]	
Group AB				
First choice	AB	A[§]	AB	AB
Second choice	A or B	0[§]	A[§]	A or B
Third choice	0[‡]		B[§]	0

*Group B or AB platelets are not routinely available.
[†]Group AB FFP is often in short supply.
[‡]Screening for high-titre anti-A and anti-B is not required if plasma-depleted group 0 red cells in SAG-M are used.
[§]Tested and negative for high-titre anti-A and anti-B.
FFP, Fresh frozen plasma.
Source: Joint United Kingdom Blood Transfusion and Tissue Transplantation Services Professional Advisory Committee (JPAC), 2014. Handbook of Transfusion Medicine. fifth ed. Norwich: TSO.

to be infused intravenously over 10 minutes followed by 2 mg/kg/h (maximum 125 mg/h) for at least 8 hours or until bleeding is controlled (RCPCH 2012).

TRANSFUSION COMPATIBILITY

The unintentional transfusion of ABO incompatible blood is considered a 'never event' by the Department of Health UK (National Health Service [NHS] England 2015/2016).

See Table 9.4 for blood compatibility. This is included for use more in developing countries, as in the United Kingdom it would be expected that the first choice blood compatibility for transfusion would be provided.

RHD ANTIGENS

It is reported that approximately 85% of Northern white Europeans and almost 100% of those of Chinese origin are RhD antigen positive

(JPAC 2014). People who are RhD negative and have been transfused with RhD-positive red cells and RhD negative women who have been pregnant with an RhD-positive baby will have antibodies to RhD (anti-D). These IgG anti-D antibodies may cause acute or delayed haemolytic transfusion reactions if transfused with RhD-positive red cells, which can cause haemolytic disease of the newborn and it is therefore important to avoid transfusing RhD-negative females who may become pregnant, with RhD-positive red cell transfusions except in extreme emergencies when no other group is immediately available (JPAC 2014).

SPECIAL REQUIREMENTS – IRRADIATED, CYTOMEGALOVIRUS, OR HEPATITIS E NEGATIVE

Irradiated blood products

Irradiation of blood components (red cells, platelets, and granulocyte concentrates) inactivates residual lymphocytes to prevent transfusion-associated graft-versus-host disease. It is NOT necessary to irradiate cryoprecipitate, fractionated plasma products (FFP) such as clotting factor concentrates, albumin, or intravenous immunoglobulin (BCSH Blood Transfusion Taskforce 2010).

Irradiated blood irradiated blood has shelf life of 14 days (Mintz & Anderson 1993), but both gamma and x-ray irradiation of red cells accelerate leakage of potassium and increase level of extracellular potassium (Moroff et al 1999; Janatpour et al 2005). This potential potassium load may be significant in rapid, large-volume transfusions such as neonatal exchange transfusion (NET) or IUT (BCSH Blood Transfusion Taskforce 2010).

Irradiated blood components should be requested according to local guidelines and policies, but the following key recommendations are prepared by the BCSH Blood Transfusion Taskforce (2010):

- All blood products for IUT should be irradiated.
- Irradiation is recommended for NET and essential if there has been a previous IUT or if the donation comes from a first- or second-degree relative. For IUT and NET, blood should be transfused within 24 hours of irradiation and within 5 days of collection.
- It is not necessary to irradiate red cells for routine 'top-up' transfusions of premature or term infants unless there has been a previous IUT, and in that case, irradiated products should be administered until 6 months after expected date of delivery.
- All severe T-lymphocyte immunodeficiency syndromes should be considered as indicators for irradiated products.
- There is no need to irradiate blood products for infants undergoing cardiac surgery unless there is a confirmed or suspected coexisting T-lymphocyte immunodeficiency syndrome (includes DiGeorge, severe combined immunodeficiency, CHARGE).
- All children with Hodgkin lymphoma should receive irradiated products for life.

- All recipients of allogenic haemopoietic stem cell transplantation must receive irradiated products from the time of initiation of conditioning chemotherapy and while the patient continues to receive graft-versus-host disease prophylaxis.
- Patients receive human leucocyte antigen (HLA)-selected components.
- Patients undergoing autologous bone marrow transplant or peripheral blood stem cell transplant should receive irradiated products.
- Patients treated with purine analogue drugs (fludarabine, cladribine, deoxycoformicin) should receive irradiated products.
- Aplastic anaemia patients on rabbit antithymocyte globulin should receive irradiated products.
- Irradiated products are recommended for patients receiving the immunosuppressive agent alemtuzumab (anti-CD52) but not rituximab (anti-CD20).

IF YOU ARE UNSURE OF YOUR PATIENT'S REQUIREMENTS, ASK FOR EXPERT GUIDANCE AT YOUR TRANSFUSION SERVICE.

Further detailed recommendations can be found at www.bcshguidelines.com.

Cytomegalovirus-negative products

CMV is a type of herpes virus that can cause potentially life-threatening infection in patients who cannot mount an effective immune response (e.g., posttransplant or in utero). CMV is the commonest cause of congenital infection and can lead to neurodevelopment abnormalities including cerebral palsy and hearing loss (Peckham et al 1987). It can be transmitted through white cells contained in blood components. FFP and other plasma components have not been shown to transmit CMV.

The Advisory Committee on the Safety of Blood, Tissues and Organs (SaBTO) (2012) identified, following literature review and risk assessment, that leucodepletion is as effective as CMV IgG–negative blood components for immune-compromised patients.

CMV IgG–negative blood components SHOULD be ordered in the following circumstances:

- IUTs
- Neonates up to 28 days post estimated date of delivery
- Pregnancy
- Immune-suppressed patients known to be CMV negative (e.g., posttransplant)

See NHS Blood and Transfusion Factsheet on CMV-Negative Blood Components www.hospital.blood.co.uk for more information.

Hepatitis E virus-negative blood components

Hepatitis E virus (HEV) is found worldwide, with increasing incidence in the United Kingdom. It can be transmitted via blood transfusion, although in the United Kingdom a common route of infection is by eating raw or undercooked meat and shellfish. Most people who are infected with HEV will have no symptoms, but it will pose most risk to the immunocompromised patients. Since 2016 in the United Kingdom, HEV-negative blood products can be requested. HEV-negative blood products (blood, platelets, FFP, and cryoprecipitate) need to be requested for the following:

- Neonates and infants younger than 1 year
- Immunocompromised/immunosuppressed patients
- Patients awaiting solid organ transplant – from 3 months prior to date of planned transplant
- Patients who have had a solid organ transplant – for as long as they are taking immune suppressants
- Patients with acute leukaemia – from diagnosis (unless/until a decision is made not to proceed with stem cell transplant)
- Patients awaiting allogenic stem cell transplant – from 3 months prior to date of transplant up to 6 months after/or for as long as the patient is immunosuppressed
- Extracorporeal procedures – if within above indications

If the blood product is HEV negative (NEG), it will show NEG:HEV on the pack if provided by NHS Blood and Transplant (NHSBT).

 NB Non-UK plasma components issued by NHSBT (i.e., MB FFP and MB Cryoprecipitate) HAVE been tested in their country of origin as HEV negative but DO NOT show NEG:HEV on the pack.

All information on HEV from NHSBT (2016).

REFERENCES

Barras, M., 2013. Anti-Xa assays. Aust. Prescr. 36, 98–101.

Becker, K.L., Snider, R., Nylen, E.S., 2008. Procalcitonin assay in systemic inflammation, infection and sepsis: clinical utility and limitations. Crit. Care. Med. 36 (3), 941–952.

Bennett, R.L., Mahabee-Gittens, M., Chua, M.S., et al., 2011. Elevated cardiac troponin I in cases of thoracic non-accidental trauma. Pediatr. Emerg. Care. 27, 941–944.

British Committee for Standards in Haematology Blood Transfusion Task Force, 2004. Transfusion guidelines for neonates and older children. Br. J. Haematol. 124, 433–453.

British Committee for Standards in Haematology Blood Transfusion Task Force, 2010. Guidelines on the use of irradiated blood components. www. bcshguidelines.com.

Chiesa, C., Natale, F., Osborn, J.F., et al., 2011. C reactive protein and procalcitonin: reference intervals for preterm and term newborns during the early neonatal period. Clin. Chim. Acta. 412, 11–12.

Colvin, B.T., Barrowcliffe, T.W., 1993. The British Society for Haematology Guidelines on the use and monitoring of heparin 1992: Second revision. BCSH Haemostasis and Thrombosis Task Force. J. Clin. Pathol. 46, 97–103.

Dacie, J.V., Lewis, S.M., 1997. Practical Haematology, eight ed. Churchill Livingstone, Edinburgh.

Hirsh, J., Bauer, K.A., Donati, M.B., et al., 2008. Parenteral Anticoagulants: American College of Chest Physicians Evidence-Based Clinical Practice Guidelines, eighth ed. Chest 133, 1415–1459.

Ignjatovic, V., Najid, S., Newall, F., et al., 2010. Dosing and monitoring of enoxaparin (LMWH) therapy in children. Br. J. Haematol. 149, 734–738.

Janatpour, K., Denning, L., Nelson, K., et al., 2005. Comparison of X-ray vs. gamma irradiation of CPDA-1 red cells. Vox. Sang. 89, 215–219.

Joint United Kingdom Blood Transfusion and Tissue Transplantation Services Professional Advisory Committee (JPAC), 2014. Handbook of Transfusion Medicine, fifth ed. TSO, Norwich.

Lim, W., Dentali, F., Eikelboom, J.W., et al., 2006. Meta-analysis: low-molecular weight heparin and bleeding in patients with severe renal insufficiency. Ann. Intern. Med. 144, 673–684.

Lipshultz, S.E., Simbre, V.C., Hart, S., et al., 2008. Frequency of elevations in markers of cardiac myocyte damage in otherwise healthy newborns. Am. J. Cardiol. 102, 761–766.

Mayo Clinic, 2016. Pediatric Test Reference Values. Mayo Medical Laboratories. www.mayomedicallaboratories.com, Accessed 4 October 2016.

Mintz, P.D., Anderson, G., 1993. Effect of gamma radiation on the in vivo recovery of stored red cells. Ann. Clin. Lab. Sci. 23, 216–220.

Moroff, G., Holme, S., AuBuchon, J.P., et al., 1999. Viability and in vitro properties of AS-1 red cells after gamma radiation. Transfusion 39, 128–134.

NHS Blood Transfusion, 2016. Hepatitis E virus (HEV) negative blood components. Information for Healthcare Professionals. www.hospital.blood.co.uk. accessed 03/10/2016.

NHS England Patient Safety Domain (2015/2016) Never Events List. NHS England, London, www.england.nhs.uk, Accessed 10 March 2016.

O'Grady, N.P., Barie, P.S., Bartlett, J.G., et al., 2008. Guidelines for evaluation of new fever in critically ill adult patients: 2008 update from the American College of Critical Care Medicine and the Infectious Diseases Society of America. Crit. Care. Med. 36 (4), 1330–1349.

Peckham, C.S., Stark, O., Dudgeon, J.A., et al., 1987. Congenital cytomegalovirus infection: a cause of sensorineural hearing loss. Arch. Dis. Child. 62 (12), 1233–1237.

Royal College of Paediatrics and Child Health and the Neonatal and Paediatric Pharmacists Group, 2012. Evidence Statement. Major trauma and the use of tranexamic acid in children. www.rcpch.ac.uk/medicines.

Souto, A.C.A., de Carvalho, W.B., 2008. Evaluation of serum cardiac troponin I values in children less than 1 year of age. Rev Bras. Cir. Cardiovasc. 23, 3.

The Advisory Committee on the Safety of Blood, Tissues and Organs (SaBTO), 2012. Cytomegalovirus Tested Blood Components Position Statement. www.gov.uk/government/news/provision-of-cytomegalovirus-tested-blood-components-position-statement-published. accessed 04/10/2016.

Van Rossum, A.M., Wulkan, R.W., Oudesluys-Murphy, A.M., 2004. Procalcitonin as an early marker of infection in neonates and children. Lancet. Infect. Dis. 4, 620–623.

Wackner, C., Prkno, A., Brunkhorst, F.M., et al., 2013. Procalcitonin as a diagnostic marker for sepsis: a systematic review and meta-analysis. Lancet. Infect. Dis. 13 (5), 426–435.

Whyte, R., Kirplani, H., 2011. Low versus high haemoglobin concentration threshold for blood transfusion for preventing morbidity and mortality in very low birth weight infants. Cochrane. Database. Syst. Rev. CD000512.

USEFUL WEBSITES

American Association of Blood Banks (AABB), www.aabb.org/resources
NHS Blood and Transplant, www.nhsbt.nhs.uk
Serious Hazards of Transfusion (SHOT), www.shotuk.org
The Cochrane Database of Systematic Reviews, www.cochrane.org

This chapter is intended for use as a quick reference guide, and it is not designed to replace the British National Formulary for Children, the Association of the British Pharmaceutical Industry Data Sheet Compendium, paediatric formularies, or any other sources of specialist information about drug use in children. A new chapter on pain and sedation in children focuses on analgesics and sedatives, but they are mentioned in this chapter.

Great care has been taken to ensure that the dosages given are correct at the time of writing but dose schedules do change and relevant information sources should be used to check doses when necessary.

NB Many drugs discussed in this chapter are unlicensed for use in children.

RESUSCITATION DRUGS

Drugs that may be used during resuscitation are outlined in Table 10.1.

Guidance regarding the indications for each of these drugs should be sought before use.

Table 10.1 Resuscitation drugs		
Drug	**Use**	**Intravenous dose**
Amiodarone	In supraventricular and ventricular arrhythmias	5 mg/kg (max. 300 mg) dilute to at least 600 µg/mL in glucose 5% (centrally if possible)
Adrenaline (epinephrine)	Cardiac arrest	10 µg/kg (0.1 mL/kg) of 1:10 000 (max. 1 mg)
Calcium gluconate 10%	Acute hypocalcaemia and hyperkalaemia	0.5 mL/kg (max. 20 mL)
Magnesium sulphate	Torsades de pointes	25–50 mg/kg (max. 2 g)
Sodium bicarbonate 8.4%	Hyperkalaemia and arrhythmias associated with tricyclic antidepressant overdose	1 mL/kg for infants and children

Advanced Life Support Group, 2016. Advanced Paediatric Life Support: A Practical Approach to Emergencies, sixth ed. BMJ Publishing Group, London.

Adrenaline (epinephrine) 0.1 mL of 1:1000 is no longer recommended, so subsequent doses should remain as 0.1 mL of 1:10 000. Higher doses of intravenous (IV) adrenaline may worsen the outcome (Enright et al 2012).

See Chapter 1 for details of drugs that can be given via the endotracheal route.

DRUGS FOR INTUBATION

To reduce the risk of damaging the upper airway during intubation, infants and children should be sedated and paralysed prior to the procedure. The sedatives and neuromuscular blocking drugs commonly used as premedication for intubation are outlined in Table 10.2.

Table 10.2 Drugs for intubation			
Drug	**Use**	**Dose (IV)**	**Comments**
Atracurium	Nondepolarising neuromuscular blocking agent	Initially 300–500 µg/kg	Often drug of choice in patients with renal or hepatic impairment can cause histamine release so avoid in asthma
			Short to intermediate duration of action
Pancuronium	Nondepolarising neuromuscular blocking agent	30–40 µg/kg in neonates; 50–100 µg/kg in children	Long duration of action (60–120 min)
			No histamine release but can cause tachycardia and hypertension
			Use with caution in severe renal and liver failure as duration is prolonged
Rocuronium	Nondepolarising neuromuscular blocking agent	0.6–1 mg/kg stat	Duration of action: infants 40 min, children 30 min
			Advantages over atracurium or vecuronium, include rapid onset of action within 60 s, cardiovascular stability, no drug accumulation or histamine release
			Duration prolonged in liver failure but do not adjust intubation dose. In myasthenia gravis, use smaller dose of 0.2 mg/kg (NB: long duration of action)
			NB: In emergencies, rocuronium can be given via the IM route in deltoid muscle: dose 1 mg/kg <1 year or 2 mg/kg >1 year, but onset of action takes 4 min (Fisher 1999)
Suxamethonium	Depolarising neuromuscular blocking agent	2 mg/kg in neonates and infants	Very rapid onset of action (1 min), but very short duration of action (4–6 min)

Table 10.2	Drugs for intubation—cont'd		
Drug	**Use**	**Dose (IV)**	**Comments**
		1–2 mg/kg in children Maximum dose 2.5 mg/kg	May cause bradycardia in children, especially following a second dose. Not recommended in liver disease, burns, or patients with Duchenne muscular dystrophy Can cause profound hyperkalaemia, especially in patients with burns, trauma, and renal failure
Ketamine	General anaesthetic agent	1–2 mg/kg	Contraindicated in hypertension. Risk of hallucinations is higher in older children and teenagers Coadministration of a benzodiazepine reduces the risk of hallucinations
Fentanyl	Opiate analgesic	1–5 µg/kg	Short-acting but potentially cumulative. At higher doses, risk of rigid chest syndrome
Morphine	Opioid sedative and analgesic	50–100 µg/kg in neonates; 100–200 µg/kg in infants and children	Neonates and infants show increased susceptibility to respiratory depression
Thiopentone	Used for induction of anaesthesia	2 mg/kg in neonates; 4–6 mg/kg in >1 month	Acutely reduces intracranial pressure and reduces cerebral metabolism, so it may be the drug of choice in patients with head injury (Singer & Webb 1997)

IM, intramuscular; *IV*, Intravenous.
Data from Guy's, St Thomas', King's College and University Lewisham Hospitals, 2010. Paediatric Formulary, eighth ed. Guy's, St Thomas', King's College and University Lewisham Hospitals, London.

Comprehensive prescribing information should be consulted before prescribing or administering these drugs.

QUICK-REFERENCE GUIDE FOR CALCULATING INFUSIONS

Many units use standard infusion calculations. Table 10.3 shows some of these 'rules of thumb' for frequently used drugs in paediatric intensive care.

These are not designed to replace infusion checking calculations which must always be performed when making up infusions. All infusions are made up to 50 mL.

Table 10.3 Standard preparation for common intravenous drug infusions

Drug	Quantity	Diluent up to 50 mL	Dose if run at 1 mL/h	Administration Central	Administration Peripheral
Adrenaline (epinephrine)	0.3 mg × weight (kg)	0.9% saline or 5% glucose	0.1 µg/kg/min	✓	
Aminophylline	50 mg × weight (kg)	0.9% saline or 5% glucose	1 mg/kg/h	✓	✓
Clonidine	50 µg × weight (kg)	0.9% saline or 5% glucose	1 µg/kg/h	✓	✓
Dinoprostone (prostaglandin E$_2$)	30 µg × weight (kg)	0.9% saline or 5% glucose	10 ng/kg/min	✓	✓
Dobutamine	30 mg × weight (kg)	0.9% saline or 5% glucose	10 µg/kg/min	✓	
Dopamine	30 mg × weight (kg)	0.9% saline or 5% glucose	10 µg/kg/min	✓	
Dopamine	3 mg × weight (kg)	0.9% saline or 5% glucose	1 µg/kg/min	✓	
Furosemide	10 mg × weight (kg)	0.9% saline	200 µg/kg/h	✓	✓
Glyceryl trinitrate	3 mg × weight (kg)	0.9% saline or 5% glucose	1 µg/kg/min	✓	✓
Midazolam	3 mg × weight (kg)	0.9% saline or 5% glucose	1 µg/kg/h	✓	✓
Milrinone	1.5 mg × weight (kg)	0.9% saline or 5% glucose	0.5 µg/kg/min	✓	✓
Morphine	1 mg × weight (kg)	0.9% saline or 5% glucose	20 µg/kg/h	✓	✓
Noradrenaline (norepinephrine)	0.3 mg × weight (kg)	0.9% saline or 5% glucose	0.1 µg/kg/min	✓	
Salbutamol	1.5 mg × weight (kg) (max. 25 mg/50 mL)	0.9% saline or 5% glucose	0.5 µg/kg/min	✓	✓
Sodium nitroprusside*	3 mg × weight (kg) (max. 50 mg/50 mL)	0.9% saline or 5% glucose	1 µg/kg/min	✓	✓
Vecuronium	5 mg × weight (kg)	0.9% saline or 5% glucose	100 µg/kg/h	✓	✓

*Sodium nitroprusside when made up must be protected from light and if available an amber giving set can be used.
Data from Guy's, St Thomas', King's College and University Lewisham Hospitals, 2010. Paediatric Formulary, eighth ed. Guy's, St Thomas', King's College and University Lewisham Hospitals, London.

Checking the infusion dose from the syringe concentration:
- Use the prescribed drug dose; that is, the total amount in the 50-mL syringe × 1000 to give amount in nanograms (ng) or micrograms (µg) if the units differ from the prescription
- Divide this by 50 to give the amount per millilitre
- Divide by the weight in kilograms to give amount per kilogram per millilitre
- Divide this figure by 60 if the infusion is calculated dose/kg/min.

INOTROPIC AND CHRONOTROPIC DRUGS

An inotrope is a drug that increases the force of cardiac muscular contraction.

A chronotrope is a drug that alters the heart rate, that is, the rate of contraction of the heart.

Inotropic and chronotropic drugs are used in clinical practice. The effects produced by inotropic and chronotropic drugs are largely dependent upon the receptor sites activated and the doses administered. Table 10.4 outlines the receptor selectivity and pharmacologic effects produced by commonly used agents.

DRUGS COMMONLY USED AS INTRAVENOUS INFUSIONS

All drug dosages unless otherwise referenced have been taken from the Paediatric Formulary online (2015).

Adenosine

Pharmacology: Adenosine is an endogenous nucleoside acting on coronary perfusion and myocardial conduction. It inhibits noradrenaline (norepinephrine) release from nerve endings, causes vasodilation, and has important antiarrhythmic properties. Adenosine has diverse physiologic functions mediated by receptors A_1, A_{2A}, A_{2B}, and A_3. Actions mediated by A_1 receptors include slowing the heart rate and blocking atrioventricular nodal conduction, reduction of atrial contractility, and attenuation of the stimulatory actions of catecholamine release on the heart. It also produces constriction of bronchial smooth muscle receptors by A_1 stimulation in asthmatics.

Adenosine is a rapidly acting drug with a half-life of less than 10 seconds.

Indications: Rapid reversion to sinus rhythm of supraventricular tachycardias, or as an aid to diagnosis of broad or narrow complex supraventricular tachycardias.

Monitoring: Continuous electrocardiograph (ECG) monitoring, blood pressure.

Side effects: Transient facial flush, chest pain, dyspnoea, bronchospasm, choking sensation, severe bradycardia.

Dosage and administration: Initial dose 150 µg/kg in neonates and infants up to 1 year, then increase the dose by 50–100 µg/kg and give

Table 10.4 The pharmacological effect and receptor selectivity of various inotropic and chronotropic drugs

	Receptor selectivity			Pharmacologic effect			
	α	β_1	β_2	Peripheral vascular vasodilation	Peripheral vascular vasoconstriction	Inotropic	Chronotropic
Dobutamine	+	+++	++	++	–	+++	+
Dopamine 0.5–2 µg/kg/min	–	–	–	– (renal and splanchnic dilatation)	–	–	–
Dopamine 2–5 µg/kg/min	–	+	–	+ (renal and splanchnic dilatation)	+	+	+
Dopamine >5 µg/kg/min	+	++	–	– (renal and splanchnic dilatation)	++	++	++
Enoximone	–	–	–	+	–	+++	+
Epinephrine	+	+++	++	++	–	+++	++
Isoprenaline	–	++++	+++	+++	–	+++	+++
Noradrenaline (norepinephrine)	+++	++	–	–	++++	+	+

Source: With permission from Young, L.Y., Koda-Kimble, M.A., (Eds.) 1995. Applied Therapeutics, sixth ed. Applied Therapeutics, Vancouver, BC.

every 1–2 minutes until tachycardia is terminated or the maximum single dose is reached (maximum single dose in neonates 300 µg/kg or infants 500 µg/kg). In 1- to 12-year-olds, give 100 µg/kg initially, then, if required, increase the dose by 50–100 µg/kg until tachycardia is terminated or the maximum single dose of 500 µg/kg (max 12 mg) is reached. Above 12 years, give 3 mg initially, followed by 6 mg if required and then a maximum dose 12 mg (Advanced Life Support Group 2016). Fast IV bolus injection over less than 2 seconds followed by 5–10 mL rapid bolus of 0.9% sodium chloride. Give centrally if access is available or into a large peripheral vein as it is rapidly metabolised in the peripheral circulation and administration is painful.

Contraindications

- Adenosine may not be the drug of choice in asthmatics as it can cause bronchospasm.
- It is contraindicated in a heart block.
- If the patient is on concurrent dipyridamole, the initial dose of adenosine should be quartered. The reason for this is not fully understood, but dipyridamole increases the plasma levels of endogenous adenosine by inhibiting its uptake into cells (German et al 1989).

Adrenaline (epinephrine)

Pharmacology: Adrenaline is a potent agonist of α-, β_1-, and β_2-adrenoreceptors and has very low affinity for dopamine receptors. The effects it produces are dependent upon this receptor sensitivity. β_1-receptor stimulation produces positive inotropy, increasing cardiac output and systolic blood pressure. β_2-receptor stimulation produces skeletal muscle vasodilation, which results in reduced peripheral vascular resistance and often a fall in diastolic blood pressure. At higher doses, α_1-receptor stimulation becomes increasingly significant and produces peripheral vasoconstriction, resulting in increases in peripheral resistance and diastolic blood pressure.

Indications: Inotropic therapy in cardiogenic shock.

Monitoring: Arterial blood pressure, heart rate, and continuous ECG.

Side effects: Tachycardia, arrhythmias, hypertension.

Administration: When used as an infusion, adrenaline should be infused via a central line because of the risk of vasoconstriction and extravasation injury.

Aminophylline

Pharmacology: Aminophylline is a combination of theophylline and ethylenediamine. This combination has the advantage of increased solubility compared to theophylline. Theophylline is an inhibitor of cyclic adenosine monophosphate (cAMP) phosphodiesterase and is an adenosine receptor antagonist. The most clinically useful pharmacologic effect is its potent bronchodilator activity.

Indications: Reversible airways disease, severe acute asthma.

Monitoring: Monitoring of plasma concentrations is necessary as theophylline's pharmacokinetics show large interpatient variation, its metabolism can be altered by other drugs and chemicals, and it has a very narrow therapeutic index.

Side effects: Hypokalaemia (particularly in combination with β_2-receptor agonists), tachycardia, palpitations, gastrointestinal disturbances, arrhythmias and, in overdose, convulsions.

Amiodarone

Pharmacology: Amiodarone is a class III antiarrhythmic drug that is useful in the treatment of supraventricular tachycardia and ventricular arrhythmias. Its main mechanism of action is prolongation of the refractory period. It has the advantage of causing little or no myocardial depression. It acts rapidly when given by IV infusion and has a very long elimination half-life, particularly after chronic treatment. Seek expert advice before prescribing.

Indications: Treatment of arrhythmias, particularly when other drugs are contraindicated or ineffective.

Monitoring: Liver and thyroid function tests should be performed on prolonged oral therapy and during IV therapy. ECG and blood pressure monitoring are mandatory.

Side effects: IV amiodarone can produce a drop in blood pressure, particularly if infused too rapidly. Hepatotoxicity, thyroid disturbances, peripheral neuropathy, pulmonary toxicity, corneal microdeposits, and phototoxicity may all occur during chronic therapy.

Administration: Infuse centrally if possible, as peripheral infusions are likely to cause thrombophlebitis. When diluted, amiodarone should not be diluted to below 600 µg/mL as it precipitates. **Dilute in 5% glucose, not 0.9% sodium chloride.**

Argipressin (vasopressin)

Pharmacology: Vasopressin is a hormone that is produced in the neuronal cells of the hypothalamic nuclei and stored in the posterior lobe of the pituitary gland. It can also be pharmaceutically prepared as argipressin.

Indications: It is used as a potent vasopressor in septic shock as it causes arterial smooth muscle contraction. It is also used for variceal haemorrhage because of its vasoconstrictive effects. It has antidiuretic properties. Vasopressin vasodilates the pulmonary circulation, decreasing pulmonary vascular resistance under both normal and hypoxic conditions as a consequence of V_1-receptor-mediated release of nitric oxide from endothelial cells. Pulmonary artery vasodilation occurs with low concentrations of vasopressin.

Monitoring: Arterial blood pressure, heart rate, and continuous ECG. Liver function tests (see below).

Side effects:

- Bilirubin levels may increase during vasopressin infusion (though no clear mechanisms are known), so liver function tests should be closely monitored during infusion.
- Conflicting data exist regarding vasopressin's effect on splanchnic circulation, gut hypoperfusion, and myocardial ischaemia.
- **Adult** data suggest that complications related to 'low'-dose vasopressin appear to be infrequent and minor and can be largely avoided by not administering bolus doses or infusion rates above 0.04 U/min (Mutlu & Factor 2004). (Where high-dose vasopressin was used in one study 4/6 patients had cardiac arrest [Holmes et al 2001].) No data exist, however, for the paediatric population
- May lower body temperature.

Administration: Infuse via a central line as vasopressin is a powerful skin vasoconstrictor and extravasation of even a small quantity of this could cause local skin necrosis. Has a short plasma half-life (5–15 min). Rebound hypotension can occur on discontinuation of vasopressin infusion.

Clonidine

Pharmacology: Clonidine is a partial agonist of α_2-adrenergic receptors and at high doses it can also stimulate α_1-receptors. It is traditionally used as a centrally acting antihypertensive agent. More recently it has been used as a sedative and analgesic. Brain and spinal cord α_2-receptor stimulation modulate the response to pain. Clonidine has also been used to prevent and treat drug withdrawal from opiates, benzodiazepines, and other narcotic drugs.

Clonidine has beneficial effects in reducing the catecholamine-mediated cardiovascular response to stress, surgery, or intubation. Clonidine does not depress the central respiratory drive and does not inhibit gastric motility. Clonidine presents synergistic effects with opioids and is morphine-sparing, so doses of opioids may be reduced.

Indications: Sedation, analgesia, or opioid withdrawal. Usually use oral clonidine first, then, if required, use IV clonidine and discontinue oral clonidine.

Monitoring: Blood pressure, heart rate, pain, and sedation levels.

Side effects: Hypotension and sinus bradycardia.

Oral use for sedation in paediatric intensive care unit:

- Initial dose of 3–5 µg/kg per dose every 8 hours (maximum total oral dose 300 µg/24 h)
- If clonidine is used for more than 2 weeks, it must be weaned off over a period of days to prevent rebound. If it is used to prevent or treat drug withdrawal, it should be continued for 2–3 days after the opioids have been stopped.

Dose and administration: Start IV infusion at 1 µg/kg/h (in paediatric intensive care unit [PICU] only). Increase dose if required by 0.5 µg/kg/h until adequate sedation is achieved. Most children do not require doses above 1 µg/kg/h (max. dose is 2 µg/kg/h). Do not bolus IV clonidine as it may cause acute hypotension. Reduce the dose if hypotension occurs and discontinue if marked hypotension or bradycardia occur.

Dinoprostone (prostaglandin E₂)

Pharmacology: Dinoprostone is derived from the unsaturated long-chain fatty acid arachidonic acid by the cyclo–oxygenase enzyme system, and it takes part in the inflammatory cascade. Prostaglandin E_2 has a variety of pharmacologic actions, including vascular smooth muscle relaxation, stimulation of uterine contractions, alteration in renal blood flow resulting in diuresis, and involvement in inflammatory responses.

Indications: Dinoprostone is most commonly used in paediatrics to maintain the patency of the ductus arteriosus in neonates with congenital heart defects until corrective surgery is possible. Alprostadil (prostaglandin E_1) can also be used for this purpose. Alprostadil is licensed for this indication; however, it is considerably more expensive.

Monitoring: Arterial blood pressure, oxygen saturation; facilities for intubation and ventilation should be available.

Side effects: IV dinoprostone can cause apnoea and respiratory depression. Other side effects include hypotension, flushing, fluctuation in temperature, bradycardia, tachycardia, and oedema.

Dobutamine

Pharmacology: Dobutamine stimulates β_1-adrenoreceptors to increase cardiac contractility and β_2-adrenoreceptors to cause vasodilation in mesenteric and skeletal vascular beds. It also stimulates α_1-adrenoreceptors to cause vasoconstriction. The vasodilatory and vasoconstricting effects counterbalance each other and the primary haemodynamic response during dobutamine infusion is an increase in cardiac output, with little change in blood pressure. Dobutamine has no effect upon dopamine receptors.

Indications: Inotropic support in cardiac surgery, cardiomyopathy, septic shock, and cardiogenic shock.

Monitoring: Arterial blood pressure, heart rate, and continuous ECG.

Side effects: Tachycardia, hypotension, systolic hypertension, arrhythmia, extravasation injury.

Dopamine

Pharmacology: The cardiovascular effects of dopamine are mediated by its stimulation of a number of different receptor types: dopamine D_1 and D_2 receptors; β_1-adrenoreceptors; and α_1-adrenoreceptors.

At low doses (0.5–2 μg/kg/min) the predominant action of dopamine is to stimulate vascular dopamine D_1 receptors, causing vasodilation in mesenteric, renal, and coronary vascular beds. The resulting increase in renal blood flow and glomerular filtration rate is the basis of the so-called 'renal' dopamine effect. At medium doses (2–5 μg/kg/min) the effects produced by stimulation of β_1-adrenoreceptors are added. Thus, positive inotropic and chronotropic effects usually result in increased systolic blood pressure and pulse pressure with no effect or a small increase in diastolic pressure.

At higher doses (>5 µg/kg/min) dopamine activates α_1-adrenoreceptors, causing vasoconstriction. Thus, increases in systemic vascular resistance, systolic and diastolic blood pressure, and a reduced renal dopamine effect are seen.

Indications: Inotropic therapy in cardiogenic shock, and to promote renal perfusion.

Monitoring: Arterial blood pressure, heart rate, and continuous ECG.

Side effects: Peripheral vasoconstriction, hypertension, tachycardia, and extravasation injury.

Furosemide

Pharmacology: Furosemide is a loop diuretic that inhibits electrolyte reabsorption from the ascending limb of the loop of Henle in the renal tubules. It can be useful in renal failure when other groups of diuretics are ineffective, but it can cause electrolyte disturbances, particularly hypokalaemia. It is one of the most potent diuretics.

Indications: Oedema, oliguria due to renal failure.

Monitoring: Fluid balance, blood urea and electrolytes, and blood pressure.

Side effects: Hyponatraemia, hypokalaemia, hypomagnesaemia, hypocalcaemia, hypotension, hypovolaemia, metabolic acidosis, tinnitus, and deafness (particularly in renal failure, large parenteral doses and rapid administration).

Glyceryl trinitrate

Pharmacology: Glyceryl trinitrate produces smooth muscle relaxation and as a result it is a powerful vasodilator of both arterial and venous vasculature. Its effects are mediated by nitric oxide, which is released when glyceryl trinitrate is metabolised. It is a powerful antihypertensive agent and reduces afterload in cardiac failure. Tolerance to the effects of glyceryl trinitrate often develops after continuous prolonged use.

Indications: Left ventricular failure.

Monitoring: Blood pressure, heart rate, methaemoglobin concentrations.

Side effects: Headache, hypotension, tachycardia, methaemoglobinaemia.

Administration: Nitrates are absorbed on to polyvinyl chloride (PVC) – select non-PVC syringe and giving set.

Levosimendan

Pharmacology: Levosimendan is a cardioprotective inodilator; and pharmacologic effects include increased cardiac contractility mediated by calcium sensitisation of troponin C (Haikala et al 1995; Sorsa et al 2004), vasodilation through the opening of potassium channels on the sarcolemma of smooth muscle cells in the vasculature (Kaheinen et al 2001), and cardioprotection through the opening of mitochondrial potassium channels in the cardiomyocytes (Maytin & Colucci 2005; Pollesello & Papp 2007). Levosimendan enhances left ventricular performance and reduces left ventricular filling pressure.

Indications: There are no current official indications in patients under 18 years of age, but it is currently used as a rescue drug in PICU, after cardiac surgery, in patients with acute cardiac failure, or cardiomyopathy for potentially reversible catecholamine-resistant cardiogenic shock.

Monitoring: Arterial blood pressure, heart rate, ECG.

Side effects: Hypotension – usually transient, headache, atrial fibrillation, hypokalaemia, and tachycardia.

Administration: Loading dose of 10 μg/kg over 30 minutes (consider need to reduce milrinone at commencement of loading dose or may need to stop milrinone infusion).

After loading dose, commence levosimendan infusion at 0.1 μg/kg/min for 24 hours.

This can be administered via a peripheral or central vein. If the clinical response is inadequate after 6 hours, the infusion rate can be increased to 0.2 μg/kg/min.

It is usually given as a 24-hour infusion after which the active metabolite reaches pharmacologic active plasma levels, resulting in a prolonged haemodynamic effect (Antila et al 2007), which persists for at least 7 days (Lilleberg et al 2007).

Lorazepam

Pharmacology: Lorazepam is a benzodiazepine that has a fast speed of onset and anticonvulsant effects that last up to 24 hours. Other effects include sedation, anxiolysis, and amnesia. It does not convert to active metabolites, unlike midazolam. Effects may be reversed by the benzodiazepine antagonist flumazenil, although this is rarely necessary.

Indications: Premedication, sedation with amnesia, status epilepticus.

Monitoring: Blood pressure and oxygen saturation.

Side effects: Hypotension and apnoea – therefore resuscitation facilities should be available.

Administration: IV bolus may be given centrally or peripherally. Also, it may be given neat by slow injection.

Midazolam

Pharmacology: Midazolam is a short-acting benzodiazepine that binds to benzodiazepine receptors in the central nervous system to produce a variety of effects, including sedation, anxiolysis, anticonvulsant effects, and amnesia. Effects may be reversed by the benzodiazepine antagonist flumazenil, although this is rarely necessary.

Indications: Sedation, premedication, treatment of epilepsy.

Monitoring: Arterial blood pressure, oxygen saturation.

Side effects: Respiratory depression and severe hypotension after IV administration, acute withdrawal syndrome after prolonged use (1–2 weeks). Patients can develop tolerance in 48–72 hours.

Milrinone

Pharmacology: Milrinone is a selective inhibitor of phosphodiesterase III, an enzyme responsible for catalysing the breakdown of cAMP. Phosphodiesterase is found in high concentrations in cardiac and vascular smooth muscle. The inhibition of phosphodiesterase results in an accumulation of cAMP, which causes positive inotropy and vasodilation. Milrinone is excreted primarily via the kidneys (dose should be reduced in renal failure to avoid accumulation).

Indications: Congestive cardiac failure where cardiac output is reduced and filling pressures are increased. Milrinone acts as an inotrope and afterload reducer.

Monitoring: Arterial blood pressure, heart rate, and continuous ECG.

Side effects: Arrhythmias, hypotension.

Dose and administration: Loading dose 50 μg/kg over 10–20 minutes then infusion rate range 0.3–0.75 μg/kg/min (0.5 μg/kg/min is adequate to maintain therapeutic levels [Bailey et al 1999]). Do not infuse milrinone with furosemide as precipitation occurs. Unlike enoximone, milrinone cannot be given orally.

Morphine

Pharmacology: Morphine is an agonist of a number of morphine receptor subtypes. The most important therapeutic and adverse effects are thought to be mediated via μ and κ opioid receptors. Morphine produces a wide range of pharmacologic effects, including analgesia, sedation, respiratory depression, euphoria, inhibition of gut motility, miosis, nausea, and vomiting.

Indications: Analgesia, sedation.

Monitoring: Sedation, respiratory rate, oxygen saturation.

Side effects: Nausea and vomiting, constipation, respiratory depression (especially neonates), hypotension, miosis, hallucinations, acute withdrawal syndrome after prolonged use.

Noradrenaline (norepinephrine)

Pharmacology: Noradrenaline is a potent agonist of α-adrenergic receptors. It produces vasoconstriction with an increase in systemic vascular resistance and an elevation of both systolic and diastolic blood pressure. Cardiac output is usually unchanged or reduced. Blood flow to most vascular beds is reduced, including the kidney and the liver.

Indications: Acute hypotension.

Monitoring: Arterial blood pressure, heart rate, and continuous ECG.

Side effects: Hypertension, arrhythmias, peripheral ischaemia.

Administration: Administer via a central line.

Propofol

Pharmacology: Propofol is a short-acting general anaesthetic agent with a rapid onset of action of approximately 30 seconds. Propofol reduces cerebral blood flow, intracranial pressure, and cerebral metabolism.

Propofol has a rapid distribution with a half-life of 2–4 minutes and rapid elimination. It is cleared by metabolic processes mainly in the liver, and is excreted in the urine.

Indications: Sedation, anaesthesia.

Monitoring: Continuous ECG, oxygen saturations, and blood pressure. Propofol is formulated in intralipid, so monitor the blood lipid levels of all patients.

Side effects: Bradycardia, hypotension, desaturation. Propofol syndrome is a rare and often fatal condition described in children treated with propofol for more than 2–3 days at high doses (>4 mg/kg/h). Symptoms include cardiac failure, rhabdomyolysis, severe lactic acidosis, renal failure, and coma.

Administration: IV infusion is not recommended by the Committee on Safety of Medicines; however, if strictly necessary, IV infusion for sedation can be cautiously administered at 2–3 mg/kg/h or adjust dose according to response. Infusion should not continue for more than 2 days and should not exceed 5 mg/kg/h.

 Propofol should be avoided in any patient who is allergic to eggs, peanuts, and soybean oil as there is a risk of anaphylaxis.

Prostaglandin E$_2$

See dinoprostone.

Salbutamol

Pharmacology: Salbutamol is a selective β$_2$-adrenergic receptor agonist. It is useful principally as a bronchodilator, although other effects, such as reducing serum potassium, are clinically beneficial.

Indications: Acute asthma, renal hyperkalaemia.

Monitoring: ECG, serum potassium, heart rate, oxygen saturation.

Side effects: Peripheral vasodilation, tachycardia, hypokalaemia.

Sodium nitroprusside (nipride)

Pharmacology: Sodium nitroprusside produces smooth muscle relaxation and as a result it is a powerful vasodilator of both arterial and venous vasculature. It is effective as an antihypertensive and to reduce preload in cardiac failure. Tolerance is less likely to develop after prolonged use of nitroprusside than with other nitrates. Breakdown of nitroprusside results in the production of thiocyanate, which may accumulate after prolonged infusion (after 3 days or earlier in renal failure).

Indications: Hypertensive crisis, left ventricular failure.

Monitoring: Blood pressure, heart rate, methaemoglobin concentrations, serum thiocyanate levels (after 72 hours of infusion).

Side effects: Hypotension, headache, tachycardia, symptoms of rapid blood pressure reduction.

Administration: Maximum concentration 1 mg/mL. Protect infusion from light and use an amber giving set.

Vecuronium

Pharmacology: Vecuronium bromide is a nondepolarising neuromuscular blocking agent with a high degree of selectivity for the nicotinic acetylcholine receptors. Its effects may be reversed by the use of an anticholinesterase drug, such as neostigmine. Following an IV bolus dose, it has an onset of action of about 2 minutes and lasts for 15–20 minutes in children and 30–40 minutes in infants. It rarely causes histamine release and has good cardiovascular stability. Use caution in liver and renal impairment.

Indications: Neuromuscular blockade.

Monitoring: Peripheral nerve stimulator; ventilation is mandatory.

Side effects: Recovery time is increased after prolonged use; very rare hypersensitivity reactions.

THERAPEUTIC DRUG MONITORING

Measurement of plasma levels is necessary for a range of drugs with a narrow therapeutic index. These drugs have a minimum therapeutic concentration that is close to their minimum toxic concentration. The target ranges of concentrations for these drugs are displayed in Table 10.5. The receptor selectivity and pharmacologic effects produced by commonly used agents are shown in Table 10.4. It may be necessary at times to run IV infusions concurrently and, while this should only be practised where absolutely essential, Fig. 10.1 shows the known IV compatabilities.

Reversal agents

Reversal agents are utilised to reverse the effects of anaesthetics, narcotics, or potential toxic agents (see Table 10.6). They are either receptor-specific antagonists or nonspecific analeptic agents (Anderson 1988). Some of the reversal agents may be short acting; therefore, they may need to be administered more than once.

Table 10.5 Therapeutic drug monitoring

Drug	Recommended sample time	Target range	Time to steady state (approx.)	Sample bottle	Notes
Aminophylline	At least 8 h after starting IV dose	10–20 mg/L	24–48 h	Plain (clotted)	Assay is for theophylline
Carbamazepine	Immediately prior to next dose	4–14 mg/L	2–4 weeks after starting then 3–4 days after each dose change	Plain (clotted)	
Digoxin	6 h postdose	0.8–2.2 µg/L	5–10 days	Plain (clotted)	
Gentamicin 'once daily'	18 h postdose	<1 mg/L trough	24 h	Plain (clotted)	Resample after 6–12 h if >1 mg/L
Phenobarbital	Before dose	9–25 mg/L in epilepsy	10–14 days	Plain (clotted)	
Phenytoin	IV: 1 h after of infusion; orally: before dose	10–20 mg/L infants; 6–15 mg/L neonates	1–2 weeks (variable)	Plain (clotted)	Seek advice if albumin binding is altered
Vancomycin	Trough: before dose; peak: 1 h after completing infusion	Trough: 5–10 mg/L; peak: 15–30 mg/L	24–36 h	Plain (clotted)	

IV, Intravenous

Data from Guy's, St Thomas', King's College and University Lewisham Hospitals, 2010. Paediatric Formulary, eighth ed. Guy's, St Thomas', King's College and University Lewisham Hospitals, London.

Fig. 10.1 Intravenous compatabilities. *TPN*, Total parenteral nutrition. (With permission from Guy's, St Thomas', King's College and University Lewisham Hospitals, 2015. Paediatric Formulary, ninth ed. Guy's, St Thomas', King's College and University Lewisham Hospitals, London.)

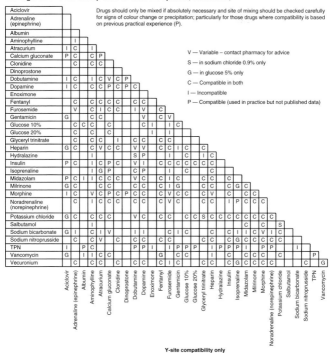

Drugs should only be mixed if absolutely necessary and site of mixing should be checked carefully for signs of colour change or precipitation; particularly for those drugs where compatibility is based on previous practical experience (P).

V — Variable – contact pharmacy for advice

S — in sodium chloride 0.9% only

G — in glucose 5% only

C — Compatible in both

I — Incompatible

P — Compatible (used in practice but not published data)

Y-site compatibility only

Table 10.6	Reversal agents	
Drug	**Dose**	**Effect**
Flumazenil	10 µg/kg – may be repeated at 1-min intervals to a maximum of 40 µg/kg (2 mg)	Reverses effects of benzodiazepines. After IV administration, has half-life of 1 h and duration of clinical effect 30–60 min. (Flumazenil may precipitate seizures in epileptic patients who are on benzodiazepines for seizure control, as it may induce withdrawal.)

Continued

Drug	Dose	Effect
Neostigimine	Slow IV injection 50–80 µg/kg in combination with a slow IV injection of atropine 10–20 µg/kg (max. 600 µg) over 1 min	Helps reverse the effects of nondepolarising muscle relaxants but should be used with train of four monitoring
Naloxone	Neonates IV injection 10 µg/kg – repeat every 2 min as necessary Children IV injection 4–10 µg/kg (max. 2 mg)	Reverses the effects of opioids. Half-life 1 h. May need repeat dose
Sugammadex	Child 2–18 years 2 mg/kg consult product literature*	Binds to rocuronium or vecuronium, terminating action
Protamine	Dose dependent on time since heparin given – see Paediatric Formulary	Reverses effect of unfractionated heparin
Dantrolene	IV injection 2–3 mg/kg followed by 1-mg/kg doses if necessary to maximum cumulative dose of 10 mg/kg.	Treatment for malignant hyperthermia caused by general anaesthetic agents

Table 10.6   Reversal agents—cont'd

* NICE BETA BNF, 2017. Drugs for reversal of neuromuscular blockade. Sugammadex. <http://www.evidence.nhs.uk/> (accessed 06.04.17).
IV, Intravenous.
Paediatric Formulary online 2015. Ninth ed. Guy's and St Thomas', Kings College and University Lewisham Hospitals. <http://www.cms.ubqo.com/> (accessed 05.08.17).

REFERENCES

Advanced Life Support Group, 2016. Advanced Paediatric Life Support: A Practical Approach to Emergencies, sixth ed. BMJ Publishing Group, London.

Anderson, J.A., 1988. Reversal agents in sedation and anaesthesia: a review. Anesth Prog 35, 43–47.

Antila, S., Sundberg, S., Lehtonen, L.A., 2007. Clinical pharmacology of levosimendan. Clin Pharmacokinet 46, 535–552.

Bailey, J.M., Miller, B.E., Lu, W., et al., 1999. The pharmacokinetics of milrinone in pediatric patients after cardiac surgery. Anesthesiology 90, 1012–1018.

Enright, K., Turner, C., Roberts, P., et al., 2012. Primary cardiac arrest following sport or exertion in children presenting to an emergency department: chest compressions and early defibrillation can save lives, but is intravenous epinephrine always appropriate? Pediatric Emerg Care 28, 336–339.

Fisher, D.M., 1999. Neuromuscular blocking agents in paediatric anaesthesia. Br J Anaesth 83, 58–64.

German, D.C., Kredich, N.M., Bjornsson, T.D., 1989. Oral dipyridamole increases plasma adenosine levels in human beings. Clin Pharmacol Ther 45, 80–84.

Haikala, H., Kaivola, J., Nissinen, E., et al., 1995. Cardiac troponin C as a target protein for a novel calcium sensitizing drug, levosimendan. J Mol Cell Cardiol 27, 1859–1866.

Holmes, C.L., Walley, K.R., Chittock, D.R., et al., 2001. The effects of vasopressin on hemodynamics and renal function in severe septic shock; a case series. Intensive Care Med 27, 1416–1421.

Kaheinen, P., Pollesello, P., Levijoki, J., et al., 2001. Levosimendan increases diastolic coronary flow in isolated guinea-pig heart by opening potassium channels. J Cardiovasc. Pharmacol 37, 367–374.

Lilleberg, J., Laine, M., Palkama, T., et al., 2007. Duration of the haemodynamic action of a 24 hour infusion of levosimendan in patients with congestive heart failure. Eur J Heart Fail 9, 75–82.

Maytin, M., Colucci, W.S., 2005. Cardioprotection: a new paradigm in the management of acute heart failure syndromes. Am J Cardiol 96, 26–31.

Mutlu, G.M., Factor, P., 2004. Role of vasopressin in the management of septic shock. Intensive Care Med 30, 1276–1291.

NICE BETA BNF, 2017. Drugs for reversal of neuromuscular blockade. Suggammadex. www.evidence.nhs.uk.

Paediatric Formulary online, 2015. ninth ed. Guy's and St Thomas', Kings College and University Lewisham Hospitals. www.cms.ubqo.com.

Pollesello, P., Papp, Z., 2007. The cardioprotective effects of levosimendan: preclinical and clinical evidence. *J Cardiovasc.* Pharmacol 50, 257–263.

Singer, M., Webb, A., 1997. Oxford Handbook of Critical Care. Oxford University Press, Oxford, p. 232.

Sorsa, T., Pollesello, P., Solaro, R.J., 2004. The contractile apparatus as a target for drugs against heart failure: interaction of levosimendan, a calcium sensitizer, with cardiac troponin C. Mol Cell Biochem 266, 87–107.

FURTHER READING

Ambrose, C., Sale, S., Howells, R., et al., 2000. Intravenous clonidine infusion in critically ill children: dose-dependent sedative effects and cardiovascular stability. Br J Anaesth 84, 794–796.

Arenas-Lopez, S., Riphagen, S., Tibby, S.M., 2004. Use of oral clonidine for sedation in ventilated paediatric intensive care patients. Intensive Care Med 30, 1625–1629.

Royal College of Paediatrics and Child Health, 2003. Medicines for Children, second ed. Royal College of Paediatrics and Child Health, London.

PAIN AND SEDATION

11

An important aspect of caring for critically ill infants and children is to minimise stress and to reduce pain whilst ensuring that children are not kept muscle relaxed and sedated for inappropriately long periods. Prolonged periods of sedation and muscle relaxation may lead to increased length of ventilation and risk a chance of drug withdrawal, predominantly benzodiazepine. It is important to consider developmental age and concept of pain, self-reporting of pain intensity using an appropriate rating scale if possible, parent's opinion, observation of behaviour, clinical observations, and information on social environment when assessing pain and level of comfort (Baeyer 2006; Craig & Badali 2004). Developmental concepts of pain are considered in Chapter 16 on child development. The importance of using pain ratings scales may be underestimated, but it has been shown that regular pain measurement improves pain management (Treadwell et al 2002). Language, ethnicity, and cultural factors may all influence the expression and assessment of pain (RCN 2009).

For pain assessment, use the Pain Recognition and Assessment Cycle (RCN 2009) (Fig. 11.1).

It is important that pain scales are not only appropriate for age and cognitive ability, but also that they are reliable and valid. Below are some referenced age-appropriate pain assessment scales, a few shown in greater detail.

Pain must be anticipated and assessed, and analgesia provided where necessary; then the pain must be reassessed. If the child is admitted to the paediatric intensive care unit (PICU) following surgery, then pain is expected at the surgical site; however, we as health care professionals must also be competent to manage chronic pain, procedural pain, recurring pain, and end-of-life pain.

It is vital to remember that for ventilated patients, muscle relaxation and sedation do not provide ANY pain control, so pain assessment and appropriate analgesia should be utilised.

ASSESSING PAIN AND SEDATION

Pain and sedation ratings scales for term neonates

All these examples of neonatal pain assessment tools require training for health care professionals; some include physiologic measures whilst others are just observer rated.

Fig. 11.1 Pain recognition and assessment cycle. (Royal College of Nursing, 2009. The recognition and assessment of acute pain in children. Update of full guideline. RCN, London.)

Pain Recognition and Assessment Cycle

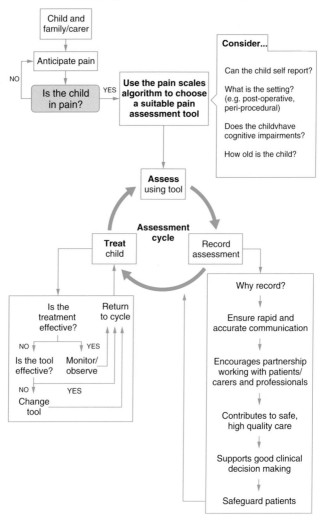

Table 11.1 Comfort score

Characteristic	Score	Evaluate
Alertness	1	Deeply asleep
	2	Lightly asleep
	3	Drowsy
	4	Awake and alert
	5	Hyperalert
Agitation	1	Calm
	2	Slightly anxious
	3	Anxious
	4	Very anxious
	5	Panicky
Respiratory response	1	No coughing
	2	Spontaneous respiration with little response to ventilation
	3	Occasional coughing with little resistance to the ventilator
	4	Active breathing against the ventilator
	5	Actively fighting the ventilator and coughing
		None
Physical movements	1	Occasional, slight movements
	2	Frequent, slight movements
	3	Vigorous movements or extremities only
	4	Vigorous movements of extremities, torso, and head
Blood pressure (mean)	1	Below baseline
	2	Normal
	3	Infrequent elevations of 15% or more
	4	Frequent elevations of 15% or more
	5	Sustained elevation greater than or equal to 15%
Heart rate	1	Below baseline
	2	Normal
	3	Infrequent elevations of 15% or more
	4	Frequent elevations of 15% or more
	5	Sustained elevation greater than or equal to 15%
Muscle tone	1	Relaxed/none
	2	Reduced muscle tone
	3	Normal muscle tone
	4	Increased tone/flexion–fingers/toes
	5	Extreme rigidity/flexion–fingers/toes
Facial tension	1	Facial muscles relaxed
	2	Normal tone
	3	Some tension
	4	Full facial tension
	5	Facial grimacing

Excessive sedation 8–16; adequate sedation 17–26; insufficient sedation 27–40.

- Comfort – a pain and sedation assessment using six behavioural and two physiologic factors to assess distress of critically ill children (Ambuel et al 1992), and reliability and validity are assessed (Van Dijk et al 2000) (Table 11.1).
- Cries – a pain assessment using five criteria assigned a score of 0–2, and if the total score is ≥5, then analgesia should be administered (Krechel & Bildner 1995).
- Neonatal Infant Pain Scale for ages 0–1 year – uses six criteria assigned a score of 0–2; a score over 3 indicates pain (Lawrence et al 1993).

This COMFORT scale assesses behavioural characteristics – alertness, agitation, respiratory response, physical movements, blood pressure, heart rate, muscle tone, and facial tension, with each scoring between 1 and 5 and the points are added for a total score. If the child scores:

8–16: sedation is excessive
17–26: sedation adequate
27–40: insufficient sedation

Pain ratings scales for children

There are over 30 pain assessment tools that have been found to be reliable and valid for use in children; however, it is also necessary to consider the context of use. For example, it is not useful to use a tool where facial expression needs to be assessed in an intensive care environment where many children are likely to have either masks or endotracheal tubes and tapes covering large parts of their face. Detailed below are a selection of paediatric pain ratings scales that may be of use in the PICU or high-dependency unit (HDU) in children without cognitive impairment.

- Cardiac Analgesic Assessment Tool – this is a pain assessment tool for intubated and ventilated children after cardiac surgery, which uses the assessment of pupil size, heart rate, blood pressure, and respiratory/motor response. A score of 4 or more leads to the assumption of pain, so analgesia is required (cardiac analgesia assessment scale [CAAS]) (Suominen et al 2004) (Table 11.2).
- Children's Hospital of Eastern Ontario Pain Scale (CHEOPS) (McGrath et al 1985).
- Wong–Baker Faces scale (Wong et al 2001) – this is a self-reporting scale that can be used in children aged 3–18 years where:
  - face 0 is happy as there is no pain
  - face 2 may have a little pain
  - face 4 hurts a little more
  - face 6 hurts even more
  - face 8 hurts a lot
  - face 10 hurts as much as you can imagine (validated by Bieri et al 1990)
- Visual Analogue Scale – this is a scale of numbers 0–10 where 0 is no pain and 10 is the worst pain; either the child may self-report or it is reported by an observer (self- or observer rated).

The Yale Visual Analogue scale is interesting to observe as it provides a correlation between the visual and verbal scales. It has been used mainly in adults in palliative care, but provides information about the impact on daily living (Fig. 11.2).

Assessing pain in children with cognitive impairment

Pain in children with a cognitive impairment can reduce functioning ability in several domains, which include communication, activities of daily living, motor skills, and socialisation (Breau et al 2007), so it is

Table 11.2 Cardiac Analgesic Assessment Scale (CAAS) (Suominen, 2004)

	Scoring		
Variables	*0*	*1*	*2*
Pupillary size[a]	≤2 mm (pinpoint)	3–4 mm (midsize)	>4 mm (dilated)
Heart rate[b]	Within baseline[c]	5–15% increase	>15% increase
Blood pressure (mean)	Within baseline[c]	5–15% increase	>15% increase
Respiratory and motor response[d]	No response	Cough and minimal movement settles after removal of stimulus	Cough and/or excessive movement >1 min after removal of stimuli

Response to suctioning or turning:
[a]Pupils: score to the nearest size.
[b]Patients with pacemaker on fixed rate or with junctional ectopic tachycardia (JET) are scored 1.
[c]Within baseline of <5% increase of BP or heart rate.
[d]Paralysed patients are scored 1.

Fig. 11.2 Yale visual analogue scale. (Wong-Baker FACES Foundation, 2016. Wong-Baker FACES Pain Rating Scale. Retrieved 10/01/2018 with permission from http://www.WongBakerFACES.org. Originally published in Whaley & Wong's Nursing Care of Infants and Children. Elsevier Inc.)

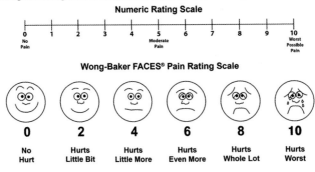

Numeric Rating Scale

0	1	2	3	4	5	6	7	8	9	10
No Pain					Moderate					Worst Possible Pain

Wong-Baker FACES® Pain Rating Scale

0	2	4	6	8	10
No Hurt	Hurts Little Bit	Hurts Little More	Hurts Even More	Hurts Whole Lot	Hurts Worst

vital that these children are carefully assessed for signs of pain, and that appropriate analgesia is given. Children with additional needs for long-term conditions may be living with:

- Dystonia, spasms
- Difficulty in positioning/pressure areas
- Reflux
- Bowel problems
- Late diagnosis due to difficulty in communication
- Fear and anxiety

Fig. 11.3 FLACC assessment tool. (Merkel, S.I., Voepel Lewis, T., Shayevitz, J.R., Malviya, S., 1997. The FLACC: a behavioural scale for scoring postoperative pain in young children. Pediatr. Nurs. 23, 293–297.)

	0	1	2
Face	No particular expression or smile	Occasional grimace or frown, withdrawn, disinterested	Frequent to constant frown, clenched jaw, quivering chin
Legs	Normal position or relaxed	Uneasy, restless, tense	Kicking, or legs drawn up
Activity	Lying quiently, normal position, moves easily	Squirming, shifting back and forth, tense	Arched, rigid,or jerking
Cry	No cry (awake or asleep)	Moans or whimpers, occasional complaints	Crying steadily, screams or sobs, frequent complaints
Consolability	Content, relaxed	Reassured by occasional touching, hugging or 'talking to', distractable	Difficult to console or comfort

The carers of these children are usually the best advocates – so do ask their opinions.

Three tools for use with nonverbal children were recommended by the Royal College of Nursing (RCN 2009) and these were:

1. Face, Legs, Arms, Cry, Consolability (FLACC) suitable for ages 2 months to 18 years and uses the patient's behaviour to assess pain (Fig. 11.3) (Merkel et al 1997).
2. Paediatric pain profile (PPP) – suitable for 1–18 years (Hunt et al 2007).
3. Non-communicating Children's Pain Checklist (NCCPC) – suitable for 3- to 19-year-olds (Breau et al 2002).

To use the tool, assess the scores in each category and add them together, so the total score is from 0 to 10. The numeric rating scale where 0 is no pain and 10 is severe pain is then utilised to assess the level of pain so that appropriate intervention may be made.

TREATING CHILDREN IN PAIN

In Together for Short Lives (2016) there is a model of integrated pharmacologic and nonpharmacologic approaches to controlling children's pain (Fig. 11.4), which is as relevant in palliation as it is in intensive

Fig. 11.4 A model of integrated pharmacologic and nonpharmacologic approach for controlling children's pain. *NSAIDs*, Non-steroidal anti inflammatory drugs. (Courtesy Dr Renée McCulloch and Dr Satbir Jassal. From Together for Short Lives (2016))

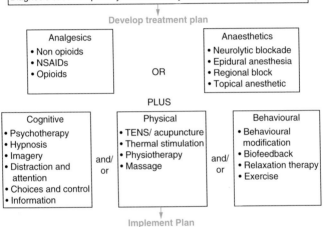

care. It is important to note that fear, or resultant unpleasant outcome, may affect whether the child discloses pain.

The World Health Organisation (WHO) 2012 guideline identified five key principles in the pain management of children:
1. Conduct a detailed assessment.
2. When pain is constant, provide regular analgesia ('by the clock').
3. Ensure there is medication prescribed for breakthrough pain.
4. Use the simplest route of administration.
5. Provide tailormade treatment for the child.

Even in paediatric intensive care, there is a place for play therapy and distraction to try to help relax the ventilated child.

Neuropathic pain

Neuropathic pain should be considered in children who have any of the following conditions, and the pain should be treated early on:

- Guillain-Barré syndrome
- Solid tumour
- Epidermolysis bullosa
- Rapidly progressing spinal curvature
- Dislocated/displaced hip and also in children with encephalocele or hypoxic ischaemic encephalopathy (Together for Short Lives 2016)

Pharmacologic management of pain in children

The WHO (2012) have modified their recommendations to a two-step analgesic approach: mild pain (treat with paracetamol and ibuprofen), then moderate to severe pain (opioids), excluding the use of tramadol and codeine (Tables 11.3 and 11.4).

Antispasmodic Medication – Check doses with formulary or local guidelines. Most of these medicines are unlicensed for children and should be prescribed by specialists.

Baclofen – used in chronic severe spasticity of voluntary muscle (considered a third-line neuropathic agent). There is a risk of toxicity in renal impairment, so administer with or after food to minimise gastric irritation. Withdraw the drug over 1–2 weeks.

Dantrolene – a skeletal muscle relaxant, used for chronic, severe muscle spasm. Liver function tests are required as the drug associated with symptomatic hepatitis. Use with caution in patients with cardiac and pulmonary disorders. Therapeutic action may take a few weeks.

Diazepam – relief of muscle spasm. Paradoxic reactions may occur in children (restlessness and agitation).

Gabapentin – adjuvant in neuropathic pain. Gabapentin is very bitter–capsules can be opened and mixed with strong tasting liquid, that is, blackcurrant juice immediately before administration.

Sedation

Chloral hydrate – used for sedation. Use with caution in children with obstructive sleep apnoea as they could be at risk of life-threatening respiratory obstruction. Use with caution in patients with renal, liver, or cardiac impairment.

Clonidine – used for anxiety/sedation/pain/opioid sparing. The administration is usually oral, but it can be given as an intravenous infusion.

Midazolam – can be used as a continuous intravenous infusion for sedation of the ventilated patient (not recommended for prolonged sedation in neonates as drug accumulation is likely to occur).

Propofol – is not recommended as a sedative by intravenous infusion for children under 16 years of age in intensive care as it is associated with a risk of propofol infusion syndrome, which has potentially fatal effects including metabolic acidosis, arrhythmias, cardiac failure,

Table 11.3 Analgesics for mild pain

Drug	Indication	Route	Age	Loading dose	Maintenance dose	Maximum daily dose	Notes
Paracetamol	Mild pain/ antipyretic	Oral	0–12 years	15 mg/kg	15 mg/kg	60 mg/kg	
			12–18 years	1 g	500 mg–1 g max	60 mg/kg or 4 g max.	
		Rectal	1–3 months	30 mg/kg	15–20 mg/kg	60 mg/kg or 4 g/day	
			>3 months	40 mg/kg			
		Intravenous	Term–1 month		7.5 mg/kg	<10 kg 30 mg/kg	Give intravenous dose over 15 min
			10–50 kg		10 mg/kg	10–50 kg 60 mg/kg	
			>50 kg		1 g	>50 kg	
						4 g	
Ibuprofen	Mild pain/anti pyretic	Oral	1–24 months	5 mg/kg		20 mg/kg/day up to max.	Avoid if history of hypersensitivity and in dehydration (as risk of renal failure)
			1–2 years	50 mg		2.4 g/day	
			3–7 years	100 mg			
			8–12 years	200 mg			
			12–18 years	200–600 mg			

Advanced Life Support Group, 2016. Advanced paediatric life support. A Practical Approach to Emergencies, sixth ed. BMJ Books, Wiley and Sons, Chichester.

Table 11.4 Opioid analgesic for moderate to severe pain

Drug	Indication	Route	Age	Loading dose	Maintenance dose	Maximum daily dose	Notes
Morphine	Moderate – severe pain	Oral	1–3 months	–	50–100 µg/kg		Adjust doses according to response. Doses may be given up to six times in 24 h.
			3–6 months		100–150 µg/kg		
			6–12 months		200 µg/kg		
			1–2 years		200–300 µg/kg		
			2–12 years		200–500 µg/kg (max. 10 mg)		
Morphine	Severe pain	Intravenous	12–18 years	50 µg/kg	5–10 mg		Respiratory monitoring mandatory. Give IV over 5–10 min <1 year use lower stated dose and consider oxygen saturation monitoring.
			Term–1 month	100 µg/kg	10–20 µg/kg/h		
			1–24 months	5 mg	10–30 µg/kg/h		
			12–18 years				

IV, Intravenous.
Advanced Life Support Group, 2016. Advanced paediatric life support. A Practical Approach to Emergencies, sixth ed. BMJ Books, Wiley and Sons, Chichester.

rhabdomyolysis, hyperlipidaemia, hyperkalaemia, hepatomegaly, and renal failure (BNFC 2015–2016).

Means of analgesic administration

There are many routes of administration for providing analgesia in children. The simplest route should be the first option, but in an awake child, the medicine needs to be palatable if it is for oral consumption. Other routes include nasogastric, nasojejunal, gastrostomy, percutaneous endoscopic gastrostomy (PEG), subcutaneous, intramuscular (avoid if possible), intravenous, rectal, epidural, topical or inhaled.

Epidural analgesia

Epidural analgesia is infused through a very small epidural catheter into the epidural space. The epidural catheter is sited by the anaesthetist to augment analgesia during the operation and to maximise pain control after the surgical procedure has been completed.

The preparation of epidural analgesic infusions is carried out in a sterile pharmacy unit. The drugs used include local anaesthetic, for example, levobupivacaine and preservative free morphine. Levobupivacaine is available in different strengths and it works by blocking sodium channels on the nerve axon. Preservative-free morphine is sometimes used as an epidural analgesic; it diffuses slowly into the subarachnoid space and circulates in the cerebrospinal fluid.

The following are basic guiding principles but detailed information is available from The Royal College of Anaesthetists/Faculty of Pain Medicine (www.rcoa.ac.uk/fpm).

Epidural lines must be clearly labelled and may be colour coded to differentiate from enteral, intravenous, or arterial lines. They should be secured with a dressing that allows clear visibility of the infusion site. Antibacterial filters should be used, no access ports should be available, the epidural sets should not connect with any other type of infusion, and epidural infusions should be prepared under sterile conditions, labelled for epidural use only, and stored separately. Epidural infusion pumps should be stored separately from other types of infusion pumps. Designated personnel and clear protocols should be in place to support the safe and effective use of epidural analgesia. Patients with epidural analgesia must be monitored closely by trained staff who can recognise and respond appropriately to abnormal values. Monitoring should include hourly:

- Heart rate and blood pressure readings
- Pain and sedation scores
- Respiratory rate and oxygen saturations
- Temperature
- Degree of motor and sensory blockade
- Urine output
- Pressure area assessment
- Epidural site inspection
- Documentation of epidural infusion rate and the volume infused, and all observations must be documented

It is vital to assess both the level and range of sensory blockade on both sides of the body and the degree of motor nerve blockade at frequent intervals according to local policy.

Assessing sensory blockade in epidural analgesia

The means of assessing sensory block is by dermatome assessment (Fig. 11.5). A dermatome is an area of skin that is supplied by a single spinal nerve. Local anaesthetics will block nerve impulses on autonomic

Fig. 11.5 Dermatome assessment. (Republished with permission from the Children's Pain Management Service, The Royal Children's Hospital, Melbourne, Australia. Image subject to copyright.)

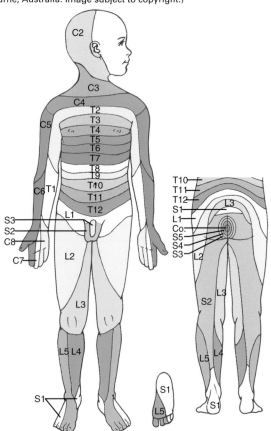

fibres first, followed by sensory then motor fibres. Sensory fibres respond to pain, temperature, touch, and pressure so the area of sensory block can be assessed using cold sensation (ice) to establish which dermatome levels are covered, and to ensure the epidural is proving adequate pain relief at an appropriate level.

Procedure (adapted from The Royal Children's Hospital, Melbourne 2015):

- Provide full explanation to the child and family.
- Use an ice cube and place it on an area, for example face or forearm, which will not be covered by sensory blockade and ask the child to tell you how cold it feels.
- Then apply the ice to an area likely to be blocked on the same side of the body and ask the child 'does this feel the same cold as you felt on your face/forearm?'
- Apply the ice to areas above and below this point until it is clear at which level the top and bottom of the block occurs.
- Repeat the procedure on the opposite side of the body (as blocks may be unilateral or uneven).
- Document the blocked dermatomes – recording both the upper and lower limits of the block; for example, T7–L1 L = R or R:T7–L1 and L:T10–L2.

In nonverbal children, observe facial expression or flinching to try to assess blocked or unblocked dermatomes.

If the epidural block is higher than T3, there is no evidence of any block or you feel that there is insufficient block to relieve pain, please inform a senior anaesthetist/member of the Pain Service.

Assessing motor nerve blockage in epidural analgesia

It is very important to assess motor nerve block to gauge the risk of pressure areas, to ensure the child is safe to walk, and to try to detect any signs of complications; for example, epidural haematoma, abscess, high block, or any other neurologic sequelae.

 Epidural haematoma or abscess can cause spinal cord compression, which is a NEUROSURGICAL EMERGENCY.

Procedure to assess motor nerve block in lower limbs (Bromage score 1978):

- Provide full explanation to the child and family.
- Ask the child to move his or her feet and bend the knees. For younger children you could gently tickle toes to try to elicit movement.
- Assess the movement observed and rate it using the Bromage score (Fig. 11.6).
- Document the degree of motor block.
- Observe for motor nerve block of both legs.

Fig. 11.6 Bromage score. (Bromage, P.R., 1978. Epidural Analgesia. WB Saunders, Philadelphia.)

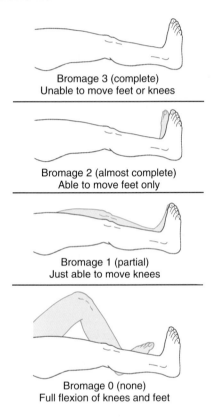

Bromage 3 (complete)
Unable to move feet or knees

Bromage 2 (almost complete)
Able to move feet only

Bromage 1 (partial)
Just able to move knees

Bromage 0 (none)
Full flexion of knees and feet

- The density of motor nerve block will be indicated by loss of movement.
- Contact a senior anaesthetist/member of the pain team if the Bromage score is ≥2 and if the block does not recede within an hour of reducing the infusion rate.

Procedure to assess motor nerve block in the upper limbs (for thoracic epidural) as well as above procedure for lower limbs:
- Provide full explanation to the child and family.
- Ask the child to grip your hand and then to lift up his or her arms.
- Assess for any loss of sensation or numbness in hands or arms.
- An unduly high motor block will be indicated by loss of power, voluntary movement, or sensation.

- Document the degree of motor nerve block.
- If there are any signs of paraesthesia or loss of motor function, stop the infusion and inform the Pain Team.

 Other signs of high motor block include shallow respiration, dilated pupils, drooping of facial muscles; if any of these signs occur, stop the infusion and inform the Pain Team or senior anaesthetist.

RED FLAGS

The following situations warrant an immediate referral to a senior appropriate anaesthetist and should be considered for neuroimaging:
1. Significant motor block with thoracic epidural
2. Unexpectedly dense motor block, including unilateral blocks
3. Markedly increasing motor block during epidural infusion
4. Motor block that does not regress when an epidural is stopped
5. Recurrent unexpected motor block after restarting an epidural infusion that was stopped because of motor block (RCA 2009)

An increasing degree of motor weakness usually indicates excessive epidural drug administration, but it could also indicate serious complications, such as dural penetration of the catheter or epidural haematoma.

Compartment syndrome is a possible complication, particularly following prolonged procedures, lower limb surgery, and when the child has been positioned any way but supine during the surgery (Llewellyn & Moriarty 2007).

Other complications of epidural analgesia include hypotension, respiratory depression (opioid use), motor block, and urinary retention and pruritis. Infrequent complications include cardiovascular collapse, respiratory arrest, unexpected development of high block (e.g., catheter migration), postdural puncture headache, drug administration errors, pressure sores, infection, haematoma or abscess, meningitis, spinal cord ischaemia, and permanent harm (e.g., paraplegia) (Royal College of Anaesthetists/Faculty of Pain Medicine 2010).

PAIN SUMMARY

To summarise – the RCN (2009) identified four recommendations:
1. Be vigilant for any indication of pain. Pain should be anticipated in neonates and children at all times.
2. Children's self-report of their pain, where possible, is the preferred approach. For children who are unable to self-report, an appropriate behaviour or composite tool should be used.
3. If pain is suspected or anticipated, use a validated pain assessment tool; do not rely on isolated indicators to assess pain. Examples of signs that may indicate pain include changes in children's behaviour, appearance, activity level, and vital signs. No individual tool can be

broadly recommended for pain assessment in all children and across all contexts.

4. Assess, record, and reevaluate pain at regular intervals; the frequency of assessment should be determined according to the individual needs of the child and the setting. Be aware that language, ethnicity, and cultural factors may influence the expression and assessment of pain.

 The infants and children in our care deserve to have optimal pain management, so it is our responsibility to assess, provide analgesia, and reassess their pain frequently.

REFERENCES

Advanced Life Support Group, 2016. Advanced Paediatric Life Support. A Practical Approach to Emergencies, sixth ed. BMJ Books, Wiley and Sons, Chichester.

Ambuel, B., Hamlett, K.W., Marx, C.M., et al., 1992. Assessing distress in pediatric intensive care environments: the COMFORT scale. J Pediatr Psychol 17 (1), 95–109.

Baeyer, C.L., 2006. Children's self-reports of pain intensity: scale selection, limitations and interpretation. Pain Res Manag 11 (3), 157–162.

Bieri, D., Reeve, R.A., Champion, G.D., et al., 1990. The faces pain scale for the self-assessment of the severity of pain experienced by children: development, initial validation and preliminary investigation for ratio scale properties. Pain 41 (2), 139–150.

Breau, L.M., Camfield, C.S., McGrath, P.J., et al., 2007. Pain's impact on adaptive functioning. J Intellect Disabil Res 52 (2), 125–134.

Breau, L.M., Finley, G.A., McGrath, P.J., et al., 2002. Validation of the non-communicating children's pain checklist postoperative version. Anesthesiology 96, 528–535.

Bromage, P.R., 1978. Epidural Analgesia. WB Saunders, Philadelphia.

Craig, K.D., Badali, M.A., 2004. Introduction to the special series on pain deception and malingering. Clin J Pain 20, 377–382.

Hunt, A., Wisbeach, A., Seers, K., et al., 2007. Development of the paediatric pain profile: role of video analysis and saliva cortisol in validating a tool to assess pain in children with severe neurological disability. J Pain Symptom Manage 33 (3), 276–289.

Krechel, S.W., Bildner, J., 1995. CRIES; a new neonatal postoperative pain measurement score. Initial testing of validity and reliability. Paediatr Anaesth 5 (1), 53–61.

Lawrence, J., Alcock, D., McGrath, P., et al., 1993. The development of a tool to assess neonatal pain. Neonatal Netw 12 (6), 59–66.

Llewellyn, N., Moriarty, A., 2007. The national pediatric epidural audit. Pediatr Anesth 17, 520–533.

McGrath, P.J., Johnson, G.I., Goodman, J.T., et al., 1985. CHEOPS: a behavioural scale for rating postoperative pain in children. In: Fields, H.L., Dubner, R., Cervero, F. (Eds.), Advances in Pain Research and Therapy, vol. 9. New York: Raven Press, pp. 395–402.

Merkel, S.I., Voepel Lewis, T., Shayevitz, J.R., et al., 1997. The FLACC: a behavioural scale for scoring postoperative pain in young children. Pediatr Nurs 23, 293–297.

Paediatric Formulary Committee. BNF for Children (2015–2016). London. BMJ Group, Pharmaceutical Press and RCPCH Publications 2015.

Royal College of Anaesthetists, 2009. The 3rd National Audit Project of the Royal College of Anaesthetists. Major complications of central neuraxial block in the United Kingdom, RCA London. www.rcoa.ac.uk. Accessed 1 August 2017.

Royal College of Anaesthetists/Faculty of Pain Medicine, 2010. Best practice in the management of epidural analgesia in the hospital setting. RCA, London. www.rcoa.ac.uk/fpm. Accessed 29 July 2017.

Royal College of Nursing, 2009. The Recognition and Assessment of Acute Pain in Children. Update of Full Guideline. RCN, London.

Suominen, P., Caffin, C., Linton, S., et al., 2004. The cardiac analgesic assessment scale for intubated and ventilated children after cardiac surgery. Paediatr Anaesth 14 (4), 336–343.

The Royal Children's Hospital, Melbourne, 2015. Anaesthesia and Pain Management. Assessment of sensory block. www.rch.org.au. Accessed 2 August 2017.

Together for Short Lives, 2016. Basic Symptom Control in Paediatric Palliative Care. The Rainbows Children's Hospice Guidelines, 9th ed. www.togetherforshortlives.org.uk. Accessed 6 May 2017.

Treadwell, M.J., Franck, L.S., Vichinsky, E., 2002. Using quality improvement strategies to enhance pediatric pain assessment. Int J Qual Health Care 14, 39–47.

Van Dijk, M., de Boer, J.B., Koot, H.M., et al., 2000. The reliability and validity of the COMFORT scale as a postoperative pain instrument in 0-to 3-year-old infants. Pain 84, 367–377.

Wong, D.L., Hockenberry-Eaton, M., Wilson, D., et al., 2001. Essentials of Paediatric Nursing, sixth ed. Mosby, St Louis, MO, 1301.

World Health Organisation, 2012. WHO Guidelines on the Pharmacological Treatment of Persisting Pain in Children with Medical Illnesses. WHO, Geneva.

Yale University, www.assessment-module.yale.edu. Accessed February 8, 2017.

There are some occasions when children present to the emergency department, a high dependency unit, or paediatric intensive care unit (PICU) when their life may hang in the balance, and it is often helpful to have some general guidance to hand that, as far as possible, follow national recommendations. We strongly recommend being guided by local policies, but the following general principles may be helpful. Some centres will also care for children postsurgery and whilst congenital cardiac disease warrants a whole chapter, it is also relevant to include here the key points of caring for children following spinal surgery. Other chapters include guidance, for example, Chapter 2: airway obstruction, acute asthma, bronchiolitis, pertussis; Chapter 4: haemolytic uraemic syndrome; Chapter 6: status epilepticus, Guillain-Barré syndrome, spinal muscular atrophy.

This chapter will cover:

- Sepsis
- Necrotising fasciitis
- Stevens–Johnson syndrome (SJS) and toxic epidermal necrolysis (TEN)
- Neonatal collapse (including parechovirus)
- Sickle cell crisis
- Diabetic ketoacidosis (DKA)
- Syndrome of inappropriate antidiuretic hormone secretion (SIADH)
- Burns
- Postoperative care following spinal surgery

SEPSIS

International definitions for childhood sepsis from the International Consensus Conference on Pediatric Sepsis (Goldstein et al 2005):

- Sepsis is a systemic inflammatory response syndrome in the presence of infection
- Severe sepsis – sepsis in the presence of cardiovascular dysfunction, acute respiratory distress syndrome or dysfunction of two or more organ systems
- Septic shock – sepsis with cardiovascular dysfunction persisting after at least 40 mL/kg of fluid resuscitation in 1 hour
- Refractory septic shock – fluid refractory septic shock – shock persisting after ≥60 mL/kg of fluid resuscitation
- Catecholamine resistant septic shock – shock persists despite treatment with catecholamines (dopamine, adrenaline, noradrenaline)

Severe sepsis kills. Its incidence in children is rising, but compliance with previous guidelines (associated with improved outcomes) was poor

(Oliveira et al 2008). One study showed that children who presented in septic shock who received less than 20 mL/kg of fluid resuscitation in the first hour of treatment had a mortality rate of 73% (Oliveira et al 2008). The Paediatric Sepsis 6 initiative is a quality improvement toolkit that facilitates prompt recognition of severe sepsis and delivery of six simple elements of care in a time-critical manner. See Fig. 12.1 for guidance.

Fig. 12.1 Paediatric Sepsis 6. (With permission from Tong, J., Plunkett, A., Daniels, R., 2014. G218(P) The Paediatric Sepsis 6 Initiative. Arch. Dis. Child 99 [Supp. 1]). *AVPU*, *A*-alert, *V*-responds to voice, *P*-responds to pain, *U*-unresponsive; *CRP*, C-reactive protein; *FBC*, full blood count; *IO*, intraosseus; *IV*, intravenous; *PCR*, polymerase chain reaction.

Recognition of a child at risk:
If a child with suspected or proven infection AND has at least 2 of the following:
- Core temperature < 36°C or > 38.5°C
- Inappropriate tachycardia (Refer to local criteria / APLS Guidance)
- Altered mental state (including: sleepiness / irritability / lethargy / floppiness)
- Reduced peripheral perfusion / prolonged capillary refill

Lower threshold of suspicion for: age < 3 months, chronic disease, recent surgery, or immunocompromised

THINK: Could this child have SEVERE SEPSIS, SEPTIC SHOCK or RED FLAG SEPSIS* - Ask for review by an experienced clinician.

High certainty of Sepsis Respond with Paediatric Sepsis 6:	High certainty NOT Sepsis or Unsure

Complete all elements within 1 hour   Date/Time   Sign

Not Sepsis
Document reasons
Unsure

1. Give high flow oxygen:

Review within 1 hour

2. Obtain IV / IO access & take blood tests:

Not Sepsis
Document reasons
Sepsis
Start Sepsis 6
Unsure

   a. Blood cultures
   b. Blood glucose - treat low blood glucose
   c. Blood gas (+ FBC, lactate / CRP as able)   Date/Time   Sign

3. Give IV or IO antibiotics: Date/Time   Sign

   - Broad spectrum cover as per local policy

Review within 1 hour
Not Sepsis
Document reasons
Sepsis
Start Sepsis 6
Unsure

4. Consider fluid resuscitation:

   - Aim to restore normal circulating volume and physiological parameters
   - Titrate 20 ml/kg Isotonic Fluid over 5 - 10 min and repeat if necessary
   - Caution with fluid overload: Examine for crepitations & hepatomegaly   Date/Time   Sign

Review within 1 hour
Not Sepsis
Document reasons
Sepsis
Start Sepsis 6
Unsure

5. Involve senior clinicians / specialists early:

6. Consider inotropic support early:

   - If normal physiological parameters are not restored after ≥ 40 ml/kg fluids
   - NB adrenaline or dopamine may be given via peripheral IV or IO access

Review within 1 hour
Not Sepsis
Document reasons
Sepsis
Start Sepsis 6

Document reason(s) for variation overleaf

Fig. 12.1, cont'd

Definitions (adapted from the international paediatric sepsis consensus conference definitions):

1. **Infection** - Proven infection by positive culture, microscopy, or PCR test caused by any pathogen **OR**
   - Clinical syndrome associated with a high probability of infection, as evidenced from clinical examination, imaging, or laboratory tests

2. **Sepsis** - Infection + Systemic Inflammatory Response Syndrome (tachycardia, tachypnoea, core temperature >38.5°C or <36°C, white cell count elevated or depressed for age)

3. **Severe sepsis** - Sepsis + one of the following: cardiovascular dysfunction OR acute respiratory distress syndrome **OR**
   - Two or more other organ dysfunctions (respiratory, renal, neurologic, hematologic, or hepatic).

4. **Septic shock** - Severe Sepsis with cardiovascular dysfunction.

> *** Red Flag Sepsis -** is an operational solution to the complexities in recognition of sepsis in children according to established consensus definitions, measurable at the bedside. Criteria are based on sepsis definitions described above coupled with the NICE traffic light system from the Feverish Illness guideline (CG160) and excludes time consuming tests. It aims to provide a pragmatic framework for timely decisions and interventions.

- Appearance: Pale/ mottled/ ashen/ blue or non-blanching (purpuric) rash.
- Cardiovascular dysfunction: Hypotension, tachycardia/ bradycardia, prolonged capillary refill time >5 seconds, or blood gas lactate > 2X upper limit of normal.
- Respiratory dysfunction: Tachypnoea/ bradypnoea/ apnoea, grunting, or oxygen required to maintain saturations >92%.
- Neurological dysfunction: AVPU = V, P or U; lack of response to social cues; significantly decreased acitivity; or weak, high-pitched or continuous cry.
- Renal dysfunction: Reduced urine output/ parents report excessively dry nappies.

In children with severe sepsis who present with fluid refractory, catecholamine-resistant shock, or suspected or proven adrenal insufficiency, hydrocortisone therapy may be beneficial (UK Sepsis Trust 2015). (Do not use corticosteroids in babies ≤3 months of age, NICE 2015b.)

> NB Prompt recognition of severe sepsis and timely and appropriate care save lives. If concerned, call immediately for the most experienced clinician's assistance. Give appropriate antibiotics within the first hour.

Meningococcal bacteria (*Neisseria meningitides*) commonly causes symptoms of both meningitis and meningococcal sepsis and although the incidence has fallen since the meningococcal C vaccination programme in the United Kingdom (the effects of the meningitis B, and meningitis A, C, W and Y vaccines are not yet published), it remains the leading infectious cause of death in UK children (NICE 2015b). For this reason, specific guidance for early management of sepsis (including meningococcal sepsis) is shown in Fig. 12.2

NECROTISING FASCIITIS

Necrotising fasciitis is a severe, life-threatening bacterial infection of the soft tissues characterised by rapidly spreading necrosis of the fascia and subcutaneous tissue; it is most commonly caused by *Streptococcus pyogenes*. Its incidence in children has increased, and predisposing factors include varicella lesions, intramuscular injections, application of cream containing menthol to the cervical region, penetrant gluteal

Fig. 12.2 Early management of sepsis. (STRS, 2017c. Sepsis early management guidelines. www.strs.nhs.uk.) This guideline was up to date at time of submission, but to ensure you are using the most up to date guideline, please go to www.strs.nhs.uk and check clinical guidelines for any changes or updates.

Paediatric Critical Care
Sepsis (early management)

Guideline for management of sepsis: patients may have shock +/– meningitis. Focus may be clear (purpura of meningococcal) or occult.

Initial Intervention
- Intravenous access x 2 quickly, Intraosseous if iv difficult
- Gas, sugar[1], B/C, FBC, clotting, U&E, CRP, Xmatch, PCR
- ✦ **Antibiotics early:**
  - < 1 month - Cefotaxime & amoxicillin & aciclovir
  - > 1 month - Ceftriaxone 80 mg/kg over 30 min
  - Travel outside UK/ risk of Abx resistance – consult I.D
- Evaluate level of consciousness and pupils

Initial resuscitation
Shock – tachycardia / poor pulses / obtunded / low BP
- High flow O_2. Maintain saturation >95%
- Push 20 mL/kg crystalloid[2] bolus and review HR / BP
- Repeat 20 mL x 2 crystalloid bolus if no response

*Fluid refractory shock (shock despite ≥60 mL/kg)
- Start peripheral **dopamine** 10 mcg/kg/min
- Titrate to response (max 15 mcg/kg/min)
- Intubate and ventilate - anticipate decompensation ✦
- Continue fluid resuscitation

Intubation: other indications
- Hypoxia (sats<92% despite oxygen)
- Altered level of consciousness
- Signs of raised ICP

INTUBATION
- **Early intubation for shock improves outcome**[3]
- Most experienced operator to intubate
- Induction of anaesthesia may cause cardiovascular instability : consider ketamine, avoid propofol
- NG tube and aspirate stomach
- Pre-oxygenate for 3 min
- Ongoing volume resuscitation throughout
- Peripheral dopamine 10 mcg/kg/min infusing
- Cardiac arrest drugs available
- Avoid nasal intubation if coagulopathic or low platelets
- May require high PEEP if pulmonary oedema

Gain CVL (USS guidance preferable)
Infuse dopamine centrally
If dopamine >10 mcg/kg/min then add 2nd agent

Warm shock	Cold shock
Wide pulse pressure	Narrow pulse pressure
Start **noradrenaline** 0.1 mcg/kg/min Titrate to response (max 1 mcg/kg/min)	Start **adrenaline** 0.1 mcg/kg/min Titrate to response (max 1 mcg/kg/min)

No or minimal response = catecholamine resistant shock
- Ensure inotrope dose/delivery correct
- Exclude other causes (pericardial effusion, pneumothorax, ongoing blood loss, intracranial event)
- Give hydrocortisone IV 2 mg/kg/bolus[4]

Low BP, warm shock	Low BP, cold shock
• Add adrenaline	• Maximise adrenaline • consider 3rd agent

Risk factors and alerts
- Age < 12 months
- Extensive/ rapidly spreading rash[5] (20% with mening, sepsis have no rash)
- Recent history of varicella/ burns (consider toxic shock)
- Low platelets/ low wbc / coagulopathy :may be normal initially & rapidly change
- Persistent tachycardia despite fluid therapy
- Hypotension is late sign
- Obtundation and depressed level consciousness

Persistent tachycardia usually = under-resuscitation

Aggressive reversal of shock improves outcome

Urgent intervention & reassessment is key

Exclude cardiac cause (hepatomegaly, cardiomegaly, ECG)

If indwelling line/VP shunt= potential focus- add vanc

Features of Toxic shock- add clindamycin

DO NOT PERFORM LUMBAR PUNCTURE[6]

Depressed level of consciousness (LOC)
Differential: shock, meningitis, raised ICP
- Treat seizures (phenytoin). Correct hyponatraemia and low sugar

Raised ICP: relative bradycardia, posturing/seizures, abnormal pupils - may mask shock with relative bradycardia/ hypertension
- Give osmotherapy: 3% saline 3–5 mL/kg
- Impending herniation: hyperventilate, give further 3 mL/kg 3% saline. Consider steroids (Dexamethasone 0.15 mg/kg Max 10 mg QDS x 4 days) if <12 h since first antibiotics and clinical signs of bacterial meningitis[7]

Ongoing support
- Ventilation: may need to ↑ PEEP if pulmonary oedema/ poor oxygenation
- Monitor central temp, invasive BP, CVP, ABG, lactate & central venous sats
- Ongoing large volume resuscitation often required in addition to inotropes
- Consider milrinone if cold shock
- Optimise haemoglobin (maintain Hb > 10 g/dL; oxygen delivery) and correct clotting abnormalities
- Consider actively cooling to 36–37 C using surface cooling or IVI saline (boluses can be cooled to 4 degrees - produces rapid cooling)
- Observe urine output, electrolytes and check CK. Correct electrolyte abnormalities
  - May require urgent CVVH on arrival on unit
- Exclude other sites of infection (e.g. necrotising fasciitis)
- A risk of pressure sores-consider Huntleigh mattress on admission
- Consider immunoglobulin in toxic shock

Public Health
- Refer to website (see below) regarding notifiable diseases[8] and prophylaxis
- Common notifiable diseases: invasive group A Strep, meningococcal, acute meningitis/encephalitis
- Prophylaxis if meningococcal probable:
  - Household contacts
  - Health workers exposed to respiratory secretions in first 24 h of Rx
  - Treat with ciprofloxacin (all ages and in pregnancy)
- If meningococcal, patient no longer infectious after 24 h of Rx[9]

1. Van den Berghe: Crit Care Med 2003 31, 2, 359–366, 2. Carcillo: Crit Care Med 2002:30, 6 1365–783, 3. Dellinger: Crit Care Med 2004 32 (3) 858–73,
4. Baines:Arch Dis Child:2008: 83, 510–13, 5. Baines: Br J Anaesth 2003:90 1, 72–83, 6. Rennick: BMJ 1993: 306, 6883, 953–955,
7. NICE Clinical Guideline CG102, 2010.
8. https://www.gov.uk/government/collections/notifications-of-infectious-diseases-noids
9. https://www.gov.uk/government/uploads/system/uploads/attachment_data/file/322008/Guidance_for_management_of_meningococcal_disease_pdf.pdf

trauma, omphalitis, dental abscess, and streptococcal toxic shock (Bingol-Kologlu et al 2007).

Initial skin presentation – induration, cellulitis, erythema, oedema, which lead to skin discolouration and bullae formation.

Clinical features – fever, tachycardia, intense pain at site; may develop diarrhoea and vomiting.

Treatment – antibiotics, urgent surgical debridement, supportive therapy. The role of intravenous immunoglobulin (IVIG) for modulation of immune response to the streptococcal super-antigens is not conclusive (Norrby-Teglund et al., 1996).

Stevens–Johnson Syndrome and Toxic Epidermal Necrolysis

These are variants of the same condition. This is an immune-complex-mediated hypersensitivity reaction that typically involves skin and mucosa. SJS applies to the disease when less than 10% of the total body surface is involved; the term TEN applies when more than 30% of the body surface area is involved; and for those patients who have 10–30% involvement it is known as SJS/TEN overlap. Mortality is around 5% for SJS and 25% for TEN (Fernando 2012). It is more common in association with the human immunodeficiency virus. It is rarely associated with vaccination.

It is normally caused by a reaction to a drug and more than 200 have been reported including allopurinol, antibiotic sulfa drugs, anticonvulsants (carbamazepine, lamotrigine, phenytoin, phenobarbitone), and nonsteroidal anti-inflammatory drugs (naproxen and ibuprofen). The mechanism of this unpredictable reaction is complex and not well understood.

Clinical features often start within a week of taking antibiotic therapy; for most other drugs it is between a few days and 1 month, but with the anticonvulsants, this may occur up to 2 months after starting therapy.

This is a rare and serious condition in which patients display symptoms of malaise, myalgia, fever, and painful erythema with blisters, which progresses to include large areas of confluent erythema with sheetlike skin loss, mucosal involvement (including eyes, lips, mouth, oesophagus), respiratory tract causing cough and respiratory distress, gastrointestinal tract resulting in diarrhoea, and genital ulceration. The maximum extent of the skin lesions is usually reached by 4 days.

DIAGNOSIS

A skin biopsy is taken to confirm the diagnosis and to exclude other potential diagnoses, such as staphylococcal scalded skin syndrome.

TREATMENT

- These patients should ideally be cared for in a specialist burn unit or an intensive care environment
- They should have immediate assessment by a dermatologist. The offending drug needs to be stopped as soon as possible as this will improve the chances of survival

- Protective isolation
- Skin care
- Eye care
- Mouth care
- Pain relief
- Temperature maintenance
- Nutritional and fluid replacement
- Respiratory support in some cases – even intubation and ventilation if trachea and bronchi are involved
- Physiotherapy

Various drug therapies have been reported in isolated cases but remain controversial; these include cyclosporine, infliximab, heparin, IVIG, and steroids.

Patients who have survived SJS/TEN will have to avoid the causative drug or any medicines structurally similar in the future.

(SJS/TEN support: www.sjsawareness.org.uk)

NEONATAL COLLAPSE

In the first 28 days after birth, presenting collapsed neonates may have nonspecific symptoms including respiratory distress, tachycardia, hypothermia, and poor pulses – all of which require rapid assessment of airway, breathing, circulation, disability, exposure (ABCDE) examination and resuscitation. See Fig. 12.3 for common causes of neonatal collapse. The differential diagnosis includes:

- Sepsis
- Cardiac
- Metabolic
- Trauma

For all babies

ABCD assessment and resuscitation
- Start high flow oxygen → if grunting or apnoea, acidotic or preductal saturations ≤70% intubate and ventilate (hypoxia without CO_2 retention in a neonate suggests cyanotic heart disease)
- Tachycardia, poor pulses, hypotension, obtunded = SHOCKED BABY = call for senior assistance
- Obtain intravenous access or I/O and send blood for culture, urea and electrolytes, C-reactive protein (CRP), blood glucose, arterial blood gas, liver function tests, full blood count and clotting (if neonate also presents with seizures, send an ammonia)
- 20 mL/kg fluid bolus 0.9% saline and repeat if heart rate >160/min
- Give intravenous antibiotics benzylpenicillin and gentamycin (NICE 2012)
- Chest x-ray, electrocardiogram, 4 limb blood pressure (and consider lumbar puncture [LP] if no contraindications)
- Consider duct-dependent cardiac lesion
  - Measure pre- and postductal saturations
  - Observe if cyanosis is responding to oxygen therapy

- Check if femoral pulses poor or absent
- Is there a heart murmur or cardiomegaly?
- Refer for urgent cardiology review/and contact PICU to refer
- Start prostin at 5 ng/kg/min if clinically well or at 20 ng/kg/min if unstable or absent femoral pulses (NB high-dose prostin may lead to apnoea and hypotension, but may be required to open/maintain patency of the duct)

Fluid refractory shock = hypotension after 40 mL/kg fluid
- Continue giving fluid boluses if responsive
- Start peripheral dopamine at 5–10 mcg/kg/min
- Intubate and ventilate
- Gain central access or input/output
- Reassess heart rate and blood pressure

Dopamine resistant shock (need second-line inotropes)
- Start adrenaline if poor pulses, cold, and low cardiac output
- Start noradrenaline if vasodilated with bounding pulse and wide pulse pressure
- If adrenaline or noradrenaline >0.5 mcg/kg/min, consider possible Addisonian crisis (low glucose, ↓Na+, ↑K+), consider hydrocortisone 2 mg/kg intravenously

See Fig. 12.4 for further detailed guidance.

Parechovirus

Parechovirus is an enterovirus with 16 different human parechovirus types (HPeV). It is easily spread through contact with someone infected, by respiratory droplets, saliva, or faeces. It usually causes mild gastroenteritis and respiratory infection, but several clusters of HPeV sepsis have been reported in neonates and infants (Khatami et al 2015; Tang et al 2016). Common presenting symptoms in HPeV sepsis include:
- Pyrexia – up to 40°C
- Lethargy or drowsiness
- Tachycardia – may be >200 beats/min
- Grunting
- Irritability
- Mottled or petechial/erythrodermic rash
- Diarrhoea
- Abdominal distension
- Oedema
- Hepatitis
- Myoclonic jerks

Seizures, encephalitis, myocarditis, and dilated cardiomyopathy have also been reported (Sun et al 2012; Wildenbeest et al 2013).

Diagnosis – HpeV can be tested for in cerebrospinal fluid, stool, blood, respiratory samples, and throat swabs, and it is important to try to establish if it is the cause so that this may reduce or prevent unnecessary antibiotic therapy.

Fig. 12.3 Causes of neonatal collapse. (STRS, 2017b. Neonatal collapse. <www.strs.nhs.uk>) This guideline was up to date at time of submission, but to ensure you are using the most up to date guideline, please go to www.strs.nhs.uk and check clinical guidelines for any changes or updates.

Paediatric Critical Care
Neonatal Collapse

- Non specific presentation: hypothermia, respiratory distress, poor pulses
- Sepsis and cardiac disease commonest cause (both present as shock)
- General supportive measures will improve outcome

1. EARLY VENTILATORY SUPPORT
2. ANTIBIOTICS (presume sepsis)
3. EARLY PROSTIN (exclude cardiac lesion)
   (prostaglandin E2)

1. Initial evaluation & resuscitation
- Tachycardia/ poor pulses/ obtunded/ low BP = SHOCK
- High flow oxygen
- Intravenous access: use intraosseous (IO) if difficult
- Push 20 mL/kg 0.9%sodium chloride(caution if signs of heart failure) (If no signs of heart failure and still signs of shock-rpt fluid bolus)
- Antibiotics: cefotaxime 50 mg/kg IV

DUCT DEPENDENT CONGENITAL HEART DISEASE[1]
- Cyanosis not responding to oxygen
- Poor or absent femoral pulses
- Heart murmur present, or cardiomegaly
(see list below regarding diagnosis of individual lesion)
Measure pre and post ductal saturations, 4 limb BP

Start prostin-dose depends on clinical state
- Discuss with STRS:
  - 5 ng/kg/min if clinically well
  - 20 ng/kg/min if unstable or absent femoral pulses
  - 50–100 ng/kg/min if no response
Apnoea common: 1st h of Rx, ↑dose
Hypotension may occur with high dose

Consider duct dependent cardiac lesion →

Lack of response = urgent cardiology review

2. Immediate investigations
- Arterial/venous gas, U+E's, blood glucose, LFTs, FBC & clotting
- Blood culture, consider LP if no contra-indications
- CXR /ECG if tachycardia (heart rate > 220 bpm, consider SVT)
- Ammonia if seizures/ encephalopathy

DO NOT DELAY TRANSFER
- Intubate and ventilate if
  1. Preductal sats < 70%
  2. Grunting / acidosis / poor pulses/ apnoea
  3. Transferring on prostin ≥ 5 ng/kg/min

3. Fluid refractory shock = hypotension despite 40 mL/kg fluid
- Continue fluid boluses if response (HR improves and liver not ↑)
- Start peripheral dopamine at 10 mcg/kg/min
- Intubate and ventilate
- Central IV access or IO.
- Central dopamine 10 mcg/kg/min
- Reassess heart rate pulses and blood pressure

ASSESSMENT OF HEART FAILURE
- Signs: gallop, cardiomegaly, hepatomegaly
- Potential diagnosis CHD, cardiomyopathy, myocarditis
- Cautious fluid resuscitation- stop if increasing liver size

4. Dopamine[4] resistant shock (use 2nd line inotrope)
- Adrenaline(ADR) if poor pulses, cold, low cardiac output
- Noradrenaline if vasodilated-bounding pulse/wide pulse pressure
- If ADR or NorADR >0.5 mcg/kg/min or possible Addisonian crisis (low glucose, ↑Na+, K+), consider hydrocortisone[2] 2 mg/kg IV

Dextrose in neonates
- Monitor regularly & aim 4–8 mmol/L
- Start 0.9% saline/10% dextrose 2 mL/kg/h
- If metabolic/hypoglycaemic- calculate:
- dextrose mg/kg/min = dextrose% x mL/h / weight x 6

Sepsis	Group B strep, E Coli	PROM, maternal GBS, fever in labour	Cefotaxime 50 mg/kg IV (add amoxicillin 100 mg/kg IV if listeria concerns (rare))
	Herpes Simplex	↓GCS, coagulopathy, ↑ALT, family cold sores	Add Acyclovir 20 mg/kg IV. High index suspicion, history may be absent
	MRSA	Unresponsive 1st line antibiotics, + contact	Add Vancomycin 15 mg/kg IV
Cardiac	Coarctation aorta	Systolic arm/leg gradient > 20 mm Hg	Urgent prostin (may need high dose) and support (ventilation/inotropes)
	Hypoplastic Left heart	Poor pulses – may be pink= pulm, overcirculation	Prostin. Avoid oxygen-can cause pulm, overcirculation. Target sats 75%
	Transposition (TGA)	Preductal sats < post ductal sats	Urgent prostin. If no response: urgent septostomy
	TAPVD (obstructed)	Shocked & cyanosed/CXR plethoric	Prostin may make worse. Need echo confirmation and surgery
	SVT	HR>220 despite fluid, fixed HR, narrow QRS	See arrhythmia guideline. Adenosine[3], if shocked: ventilate +DC shock
	Myocarditis	Cardiac failure, tachycardia, small QRS	Supportive (ventilation, inotropes). Immunoglobulin may be beneficial
Metabolic	Urea cycle defect	↓GCS, Seizures, ↑ammonia, alkalosis	Ammonia >150 mmol/L. Repeat to confirm. Metabolic opinion
	Organic acidosis	Profound metabolic acidosis, ketone negative	Supportive (inotropes, ventilation). May co-present with sepsis
	Mitochondrial	↑Lactate, seizures, cardiomyopathy	Supportive (inotropes, ventilation). May co-present with sepsis
Trauma	Intracranial bleed	Focal neuro signs, fontanellej, retinal bleeds	Head CT to exclude neurosurgical problem/ ?NAI, ?haemorrhagic disease
	Intraabdominal bleed	Unexplained anaemia, abdominal bruising	Abdominal and head CT, ?NAI, ?haemorrhagic disease of newborn

Ref: 1.Penny DJ *ADC 2001*; 84:F141-145, 2.Carmo KA *ADC 2007*; 92:F117-119 3.Dixon J ADC 2005; 90:1190-95 4. Dellinger RP CCM 2013; 41:580-637

Fig. 12.4 Inborn errors of metabolism. (STRS, 2017a. Inborn errors of metabolism.<www.strs.nhs.uk>) This guideline was up to date at time of submission, but to ensure you are using the most up to date guideline, please go to www.strs.nhs.uk and check clinical guidelines for any changes or updates.

Paediatric Critical Care
Inborn errors of metabolism

Parental history:
- Consanguinous parents
- Previous SIDS/Multiple miscarriages
- Maternal illness in pregnancy e.g. HELLP, acute fatty liver
- Increased foetal movements (seizures)

Clinical features: varied
- Dysmorphism at birth/subsequently
- Hypotonia and lethargy
- Poor feeding +/- hypoglycaemia
- Vomiting, diarrhoea, dehydration
- Seizures, encephalopathy
- Hepatomegaly, jaundice
- Cardiac failure

Differential diagnosis
- **Sepsis:** metabolic acidosis, lactate, labile glycaemic control (May be concomitant with metabolic disease)
- **Congenital heart disease:** Present with collapse e.g. coarctation aorta (as duct closes), hypoplastic left heart

Mechanism of decompensation
1) Energy insufficiency: present if delay in fuel provision or increase metabolic rate (illness)
   - **Fatty acid oxidation defects (FAOD):** MCAD/VLCAD; medium/very long chain acylcoenzyme A dehydrogenase, carnitine transport defect (CTD)
   - **Glycogen storage disease (GSD):** von Gierke disease (I), Pompe's disease (II)
   - **Gluconeogenesis defects (GD):** Glycogen syntheses (GS)/Glucose-6-phosphatase (G6P) def
   - **Ketolysis defects (KD):** 3-hydroxy-3methylgluaryl-CoA lyase deficiency
   Mitochondrial disorders (MD):(despite adequate fuel provision)
   - Respiratory chain defects (RCD), congenital lactic acidosis, pyruvate dehydrogenase (PDH), pyruvate carboxylase deficiency (PC)
2) Intoxication: Symptom free period prior to clinical signs of intoxication; acute vs. chronic
   - **Amino acid (AA):** Maple syrup urine disease (MSUD), nonketotic hyperglycinaemia (NKH)
   - **Branch chain organic acidurias (BCOA):** Methylmalonic aciduria (MMA), propionic aciduria (PA), isovaleric aciduria (IVA)
   - **Urea cycle defects (UCD):** Ornithine transcarbamoylase (OTC), citrullinaemia (CIT)
   - **Sugar intolerance:** Galactosaemia (GAL), hereditary fructose intolerance
3) Failure to make complex molecules: Disordered embyogenesis; dysmorphic at birth
   - **Peroxisomal disorders:** Zellweger's disease, neonatal adrenoleukodystrophy
4) Failure to break complex molecules: Progressive deterioration as storage accumulates
   - **Lysosomal disorders:** Mucopolysaccharidoses (MPS), Tay Sach's disease (TS)
5) Disorders of intracellular trafficking: α -1 Antitripsin, congenital defects glycosylation (CDG)

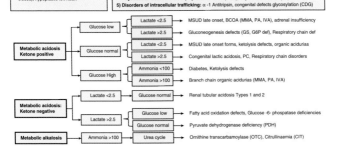

Metabolic acidosis Ketone positive	Glucose low	Lactate <2.5	MSUD late onset, BCOA (MMA, PA, IVA), adrenal insufficiency
		Lactate >2.5	Gluconeogenesis defects (GS, G6P def), Respiratory chain def
	Glucose normal	Lactate <2.5	MSUD late onset forms, ketolysis defects, organic acidurias
		Lactate >2.5	Congenital lactic acidosis, PC, Respiratory chain disorders
	Glucose High	Ammonia <100	Diabetes, Ketolysis defects
		Ammonia >100	Branch chain organic acidurias (MMA, PA, IVA)
Metabolic acidosis: Ketone negative	Lactate <2.5	Glucose normal	Renal tubular acidosis Types 1 and 2
	Lactate >2.5	Glucose low	Fatty acid oxidation defects, Glucose -6- phospatase deficiencies
		Glucose normal	Pyruvate dehydrogenase deficiency (PDH)
Metabolic alkalosis	Ammonia >100	Urea cycle	Ornithine transcarbamoylase (OTC), Citrullinaemia (CIT)

PICU Special investigations:
- **Blood:** Repeat arterial gas, lactate & ammonia
- Send acylcarnitines (FAOD), amino acids(AA/BROA)
- **Urine:** Repeat ketone dipstick, urgent organic acids for gas chromatography mass spectrometry
- **CSF:** Lactate (MD), glycine (NKH)
- **ECG, ECHO:** Cardiomyopathy (MD, FAOD, GSD II)
- **Ophthalmology:** Oil-drop cataracts (GAL), cherry red spot (TS), retinopathy (MD, FAOD)
- **EEG:** Seizure disorder (NKH), encephalopathy (UCD/BCOA)
- **CT head or MRI:** Basal ganglia changes (MD)

Definitive treatment: *Consult metabolic team at earliest opportunity*
1. Clear toxic metabolites and prevent ongoing production (promote anabolism)
2. Supplement cofactors as indicated e.g. biotin, pyridoxine, folate
3. Monitor for cerebral oedema
Disease specific treatment:[1]
FAOD: Glucose infusion 5–8 mg/kg/min, keep glucose >3 mmol/L, carnitine (only CTD)[2]
GSD/GD: Infusion of dextrose to keep glucose normal (4–7 mmol/L)
KD: High carbohydrate intake; PO or IV dextrose, moderate protein and fat restriction
MD: PDH: ketogenic diet, dichloroacetate, otherwise supportive management
AA: Stop protein intake, CVVH (hyperleucinaemia), MSUD protein formula, carnitine
BCOA: Restrict protein intake, IV rehydration, carnitine (all)[3], B12 (MMA), glycine (IVA)
UCD: Stop protein intake, alternate pathway drugs; sodium benzoate / phenylbutyrate[4], L-arginine, CVVH for hyperammonaemia, introduce low protein diet after 48–72 h. Prognosis if ammonia > 1000 μmol/L for >6 h POOR. Peritoneal dialysis if wt <3.5 kg.

Principles of continuous veno-venous haemofiltration (CVVH):
1. Clear toxic metabolites: Ammonia in BCOA/UCD, Leucine in MSUD
2. Instigate CVVH ASAP to prevent irrevocable brain damage: - Ammonia : > 350 x 4 h
   -Leucine: If elevated and encephalopathic.
3. Rapid fall of metabolites may be associated with increasing cerebral oedema
4. Peritoneal dialysis may be used due to size of infant and logistics but is not as effective as CVVH[2]

Post-mortem diagnosis:
Save: Plasma, urine for organic acid spectrometry
   Blood for chromosome/DNA store: Lith Hep and EDTA
   Biopsy: Muscle (1 flash frozen sample; one saline gauze sample), **Liver** (2 samples flash frozen –80°C freezer), **Skin fibroblasts:** 1 sample into viral culture medium (pink fluid kept in PICU fridge)
   Consent for post-mortem diagnosis/storage of tissues If not then for photographs and post-mortem MRI

References

1. Van den Berghe G, Wouters PJ, Bouillon R, Weekers C, Schetz M, Vlasselaers D, Ferdinande P, Lauwers P 2003 Outcome benefit of intensive insulin therapy in the critically ill: Insulin dose versus glycaemic control. Critical Care Medicine 31(2):359-366
2. Pierpont Am Heart J. 2000;139: S96-S106
3. Di Donato et al, Clin Chim Acta. 1984;139:13-21
4. Batshaw et al. J Pediatr. 2001;S46-54

Management – is supportive care. Antibiotics are prescribed prior to confirmation of diagnosis. May need circulatory and ventilator support. The use of IVIG where HPeV is associated with severe myocarditis and dilated cardiomyopathy is described (Wildenbeest et al 2013). There are not yet vaccines for HPeV but clinical trials using antiviral drugs continue.

SICKLE CELL CRISIS

Acute sickle cell crisis should be suspected in children with sickle cell disease who have a sudden onset of pain, infection, anaemia, stoke, or priapism. Rarely, sickle cell may be undiagnosed on admission. The most common crisis is an acute painful crisis with pain and swelling in the joints. (Also consider possibility of acute osteomyelitis.) Fever may be present with infection. Other presentations include:

- Acute chest syndrome (new onset chest or pleuritic pain, cough, shortness of breath, tachypnoea, fever, hypoxia, crepitations, rib tenderness)
- Acute splenic or hepatic sequestration (pain, pallor, tender and distended abdomen, and sometimes circulatory collapse)
- Transient red cell aplasia (due to parvovirus infection) – severe pallor, fever, headache, myalgia, arthralgia, respiratory symptoms, heart failure, abdominal pain
- Acute neurologic complications including stroke, seizures, loss of consciousness
- Acute hepatic sequestration
- Acute priapism (medical emergency after 3 hours)
- Acute abdominal pain (due to ischaemia, infarction, abscesses, thrombosis, sequestration, secondary to gall stones) and this may be difficult to distinguish from an acute surgical abdomen
  Principles of treatment include:
- Pain assessment and appropriate analgesia within 30 minutes
- Oxygen therapy if oxygen saturations ≤95%
- Fluids to prevent dehydration
- Blood transfusion or exchange transfusion
- Antibiotics
- Physiotherapy
- Incentive spirometry.

(Further information is available at https://cks.nice.org.uk/sickle-cell-diseases.)

Children may require admission to PICU for acute chest syndrome or neurologic symptoms including stroke, or posterior reversible encephalopathy syndrome – for intubation and ventilation.

DIABETIC KETOACIDOSIS

All information from BSPED Guideline for the Management of Children and Young People under the age of 18 years with DKA (BSPED 2015).

Diagnosis of DKA in children if:
- There is acidosis with blood pH <7.3 or plasma bicarbonate <18 mmol/L AND
- Ketonaemia with blood beta-hydroxybutyrate >3 mmol/L

If pH is ≥7.1 then DKA is mild or moderate.
If pH is <7.1 then DKA is severe.

The guidelines are intended for children who not only have the above features, but also may have:
- Clinical dehydration
- Nausea and/or vomiting
- And/or drowsiness
- Acidotic respirations

Children can die from DKA – from cerebral oedema (mortality around 25%), hypokalaemia, or aspiration pneumonia (BSPED 2015).

See Fig. 12.5.

General resuscitation notes – ABCDE assessment
- Seek urgent anaesthetic review if child has a reduced level of consciousness and is unable to protect the airway.
- Give 100% oxygen via facemask.
- Monitor all vital signs hourly including cardiac monitoring, half-hourly neurologic observations, hourly blood glucose, 1–2 hourly blood ketones, 2-hourly electrolytes, strict hourly fluid balance, AND REPORT CHANGES/ABNORMALITIES.
- Seek urgent advice from paediatric intensive care; discuss child's condition if hypotensive shock, as they may require inotropic support.
- DO NOT GIVE ROUTINE FLUID BOLUS – only give 10 mL/kg of 0.9% saline if there are signs of shock (poor peripheral pulses, poor capillary filling with tachycardia, and/or hypotension). Do not give a second dose without discussion with the responsible senior paediatrician.

Suspect sepsis if there is fever or hypothermia, hypotension, refractory acidosis, or lactic acidosis.

- Observe for evidence of cerebral oedema (headache, irritability, slowing pulse, rising blood pressure, reducing conscious level; NB papilloedema is a late sign).
- Observe for infection.
- Observe for ileus.

Fig. 12.5 Algorithm for the management of diabetic ketoacidosis (BSPED, 2015. Diabetic ketoacidosis guideline. www.bsped.org.uk, Accessed 14 December 2016.)

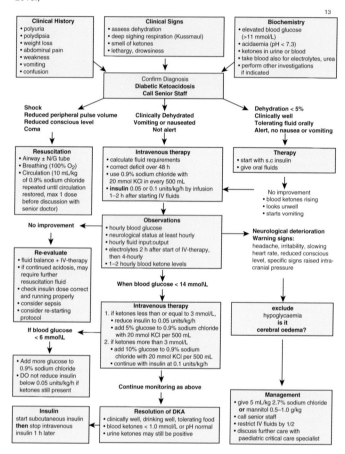

Fluid management in diabetic ketoacidosis

Accurate fluid management is vital and must be documented. If a fluid bolus has been given (10 mL/kg), it is expected that the child will no longer be in shock; however, if shock persists, discuss with a senior doctor about a further bolus. Fluid requirements in DKA are:

$$\text{Requirement} = \text{Deficit} + \text{Maintenance}$$

Deficit – it is not possible to accurately assess the degree of dehydration; therefore

Assume a 5% fluid deficit in children in mild or moderate DKA (pH 7.1 and above)
Assume a 10% fluid deficit in children in severe DKA (pH below 7.1)

Maintenance – use the following 'reduced volume rules'

Weight <10 kg, give 2 mL/kg/h
Weight 10–40 kg, give 1 mL/kg/h
Weight >40 kg, give fixed volume of 40 mL/h (NOT PER KG)

Large fluid volumes are associated with an increased risk of cerebral oedema.

(Neonatal DKA will require special consideration and possibly larger volumes of fluid – usually 100–150 mL/kg/24 hours – but seek advice from the most senior doctors.)

Resuscitation fluid – if more than 20 mL/kg of 0.9% sodium chloride has been given as an intravenous bolus, subtract any additional bolus from the total fluid calculation for the 48-hour period.

Fluid calculation

Calculate the fluid deficit (either 5% or 10% dehydration depending on the severity of acidosis), divide over 48 hours, and add to the hourly rate of maintenance, which equals the hourly fluid rate.

For example, if a child weighs 20 kg then 5% (of the body weight) dehydration = 1 kg = 1000 mL

Therefore 1000 ÷ 48 = 21 mL/h plus maintenance at 1 mL/kg/h (20 mL) = 41 mL hour total volume over 48 hours – initially intravenous fluid (until ketosis is resolving) but if oral fluids are given before the 48-hour rehydration period is complete, this must be subtracted from the intravenous hourly total.

Do not give additional intravenous fluid to replace urinary losses.

Recommended intravenous fluid is 0.9% sodium chloride with 20 mmol potassium chloride in 500 mL until blood glucose levels are less than 14 mmol/L.

Corrected sodium levels should rise as blood glucose levels fall during treatment. (See www.strs.nhs.uk/resources/pdf/guidelines/correct edNA.pdf.)

If the child is becoming hypernatraemic, this is generally not a problem and is protective against cerebral oedema, but if corrected sodium levels do not rise, discuss with the most senior doctor available.

If the child with DKA develops hypokalaemia (potassium <3 mmol/L), urgently discuss with a specialist in paediatric critical care.

INSULIN

Once rehydration fluids and potassium are running, the blood glucose level will start to fall. Cerebral oedema may be more likely to develop if insulin is started early (BSPED 2015).

DO NOT GIVE A BOLUS DOSE OF INTRAVENOUS INSULIN.

Start an intravenous insulin infusion 1–2 hours after starting intravenous fluid therapy. Use a short-acting (soluble) insulin; for example, Actrapid at a dosage between 0.05 and 0.1 units/ kg/h.

Do not give sodium bicarbonate to children with DKA.

There is a significant risk of femoral vein thrombosis in young and very sick children with DKA who have femoral lines inserted.

Continuing management of diabetic ketoacidosis

Once blood glucose has fallen to 14 mmol/L, add glucose to the fluid and think about the insulin rate as follows:
If ketone levels are less than 3 mmol/L:
- Change the fluid to 5% glucose with 0.9% sodium chloride and 20 mmol potassium chloride in 500 mL
- Reduce to or maintain an insulin infusion rate of 0.05 units/kg/h
If ketone levels are above 3 mmol/L:
- Maintain the insulin infusion rate at 0.05 to 0.1 units/kg/h to switch off ketogenesis
- Change the fluid to contain 10% glucose rather than 5% glucose to prevent hypoglycaemia when the higher dose of insulin is given
- Use 500 mL bags of 0.9% sodium chloride with 10% glucose and 20 mmol potassium chloride

---

Do not stop the insulin infusion while glucose is being given as insulin is required to switch off ketone production.

If blood glucose falls below 6 mmol/L:
- Increase glucose concentration
- And if ketosis persists, continue to give insulin at a dose of at least 0.05 units/kg/h

---

If blood glucose falls below 4 mmol/L:
- Give a bolus of 2 mL/kg of 10% glucose and increase the glucose concentration of the infusion
- Insulin can temporarily be reduced for 1 hour
If acidosis is not correcting, consider the following:
- Insufficient insulin to switch off ketosis
- Inadequate resuscitation
- Sepsis
- Hyperchloraemic acidosis
- Salicylate or other drugs.

Continually assess child for signs of cerebral oedema (headache, agitation, falling heart rate and increasing blood pressure, deteriorating level of consciousness, abnormalities in breathing pattern, oculomotor palsy, abnormal posturing, pupillary inequality, or dilatation) – and if suspected:

- Immediately treat with EITHER hypertonic saline 2.7% (2.5–5 mL/kg over 10–15 min) OR mannitol 20% (0.5–1 g/kg over 10–15 min).
- Inform the most senior staff IMMEDIATELY and seek specialist advice on further management.

SYNDROME OF INAPPROPRIATE ANTIDIURETIC HORMONE SECRETION

SIADH secretion can develop in any child who sustains injury to or compression of the pituitary or hypothalamus – this may occur as a result of:

- Head injury
- Intracranial haemorrhage
- Encephalopathies (including Guillain-Barré syndrome, meningitis, and encephalitis)
- Hydrocephalus
- Raised intracranial pressure
- Neurosurgery
- Antidiuretic hormone (ADH)-secreting tumours

ADH or arginine vasopressin is formed in the hypothalamus. It is transported to the posterior pituitary gland, where it is released in response to differences between extracellular and intracellular osmolality. ADH increases the permeability of the renal distal tubule and collecting ducts to water, so that less free water is excreted in the urine, reducing urine volume and increasing concentration. If ADH levels remain elevated, serum hypo-osmolality and hyponatraemia will develop.

In SIADH, hyponatraemia results from an excess of water rather than a deficiency of sodium.

Signs and symptoms

Urine volume is often reduced but the urine osmolality and sodium concentration will be high. If the SIADH continues, water intoxication and hyponatraemic seizures can result from the movement of water from the intravascular space into cerebral tissue. Confusion and coma can occur.

Management

- Diagnosis is confirmed when the patient responds to fluid restriction with correction of hyponatraemia.
- Fluids usually restricted to 30–75% maintenance.

- In a nonacute setting, aim to raise serum sodium by 0.5–1 mmol/L/h and not more than 10 mmol/L in the first 24 hours (to avoid neurologic complications such as central pontine myelinolysis).
- If profound hyponatraemia or signs of water intoxication are present (deterioration in level of consciousness or seizures), administration of hypertonic saline (3% sodium chloride) and a diuretic (e.g., furosemide) may be prescribed to increase serum sodium concentration and eliminate excess intravascular water.
- Close monitoring of level of consciousness, fluid balance, daily weight, and blood and urine chemistries.
- The underlying cause of the SIADH should be treated.

BURNS

There are two important factors that determine the severity of a burn and these are the temperature and the duration of contact. It is necessary to establish the history of the burn; nonaccidental injury may be considered if there are inconsistencies in the history. The most common cause of death within the first hour following burn injury is due to smoke inhalation (ALSG 2016), so airway and breathing assessment must be a priority. See Fig. 12.6 for guidance regarding burns in children.

(See www.cks.nice.org.uk. Burns and scalds guidance for need for referral to a specialist burns unit.)

CARE OF CHILD POST SCOLIOSIS SURGERY

Children may require scoliosis surgery for several reasons:
- Idiopathic
- Congenital malformation
- Neuromuscular disorder (e.g., Duchenne's muscular dystrophy)

Surgery may help with pain and positioning to prevent deterioration of lung function or less commonly for cosmetic reasons. Halo gravity traction is used in some centres prior to surgery to reduce the degree of curvature.

Type of surgical approach: posterior approach and fusion, anterior release and posterior fusion, or anterior approach and fusion. Steel rods help support the fusion of vertebrae, and bone grafts are placed to grow into the bone and fuse the vertebrae. Anterior spinal fusions often have underwater seal chest drain in situ postoperatively.

Postoperative considerations: ABCD assessment
A – AIRWAY
- The child may have a syndrome with an associated difficult airway.
- Prolonged procedure may result in airway swelling postoperatively.
- There may be limited neck extension in this group of patients.
- Halo traction may be in situ on return from surgery – a key should always be attached to the end of the patient's bed.
- The endotracheal tube (ETT) position should be noted on return to PICU.

Fig. 12.6 Early management of paediatric burns. (STRS, 2015. Early management of paediatric burns. www.strs.nhs.uk) This guideline was up to date at time of submission, but to ensure you are using the most up to date guideline, please go to www.strs.nhs.uk and check clinical guidelines for any changes or updates.

Paediatric Critical Care
Burns (early management)

- Major burns require multidisciplinary assessment[1,2]
- Contact plastic surgeons and anaesthetists in all cases
- Burns referral if Total Burn Surface Area (TBSA) ≥10%
  Burns ICU if intubated (any reason) or TBSA >20%

Airway

- Maintain patent airway
- C-spine protection if any possibility of spinal injury
- Early intubation if anticipated airway problems (oedema face/lips)
  Consider cuffed endotracheal tube (may be difficult to replace)
  Leave endotracheal tube long and uncut to allow for length if
  swelling occurs (facial burns) Consider suture, or wire to teeth in
  major facial burns if endotracheal tube unsecure
- Rapid Sequence Induction with Rocuronium (not suxamethonium)

Breathing

- Ensure adequate oxygenation and ventilation
- 15 l O_2 non-rebreathing mask/ 100% O_2 if intubated & ventilated
- Respiratory failure can be due to chest trauma, inhalational injury
  and restrictive chest wall eschar formation

Circulation

- 2x large bore cannulae or intraosseous access in first 5 min
- Baseline bloods: ABG (lactate, O_2Hb, COHb, MetHb), x-match,
  glucose, baseline electrolytes, renal function and CK
- Signs of shock, 20 mL/kg Hartmann's solution (check serum
  potassium) titrated to cardiovascular response
- Burns fluid resuscitation using Parkland Formula*
- Refractory hypotension, consider other causes e.g. trauma
- Electrical burn: Baseline 12 lead ECG & monitor for arrhythmias

*Parkland Formula

- Applicable to burns >10% TBSA
- Fluid requirement commences from time of burn
- Aim to replace fluid lost from burned surface in first 24 hours
- Total volume (first 24 h) Hartmann's solution

4 mL x weight (kg) x %TBSA
50% volume in first 8 h → 0.25 mL/kg/% TBSA/h
50% volume in next 16 h → 0.125 mL/kg/% TBSA/h

- Volume calculation is starting point
- Alter volume infused to maintain urine output 1–2 mL/kg/h[3]
- Urinalysis for myoglobinuria (rhabdomyolysis) – aim for 2 mL/kg/h
- Other trauma & ongoing bleeding will require additional
  resuscitation. No maintenance required during stabilisation

Neurological status

- Assess and document coma score and pupil size. Check glucose
- Decreased level of consciousness can be multifactorial
- May need CT head to exclude head injury

Exposure / Environment: Actively maintain normothermia

- Secondary survey: Examine head to toe, front and back.
- Check distal perfusion, temperature and colour: Consider
  escharotomy for circumferential limb burns
- Use Lund & Browder chart to document percentage and depth of
  burn. Do not count erythema (estimate if non chart: Child's palm =
  1% BSA) Cover burn area with longitudinal cling film and avoid
  circumferential dressings
- Early gastric and urinary catheter insertion (before oedema)

Anticipate airway problems: Intubate early in these settings

1) Airway burn: presence of facial or circumferential neck burn.
Burn sustained indoors. Carbonaceous debris in mouth or nose
2) Inhalational injury: Indicated by any of stridor, singed nasal hair,
carbonaceous septum, burned sustained indoors or increased
carboxyhaemoglobin (COHb)
3) Reduced or falling level of consciousness
4) Large burn ≥25% or electrical burn

Carbon Monoxide (CO) poisoning[4]

- Pulse oximetry unreliable (false high SpO_2 despite arterial hypoxia)
- Arterial blood gas (ABG) co-oximetry (normal COHb levels 1–3%)
- Use 100% O_2 as carbon monoxide clears in 3–5 h
- CO Hb level >30% may benefit from Hyperbaric Oxygen Therapy

Cyanide poisoning (aerosolisation of upholstery and fabrics)

- Metabolic acidosis (particularly if lactate >10 mmol/L) despite 100%
  O_2 & adequate fluid resuscitation in first 2 h of presentation
- Arteriovenous saturation difference <5%
- Preferred treatment: Hydroxycobalamin (Cyankit) 70 mg/kg IVI
  or 50% sodium thiosulfate 0.5 mL/kg over 10 min
- Discuss with burns centre & on call GSTT consultant toxicologist

Chest wall injury[5]: Full thickness burns to lateral and anterior chest
wall may necessitate early escharotomy

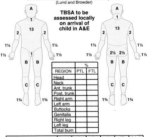

% Total Body Surface Area Burn
Be clear and accurate, and do not include erythema
(Lund and Browder)

TBSA to be assessed locally on arrival of child in A&E

REGION	PTL	FTL
Head		
Neck		
Ant. trunk		
Post. trunk		
Right arm		
Left arm		
Buttocks		
Genitalia		
Right leg		
Left leg		
Total burn		

AREA	Age 0	1	5	10	15	Adult
A = ½ of head	9½	8½	6½	5½	4½	3½
B = ½ of one thigh	2¾	3¼	4	4½	4½	4¾
C = ½ of one lower leg	2½	2½	2¾	3	3¼	3½

Analgesia: Dosing according to STRS drug calculator & formulary

- Assess and document pain score using age appropriate tool
- Use regular paracetamol: anti-pyretic and analgesic effects
- IV morphine infusion preferred to obtain baseline control of pain
- IV morphine boluses to supplement pain control for interventions
- IV ketamine can be used, with anaesthetic support, for procedures
- Oral/IV clonidine augments morphine

References 1. COBIS guidelines 2009 **2.** LSEBN guidelines 2010
3. Greenhalgh DG. Burn resuscitation, Burn care & Research 2007
4. Smollin C. Carbon monoxide poisoning Clinical evidence BMJ 2008
5. ATLS manual eighth ed. 2008 212-224

B – BREATHING

- Note ventilator settings on return to PICU as well as any intraoperative ventilator difficulties.
- Preoperative respiratory investigations are useful in determining baseline respiratory status. There may be plans in situ regarding weaning from respiratory support.
- Chest x-ray postoperatively will identify ETT position, exclude pneumothorax, and confirm position of chest drain (likely if anterior approach). A pleural drain is usually put on suction (and usually removed after 48 hours if swinging and draining cease).
- Involve physiotherapy team – may require interventions such as cough assist or noninvasive ventilation.

C – CARDIOVASCULAR

- Preexisting cardiac condition may have been identified (e.g., cardiomyopathy, pulmonary hypertension, or a structural lesion).
- Identify if any inotropic support was required intraoperatively.
- Identify intraoperative blood loss – (typical blood loss is 20% of circulating volume) and monitor for bleeding. (Disorders of coagulation are not uncommon in this population, e.g., Von Willebrand factor deficiency, or platelet dysfunction secondary to medications such as sodium valproate.)
- Routine PICU monitoring to include HR, BP, CVP, perfusion, oxygen saturations, fluid balance, and temperature.
- If any evidence of deteriorating cardiovascular status, consider an ECG to look at both systolic and diastolic function and monitor for signs of sepsis.

D – DISABILITY

- Assess preoperative baseline neurologic status.
- Intraoperatively there will have been monitoring of sensory and motor function and it is very important to assess as soon as possible in PICU that there is no deterioration in movement of the lower limbs, or new onset paraesthesia. Motor and sensory loss can occur as a result of compression of the spinal cord.

Neurovascular assessment – follow local guidelines but these must be carried out regularly (usually hourly for 48 hours and then 4-hourly for the next 48 hours) and thoroughly, and any deviation from the child's baseline must be reported.

Neurovascular assessment – Assess the Seven *P*s
Pain
Pallor – colour and temperature
Pulses
Paresis – weakness
Paraesthesia – pins and needles/tingling
Paralysis
Puffiness/swelling from oedema or haematoma; document and report any abnormal findings IMMEDIATELY.

Antiembolic stockings are usually worn until ambulatory.

Assess vision postoperatively.

Neurologic complications of spinal surgery include:

- Spinal epidural haematoma (1–2% incidence)
- Spinal cord ischaemia (1–2% incidence)
- Peripheral neuropathies and brachial plexus injuries
- Visual loss due to pressure on the eyes in the prolonged prone position; the majority of these are due to ischaemic optic neuropathy

Nutrition and hydration – These children are usually nil by mouth (NBM) until bowel sounds resume. Some children develop an ileus post spinal surgery. Intravenous fluid maintenance initially.

Postoperative pain – This is often managed using a regional infusion or an epidural in combination with a narcotic infusion or patient-controlled analgesia. See Pain chapter for guidance for assessment of the level of epidural and pain control.

Positioning – Note any specific postoperative instructions regarding positioning. Ensure adequate analgesia and reposition the child at least every 2 hours using the log rolling technique. Use pillows to support back, knees, and feet. Check skin regularly for signs of pressure areas.

Wound care and potential sepsis – Postoperative scoliosis patients are at risk of septic complications, which include surgical site infection, pneumonia, and urinary tract infection (as the child will be catheterised). The wound dressing should be observed for signs of bleeding but should be left intact until the surgeons indicate it should be changed. A wound drain may be in situ for 24–48 hours.

REFERENCES

Advanced Life Support Group (ALSG), 2016. Advanced Paediatric Life Support, sixth ed. Wiley Blackwell, Oxford.

Bingol-Kologlu, M., Yildiz, R.V., Alper, B., et al., 2007. Necrotising fasciitis in children: diagnostic and therapeutic aspects. J. Pediatr. Surg 42 (11), 1892–1897.

British Society for Paediatric Endocrinology and Diabetes (BSPED), 2015. Diabetic ketoacidosis Guideline. www.bsped.org.uk. Accessed December 14, 2016.

Deep, A., Cantle, F., Daniels, R., 2015. for UK Sepsis Trust. Clinical Toolkit 6: Emergency Department Management of Paediatric Sepsis. www.sepsistrust.org. Accessed January 31, 2017.

Fernando, S.L., 2012. The management of toxic epidermal necrolysis. Australas. J. Dermatol 53 (3), 165–171.

Goldstein, B., Giroir, B., Randolph, A., 2005. International pediatric sepsis concensus conference: definitions for sepsis and organ dysfunction in paediatrics. Pediatr. Crit. Care. Med 6 (1), 2–8.

Khatami, A., McMullan, B.J., Webber, M., et al., 2015. Sepsis-like disease in infants due to human parechovirus type 3 during an outbreak in Australia. Clin. Infect. Dis 60 (92), 228–236.

National Institute for Health and Care Excellence (NICE), 2012. Neonatal infection (early onset); antibiotics for prevention and treatment: guidance. (CG149).

National Institute for Health and Care Excellence (NICE), 2015a. Burns and scalds. www.cks.nice.org.uk.

National Institute for Health and Care Excellence (NICE), 2015b. Meningitis (bacterial) and meningococcal septicaemia in under 16s: recognition, diagnosis and management. CG102. www.nice.org.uk.

Norrby-Teglund, A., Kaul, R., Low, D.E., et al., 1996. Plasma from patients with severe group A streptococcal infections treated with normal polyspecific IgG (IVIG) inhibits streptococcal superantigen–induced T cell proliferation and cytokine production. J. Immunol 156, 3057–3064.

Oliveira, C.F., Nogueira de Sa, F.R., Oliveira, D.S., et al., 2008. Time and fluid sensitive resuscitation for hemodynamic support of children in septic shock: barriers to the implementation of the American College of Critical Care Medicine/Pediatric Advanced Life Support Guidelines in a pediatric intensive care unit in a developing world. Pediatr. Emerg. Care 24 (12), 810–815.

South Thames Retrieval Service (STRS), 2015. Early Management of Paediatric Burns. www.strs.nhs.uk.

South Thames Retrieval Service (STRS), 2017a. Inborn Errors of Metabolism. www.strs.nhs.uk.

South Thames Retrieval Service (STRS), 2017b. Neonatal Collapse. www.strs.nhs.uk.

South Thames Retrieval Service (STRS), 2017c. Sepsis early management guidelines. www.strs.nhs.uk.

Sun, G., Wang, Y., Tao, G., et al., 2012. Complete genome sequence of a novel type of human parechovirus strain reveals natural recombination events. J. Virol 86 (16), 8892–8893.

Tang, J.W., Holmes, C.W., Elsanousi, F.A., et al., 2016. Cluster of human parechovirus infections as the predominant cause of sepsis in neonates and infants, Leicester, United Kingdom, 8 May to 2 August 2016. Euro. Surveill. 21 (34). www.eurosurveillance.org.

Tong, J., Plunkett, A., Daniels, R., 2014. G218(P) The Paediatric Sepsis 6 Initiative. Arch. Dis. Child 99 (Supp. 1).

Wildenbeest, J.G., Wolthers, K.C., Straver, B., et al., 2013. Successful IVIG treatment of human parechovirus–associated dilated cardiomyopathy in an infant. Pediatrics 132 (1), 243–247.

TRANSPORT OF CRITICALLY ILL INFANTS AND CHILDREN

13

There is evidence from studies in the United Kingdom and Australia that the centralisation of paediatric intensive care unit (PICU) services improves outcomes (Pearson 1997). However, to achieve this centralisation, children need to be moved from their local hospital to a PICU. Different provision exists in countries around the world for transfer if required. This chapter contains guidance for the stabilisation and preparation for transfer of the critically ill child as well as practical advice on the safe and efficient transport of critically ill infants or children. The chapter includes information for road, fixed-wing, and helicopter transfers.

The majority (90%) of transfers in the United Kingdom are performed by specialist services. Detailed information about specialist paediatric transport services, including quality standards identified by The Paediatric Intensive Care Society, United Kingdom, is available at http://www.picsociety.uk.

This provides recommendations regarding:
- Support for children and their families
- Staffing of a specialised paediatric transport service for the critically ill
- Indemnity
- Administration, clerical, and data support
- Communication
- Emergency transport arrangements
- Equipment
- Guidelines and protocols

The information contained in this chapter will also provide useful checklists and information for intrahospital transfers; for example, if PICU patients need to be taken to magnetic resonance imaging (MRI) or computed tomography (CT) scan.

TRANSPORT TEAM COMPOSITION

The transport team composition will vary from country to country. Key personnel will include a team leader and at least two others:
- The team leader may be a doctor or an advanced nurse practitioner both of whom should have received specialised training in paediatrics, PICU, and interhospital transport of the critically ill child
- A PICU transport nurse
- An ambulance driver
- A technician
- A respiratory therapist

AWAITING THE PAEDIATRIC CRITICAL CARE TRANSPORT TEAM – WHAT CAN YOU DO TO HELP?

If a paediatric critical care transport team is on the way to come and transfer your patient to a tertiary PICU, there are many things you can do to facilitate the transfer and help prepare the child and family. The child should be continually monitored using electrocardiography (ECG), blood pressure (BP), and oxygen saturations as a minimum (plus end-tidal CO_2 if the child is intubated and ventilated), and should have either a nurse or doctor present at all times. Most paediatric transport teams have online emergency drug calculators and guides for tube sizes/equipment required, which are specific to the age/weight of your patient. It is useful to print these off (e.g., South Thames Retrieval Service [STRS] emergency drugs calculator; see http://www.strs.nhs.uk). An ABCDE approach, as always, is useful to prioritise care. (Resuscitation guidelines have changed to address catastrophic haemorrhage prior to ABCD, but in this setting, such bleeding should have been addressed by this stage [ALSG 2015]).

Airway

Most infants and children being retrieved will require intubation. Please see airway chapter for hints on the intubation procedure. Remember C-spine collars are no longer recommended, but if concerns exist about C spine, then manual inline stabilisation, including blocks and tapes, are still recommended (ALSG 2015).

- Please do not precut the endotracheal tube (ETT) or even cut after intubation.
- Please secure with long trouser leg tapes that reach from ear to ear, preferably secured on top of a hydrocolloid dressing (e.g., Duoderm) if available.
- Please take a chest x-ray after intubation (with the child's head in a neutral position) to check the position of ETT as the retrieval team requires this before departure.
- Document size and length of the ETT.

Breathing

Once intubated, try putting on an age/weight-appropriate ventilator.

- PEAK pressures – start with low peak pressures and increase peak pressures whilst closely observing the child's chest movement and stop when the child has adequate chest movement
- Positive end-expiratory pressure (PEEP) – 5 cm H_2O – for all babies and children (some children with severe obstructed airways may need a higher PEEP)
- Inspired time – 0.75 second for a baby, up to 1 second for an older child
- Rate – start at 30 breaths/min for a baby, 20–25 for a young child, 12–15 for a teenager

- Set oxygen level as required (except in babies with congenital heart defects [e.g., hypoplastic left heart syndrome] who may require ventilation in air while tolerating lower than normal saturations)

 NB Ensure end-tidal CO_2 monitoring is in use for EVERY intubated and ventilated child.

Circulation

Ideally all children should have two patent and securely fastened intravenous cannula.

- If inotropes are required, then a central venous line is needed.
- All lines should be labelled – particularly distinguishing between arterial and venous lines.
- Prepare fluid boluses and inotropic infusions before departure.
- Ensure all blood results are documented for the transport team.
- Continuous haemodynamic monitoring.

Disability/neurology

- Pupil size and reactivity should be documented as a minimum and reported if abnormal. If required, carry out full neurologic observations (use age-appropriate paediatric glasgow coma score (GCS).
- Consider if inline manual stabilisation is required.
- All children with a head injury must be nursed maintaining $ETCO_2$ 4–5 kPa, head-up tilt to 30 degrees, midline, with a good BP to maintain an adequate cerebral perfusion pressure, manage pain effectively, catheterise.
- Treat seizures.
- Adequate sedation to keep the child comfortable and safe, and consider the use of muscle relaxation (but this may mask seizures).
- Manage raised intracranial pressure (ICP) (give 3 mL/kg of 3% saline if acute deterioration with ↑ICP).
- Stabilise fractures.
- Maintain blood sugar in the normal range.

Everything else

- Drugs – ensure all drugs prescribed, particularly antibiotics, are given and signed; photocopy drug chart.
- Temperature control – aim for normothermia – may need to actively cool the septic child (fan or ice packs), or warm the neonate booties, mittens, hat, warm blankets, babytherm.
- Fluids – prepare fluid boluses, start intravenous maintenance fluid on any infants (usually normal saline plus either 5% or 10% dextrose).
- Family and communication – try to update the family as to the condition of their child and prepare them for the child being transferred to another hospital. Some transport teams have space

to allow parents to accompany their child, but it is best not to promise this option as it is down to the discretion of the team to authorise this. (There may be occasions where the ill health of a parent precludes them travelling in the ambulance [i.e., a physical or mental health issue; they may have just given birth, or be highly stressed and not able to look after themselves, or be aggressive or angry, and all these reasons could be too distracting for the team who need to focus on the critically ill child].) It is the responsibility of the referring hospital to ensure the parents are able to get to the tertiary centre even if this means providing a taxi if there are no other options; however, do not advise the parents to leave before the transport team arrive.

- Documentation – prepare all documentation, including a medical letter to the receiving team; photocopy notes, drug charts, observation charts; ensure any imaging is image-linked to the receiving hospital or have a hard copy to take; ensure the child has a name band on and any allergies clearly documented. All family contact details must be available, the name of the general practitioner (GP) and the health visitor, and any safeguarding concerns must be verbally shared as well as documented. Infectious status must be clearly stated in addition to any known exposure to infectious diseases.

ARRIVAL OF THE PAEDIATRIC CRITICAL CARE TRANSPORT TEAM

Communication – On arrival at the referring hospital and after introducing team members to referring hospital staff (and child/family), it is essential at this point, and BEFORE handover, that the transport team become SITUATIONALLY AWARE. That is, they physically see the child, the monitor, and their observations to ensure that it is appropriate to start handover or to decide whether immediate resuscitation or intervention may be beneficial.

Good communication is a key skill for a smooth and effective functioning team so that constructive relationships develop. Voicing concerns aloud can be helpful in focusing the team to deliver the same goal ('I'm worried about …'). The referring team may have been working for many hours stabilising the child, and their continued input and collaboration until the point of departure is invaluable.

Assessment of the infant/child

Following handover of the history and management of the child, examine and assess the child's condition and ascertain the following:

- Check what personal protective equipment may be required (the infection status of the child or any recent foreign travel).
- If the child is ventilated, what is the size, length, position, and mode of securing of the ETT tube?
- Is the child effectively ventilated or are there problems? Is there humidification?

- Were there any problems during intubation and is there a leak around the tube?
- Has a recent arterial blood gas analysis been undertaken?
- Where are chest and other x-rays?
- Is the child cardiovascularly stable? Are the child's heart rate and BP within reasonable ranges for his/her age and condition?
- If the child has had cardiac rhythm disturbances or a cardiac arrest, ascertain if a cause was found, and the treatment required to stabilise the child's condition.
- Has a 12-lead ECG been performed, if required?
- Assess the child's current perfusion – central and peripheral pulses, and what is the capillary refill time?
- Note peripheral and central lines, their location, patency, secureness of dressings, and the fluids/drugs running through them.
- Check and record the dosages of drug infusions/fluids in progress, paying particular attention if the patient is a child with a suspected congenital cardiac abnormality on a Prostin E_2 infusion – this drug has been known to be confused with prostacyclin, which could have serious implications and, as the dosage for Prostin E_2 is calculated in nanograms, there is increased potential for error.
- Note any allergies.
- Note blood/specimen results that may be available.
- Has a recent blood sugar level been checked?
- What is the child's urine output like? Quantity/colour/urinalysis?
- Has the child been catheterised?
- What are the core/peripheral temperatures?
- Does the child have any rash/cuts/bruises/superficial or more serious injuries (e.g., consider abdominal injury)?
- Assess and document the child's neurologic status, taking into consideration drugs that have been given or are in progress. Check pupil reaction and size.

Try to gain some space to lay out the equipment you need – ask to borrow some trolleys, as these are invaluable, enabling you to lay out drugs/equipment for any procedure you need to undertake.

When you have completed all procedures required to stabilise and treat the child, prior to preparing to leave the parents will need to be updated and see their child. They may, of course, be present throughout the stabilisation period. Some transport teams are able to accommodate one or both parents in the ambulance to travel with their child. Otherwise, check their travel arrangements – if they are very shocked/distressed, it is inadvisable for them to drive. If a friend/relative is unable to help them, involve staff at the referring hospital in making arrangements. Many teams provide maps for parents together with their information booklet, to make their journey easier. If the parents are driving, make sure they understand that under no circumstances should they attempt to follow the ambulance as it travels with blue lights at speed back to your base. If traffic is likely to be heavy or the doctor feels it is indicated for other reasons, a police escort may be required, which will need to be organised.

BEFORE TRANSFER

Safety

- Appropriately secure infant or child on the transfer trolley or in transport incubator or pod prior to departure.
- Perform appropriate continuous monitoring in situ – ECG, pulse oximetry, end-tidal CO_2, continuous/intermittent BP, respiratory rate, and heart rate.
- Set appropriate limits on transport monitor.
- Secure all equipment, including monitor and infusion pumps, prior to departure.
- Record physiologic variables as a baseline at the referring hospital and during the transfer, as well as therapeutic interventions.
- Document and report adverse incidents.
- Use adequate and appropriate sedation with or without muscle relaxant.
- Check that the portable suction is working and have appropriate-sized suction catheters to hand.
- The child must wear a hospital nameband.

Airway

- Check that airway is safe or secured by intubation.
- Assess position of endotracheal tube clinically/x-ray prior to departure and that it is well secured.
- Apply humidification in ventilator circuit.
- Consider the need to suction ET tube prior to departure.
- Pack reintubation equipment; for example, spare ET tube of the same size plus one size smaller, Magill's, laryngoscope, mask and airway to hand for transfer.
- Provide nasogastric or orogastric tube in situ.

Breathing

- Select transport ventilator appropriate for age and weight of patient (preferably with high pressure and disconnect alarms).
- Check adequate gas exchange once stabilised on the transport ventilator, confirmed by arterial blood gas if appropriate.
- Provide end-tidal CO_2 monitoring in situ.
- Provide adequate supply of oxygen in ambulance and reserve supply for emergency use.
- Provide a rebreathe bag and self-inflating bag to hand as a backup during transfer.
- Provide a supply of oxygen (and air) for ventilator use if required.
- Have a PEEP valve in use if required.

Circulation

- Provide continuous haemodynamic monitoring as previously described.
- Ideally have at least two intravenous cannulas in situ that have been checked as patent by the retrieval team.

- Ensure that intravenous and arterial lines are securely fastened and labelled, with easy access to the intravenous lines during transfer.
- If a central venous line is inserted for clinical reasons, it should be transduced.
- As far as possible, the child should be haemodynamically stable for transfer but, in situations where ongoing haemodynamic deterioration is likely (e.g., meningococcal septicaemia), appropriate anticipatory measures must be undertaken (e.g., draw up sufficient fluids and inotropic infusions).
- Ensure arterial and central venous pressure (CVP) lines are rezeroed once transducers have been attached to child.
- Ensure the most recent blood results are documented and appropriate treatment administered as required.

Neurology/trauma

- Neurologic observations including pupil size and reactivity should be carried out and documented prior to departure. Note fullness of fontanelle if applicable.
- Spinal boards must be used where appropriate and secured to the trolley.
- Use end-tidal CO_2 monitors on all head-injured patients so that CO_2 may be monitored and controlled (and adequate cerebral perfusion pressure may be addressed).
- All head-injured children should be nursed (where possible) midline with 30 degrees head-up tilt to decrease ICP.
- Investigate and appropriately manage intrathoracic and intra-abdominal injuries.
- Stabilise long bone/pelvic fractures.
- Manage raised ICP appropriately (have 3 mL/kg of 3% saline prepared in case of increasing ICP during transport).
- Control seizures.
- Take measures to maintain blood sugar in normal range if appropriate.

Temperature control

- Take measures to maintain normothermia and prevent hyperthermia in situ if appropriate.
- Take temperature at referring hospital.
- Use mittens, socks, hats, blankets, transport incubator, ambulance heater, and other available products as appropriate to maintain adequate body temperature, considering the season and length of journey as well as the child's illness.

Drugs/fluids

- Have sedation and muscle relaxant drugs infusing/to hand if intubated.
- Have drugs available and/or prepared for intubation/reintubation.
- Have normal saline flushes and volume drawn up in syringes sealed with a bung.

- Label all drugs/fluids accurately.
- Calculate and draw up resuscitation drugs, to hand if required.
- Use appropriate handling, administration, and documentation of controlled drugs.
- Have maintenance fluid if required (usually infants ≤1 year, metabolic conditions, diabetic ketoacidosis (DKA), or any child with low or unstable blood sugar).
- Maintain appropriate storage and use of blood products if required.

Family and communication

- Make good introduction to child, family, and referring team on arrival.
- Talk to family to update on child's condition.
- Ensure all essential documentation is complete (i.e., names, contact telephone numbers).
- Ensure the family knows which PICU their child will be taken to and that they have all contact details of the unit.
- If possible (i.e., if space, insurance, and retrieval policy allow), take parent/parents with the team in the ambulance – making clear the expectations of the team during the journey (i.e., parent must remain seated, seatbelt fastened, must allow team to treat child first without distraction in case of emergency) (Davies et al 2005).
- Telephone the receiving PICU prior to leaving referring hospital to update on child's condition and give estimated time of arrival (also important to let them know about any special requirements: need for cubicle, need for immediate continuous veno-venous haemofiltration (CVVH) therapy, or inotrope change on arrival, for example).
- Telephone the referring hospital on arrival in PICU to inform them of safe transfer.

DOCUMENTATION transfer details

- Name, address including post code, date of birth (Fig. 13.1)
- Next of kin, names and contact details
- Parents' marital status for purposes of consent if further treatment is required
- Any safeguarding concerns
- Name and address of GP
- Referring ward, hospital, and telephone number
- Name of referring doctor and contact details
- Receiving doctor, ward, hospital, and contact details
- Names and status of escorting personnel in retrieval team

Fig. 13.1 Documentation.

Patient name:	Destination: e.g. MRI scan first floor X Wing		
Date of Birth:	Time of scan:		
Hospital Number:	Contact number:		
Allergies:	Contact name:		
Patient weight Kg:	Consent completed:	☐ yes	☐ no

A medical summary

- Diagnosis and reason for requiring intensive care
- History and past history
- Intubation history, ventilatory support, and blood gases
- Cardiovascular status including fluid, inotrope, and vasopressor requirements
- Medication given and allergy status
- Intravenous access and monitoring lines
- Recent blood/cerebrospinal fluid (CSF) results and infectious status (e.g., carbapenem-resistant organisms (CRO), methicillin resistant staphylococcus aureus (MRSA) and respiratory syncitial virus (RSV), pertussis) or recent exposure to infectious disease (e.g., chickenpox)
- Vaccination history

A nursing summary

- Observations, documentation of vital signs during transfer
- Drugs and fluids given during transfer
- Respiratory and cardiovascular status, communication method, nutrition, pain and sedation, elimination, skin condition, social and family needs (particularly any child protection issues)
- Summary of patient's condition during transfer

Audit data

- Severity of illness
- Reason for transfer
- Response times
- Adverse incidents

IN TRANSIT

- Change from the portable O_2 cylinder to the ambulance supply.
- Check that all your emergency equipment and drugs are nearby (on charge if possible) and secured; check suction before departure.
- Check that you have a clear view of the child and all the monitors and pumps.
- Ask the crew to adjust the temperature of the ambulance according to your needs.
- Some teams carry portable blood gas analysers, others find end-tidal CO_2 monitors useful in assessing the child's ventilation requirements.
- If the ventilated child is going to be hand-ventilated for any reason, you might be able to take turns doing this with the doctor – it can be a tiring job on a long journey!
- Make sure all members of the team and any parents use their seatbelts.
- If you need to administer treatment, ask the ambulance crew to slow down and stop.
- Record observations, drug dosages, etc., according to your unit policy – commonly this is done every 15 minutes.

- Observe the child and monitor closely for signs of deterioration in vital signs/lightening level of consciousness/fitting.
- In the event of an acute deterioration, the ambulance will need to pull over and stop, and you may need to request the help of the crew (e.g., if the child has a cardiac arrest).
- In these situations, call ahead to your unit to inform them of a major problem; this will enable them to assist you immediately on arrival if required.

LOOKING AFTER YOURSELF

Retrievals can involve many hours of travelling and working in hot, stressful conditions. It is a good idea to take water and snacks with you, and the referring unit may offer tea or coffee. Some people find nausea a problem, particularly on long journeys in the back of a swaying ambulance. Many of the new ambulances have forward-facing seats, which can help, as can opening the sliding windows a little to let in some air. Some people find sweets helpful and mints are highly recommended! If nausea becomes a real problem on retrieval journeys, you may need to consider trying antinausea wrist bands or appropriate medication to relieve it. Keep vomit bowls handy for staff or parents if required.

Remember to update the referring unit regularly on the condition of the child, particularly shortly after admission and when the child leaves the unit.

Time-critical transfers

NHS England (2015) recommend a few circumstances where time-critical transfers will normally be carried out by the referring unit:
- children requiring emergency neurosurgery
- children with an acute abdomen
- where early intervention (surgery) will have a greater impact on the outcome for these children than transfer by a specialist transport team

Guidance for preparation and transfer in these time-critical circumstances are provided.

Time-critical neurosurgical transfer

Rapid identification and appropriate early management of a child with an acute neurosurgical lesion is crucial. Children of concern could include those who have suffered trauma – with altered or fluctuating levels of consciousness, unequal pupils, abnormal GCS, head injury, or focal neurologic deficit, but could also include blocked ventriculoperitoneal (VP) shunts leading to obstructive hydrocephalus, nonaccidental injury, subdural or extradural bleeds. See NICE (2014) for further guidance.

As mentioned, any infant or child who requires emergency neurosurgery should normally be transferred to the nearest neurosurgical centre by the referring hospital and not the specialist paediatric transport team, as this is likely to provide the quickest way for the child to receive the life-saving treatment required (Tasker et al 2006). In order to streamline efficiency a recommended timeline for investigations and transfer of neurosurgical emergencies has been provided by the National Institute for Clinical Excellence (Table 13.1).

Time (min)	Actions required
Table 13.1 Time line for suspected neurosurgical emergency. National Institute for Health and Care Excellence. Clinical guidance (CG176)	
0	Infant or child identified with suspected mass lesion.
0–60	CT scan should be performed within 60 min and a provisional written
60–120	radiology report should be available within 60 min of scan being
0–240	performed (NICE 2014).
	If mass lesion identified, prepare to move child to nearest neurosurgical centre within a MAXIMUM of 60 min from end of scan. Neurosurgery within 4 h if required.

CT, Computed tomography.

It is helpful to have a plan as to whose responsibility it is to organise certain tasks and each transport service should have guidelines to follow. The following guideline is based on the STRS guideline (available at http://www.strs.nhs.uk) but slightly expanded, giving rationale.

Responsibilities of referring paediatric team:

- Consultant should be present and should update parents at the appropriate time.
- Commence resuscitation and inform anaesthetic team as soon as possible.
- Organise urgent computed tomography (CT) scan and report.
- Refer to regional paediatric neurosurgeon and ask, 'Is this a time-critical lesion?' Document time of all calls.
- Refer to paediatric critical care transport service for advice.
- Ring for an emergency ambulance and state 'paediatric neurosurgical emergency critical care transfer' (and the ambulance should have a response time of 8 min in urban settings in England).
- Support the anaesthetic team and help them prepare the equipment and drugs required for transfer.
- Prepare documentation – photocopy notes, blood results, observation charts, x-rays, and CT scans.
- Print emergency drug calculator for patient weight (available on STRS website and age- and weight-based parameters; http://www.strs.nhs.uk).

Responsibilities of the anaesthetic team:

- Continue resuscitation.
- Provide respiratory support as required.
- Identify suitable transport team.
- Prepare for transfer – airway equipment, drugs, monitoring, portable ventilator.
- Monitor child closely and transfer as soon as safely possible.
- Do not delay with unnecessary procedures.

Responsibilities of regional paediatric critical care transport service:

- Facilitate neurosurgical referral and secure a bed on paediatric intensive care unit.
- Advise referring hospital on management of child.
- Encourage swift transfer.

Responsibilities of the neurosurgical team:

- Confirm diagnosis – 'this is a time-critical neurosurgical emergency'.
- Provide feedback to referring hospital within 30 min of initial referral.
- Liaise with receiving paediatric intensive care unit (PICU) to confirm acceptance of child.
- Inform referring hospital where they should take child (i.e., straight to theatre or PICU).

ABCDE transfer guidance:

A – Airway

- Consider need for intubation – indications include GCS ≤8, loss of airway reflexes, signs of raised intracranial pressure (asymmetric or unreactive pupils, hypertension with bradycardia), inadequate ventilation – hypoxaemia or hypercarbia or spontaneous hyperventilation with $PaCO_2$ < 4 kPa.
- Avoid nasal intubation if possible basal skull fracture or coagulopathy.
- Secure ETT (note correct size and position).
- Consider C spine if trauma.
- Use gastric tube on free drainage.

B – Breathing

- Monitor end-tidal CO_2 (aim for 4–5 kPa).
- Take urgent chest x-ray postintubation to ensure good position of ETT.
- Exclude ETT problems if hypoxic or hypercapnic.

C – Circulation

- Ensure two patent and secure intravenous lines in situ.
- Do not delay for difficult central or arterial access.
- Consider intraosseous route if required
- Maintain age-appropriate BP.
- Use fluid bolus and peripheral dopamine to maintain BP (to maintain adequate cerebral perfusion pressures).
- If central venous line (CVL) in situ, use noradrenaline to support BP if required.

If intracranial hypertensive crisis with bradycardia, hypertension and pupil dilatation
- **Maintain end tidal CO_2 between 4 and 5 kPa.**
- **Give 3 mL/kg of hypertonic (2.7% or 3%) saline.**
- **Sedate the patient.**
- **Do not delay – urgent transfer – keep moving.**

Age-appropriate target systolic blood pressure (BP)

<1 year >80 mm Hg

1–5 years >90 mm Hg

5–14 years >100 mm Hg
>14 years >110 mm Hg
Peripheral dopamine prescription:
3 mg × weight kg in 50 mL of
  N/S or 5%D
1 mL/h = 1 mcg/kg/min

D – Disability and E – Everything else

- Monitor pupil response (at least every 15 min).
- Do not tape over eyelids.
- Sedate adequately.

- Use phenytoin load if seizure noted.
- Trauma patients – ensure other injuries excluded, stabilised, sutured.
- Maintain temperature 36–37°C, treat hyperthermia.
- Identify and treat seizures.
- Maintain normal blood sugar.
- Maintain plasma sodium >140 mmol/l.
- Identify associated injuries (falling Hb/hypotension).

Transfer to ambulance and onward journey:
- Secure child on ambulance trolley.
- Ensure documentation to hand.
- Provide ambubag, mask, and airway on trolley.
- Provide drugs for transfer (sedation/muscle relaxation and resuscitation drugs).
- Provide full portable oxygen cylinder plus spare.
- Switch to ambulance oxygen supply when in ambulance.
- Bring parents if possible, or if parents travelling independently, ensure they have directions to destination hospital and telephone number of receiving unit, and ensure transfer team have their contact details.
- Wear seatbelts when vehicle moving.
- Request a smooth journey and avoid sudden braking.
- Record observations every 15 min.
- Inform receiving paediatric intensive care unit (PICU) of departure from referring hospital.
- Check where child is expected.
- Receiving PICU should inform neurosurgeon of imminent arrival.
- Update neurosurgeon/PICU if condition deteriorates on route.

Time-critical transfer for acute abdomen in children

Diagnosis of children who present with acute abdominal pain is vital so that appropriate and timely care may be given whether medical or surgical in origin. Please see 'Acute Abdominal Pain Pathway, Clinical Assessment Management Tool for Children' on the NHS website (NHS 2016), which provides clinicians with a pathway to follow; however, a quick guide to the most common causes of acute abdominal pain provided in this pathway can be seen in Table 13.2.

Initial management of the child with acute abdominal pain
PRIMARY SURVEY
A-Airway, B-Breathing, C-Circulation, D-Disability, E-Exposure, F-Fluids, G-Glucose
- Take a history, examination, and investigations
  Any concerns → resuscitation if required and refer immediately to a paediatrician or paediatric surgeon.
- Consider pain relief
- Treatment/referral/follow-up
  If a diagnosis of acute abdomen is made and the child has presented in a hospital where there are no specialist paediatric surgeons, then ideally, the child needs to be transferred to a more specialised centre for urgent surgical intervention by the referring hospital. There may

Table 13.2   Quick guide to most common causes of acute abdominal pain in children

	Most important features
Gastroenteritis	Diarrhoea and/or vomiting, other family members affected
Infantile colic	Young healthy infant with episodes of inconsolable cry, drawing up of knees, flatus
Appendicitis	Fever, anorexia, nausea/vomiting, migration of pain from central to RIF, peritonism, tachycardia, raised CRP (or CRP rise after 12 h)
Mesenteric adenitis	Fever, peripheral lymphadenopathy (in 20%), pain more diffuse than in appendicitis, concomitant or antecedent URTI
Intussusception	Mostly <2 years, pain intermittent with increasing frequency, vomits (sometimes with bile), drawing up of knees, red currant jelly stool (late sign)
Volvulus	Abdominal pain due to twisted intestine, bowel obstruction and ischaemia, bloody stool, bile stained vomit
Meckel's diverticulum	Usually painless rectal bleeding, symptoms of intestinal obstruction, can mimic appendicitis
Constipation	Positive history, pain mainly left sided/suprapubic, if acute look for organic causes (i.e., obstruction)
UTI	Fever, dysuria, loin/abdominal pain, urine dipstick positive for nitrites/leucocytes – send formal MC+S if age <3 years
Testicular torsion	More common after puberty. Sudden onset, swollen tender testis (no relief/increase of pain after lifting testicle suggests torsion rather than bacterial epididymitis)
Irreducible hernia	Painful enlargement of previously reducible hernia +/– signs of bowel obstruction
Henoch-Schönlein purpura	Diffuse/colicky abdominal pain, nonblanching rash (obligatory sign), swollen ankles/knees, haematuria/proteinuria
Haemolytic uraemic syndrome	Unwell child with bloody diarrhoea and triad of anaemia, thrombocytopenia, and renal failure
Lower lobe pneumonia	Referred abdominal pain + triad of fever, cough, and tachypnoea
Diabetic ketoacidosis	Known diabetic or history of polydipsia/polyuria and weight loss, BM >15, metabolic acidosis (HCO_3 <15) and ketosis
Sickle cell crisis	Nearly exclusively in black children. Refer to sickle cell disease guideline for differential with noncrisis causes
Trauma	Always consider NAI, surgical review necessary
Psychogenic	Older children with excluded organic causes

NHS Acute Abdominal Pain Pathway, 2016. Clinical assessment management tool for children. <http://www.what0-18.nhs.uk/health-professionals/front-line-hospital-staff/clinical-pathways/abdominal-pain/> (accessed 22.09.2016) with addition of volvulus with permission.
CRP, c-reactive protein; *NAI,* non-accidental injury; *RIF,* right iliac fossa; *URTI,* upper respiratory tract infection; *UTI,* urinary tract infection.

be rare occasions where the child requires life-saving and immediate surgery at the referring hospital even if there are no specialist surgeons present.

Infants and children with an acute abdomen are likely to be hypovolaemic and may be in shock, so will require timely resuscitation, analgesia, and often surgery.

'RED FLAG' indicators requiring URGENT ACTION (see NHS 2016 for detail)

If any of these signs (listed in Box 13.1) are present, call for URGENT paediatric or surgical review.

Box 13.1   Red flags (medical or surgical)
• Severe or increasing abdominal pain • Blood in stool • Abdominal distension • Bilious (green) or blood-stained vomit • Palpable abdominal mass • Child unresponsive or excessively drowsy • Child nonmobile or change in gait pattern due to pain

From NHS Acute Abdominal Pain Pathway, 2016. Clinical assessment management tool for children. <http://www.what0-18.nhs.uk/health-professionals/front-line-hospital-staff/clinical-pathways/abdominal-pain/> (accessed 22/09/16).

Also consider:
- If child could be pregnant/ectopic pregnancy/other gynaecological problem
- If there is possible liver dysfunction/obstructive jaundice
- Possible toxic ingestion

NB Bilious vomiting/aspirates is a sign of intestinal obstruction until proven otherwise!

Further investigations include abdominal x-ray, abdominal ultrasound scan (USS), abdominal CT or MRI scan – with ultrasound being a preferred modality for initial investigation as it is cheap, noninvasive, and radiation free (Saito 2012).

Most importantly – take heed of parental concerns – they know their child best.

Management of acute abdominal pain (Kim 2013)

- Treat underlying cause
- Correction of hypoxaemia
- Replacement of intravascular volume loss

- Correction of metabolic derangement
- Analgesia
- Gastric decompression using a nasogastric tube
- Consider the need for antibiotics
- Urgent transfer to paediatric surgical centre if required

Intrahospital transfer

Preparation is key to a swift and safe intrahospital transfer for emergency imaging or surgery. Most hospitals will have local policies and protocols that determine personnel required and equipment needed, so always use these. Table 13.3 is a generic checklist that includes vital equipment for any transfer but does not detail specific extra equipment that may be needed in individual circumstances.

ESSENTIAL EQUIPMENT AND MONITORING

This must be checked as being intact and functioning prior to use. Please tick the box when equipment collected together with the patient. Check it is age/weight appropriate. (See Table 13.3.).

Observations should be noted prior to transport, during the transport, and in the scan, and should reflect any deterioration. Resuscitation drug doses should be calculated prior to transfer and drawn up if required or if requirement is anticipated. Any critical

Table 13.3 Equipment and monitoring checklist	
Facemask	IV line in situ and patent
Oropharyngeal airway	Gloves
Laryngeal mask	Nasogastric tube
Endotracheal tubes—various sizes	Spare IV cannula and I/O needles (Eze I/O)
Bougie	ECG monitoring
Tracheal introducer	Pulse oximeter + spare probe
Laryngoscopes (x2)	Blood pressure monitoring
Magills forceps	End tidal monitoring
Endotracheal tube (ETT) tapes	Temperature monitoring
Self-inflating resus bag + O_2 tubing	Alarms set on monitor
Ayre's T piece	Alarms set on ventilator
Oxygen (calculate amount needed ×2)	ICP monitor (if required)
Ventilator + filter + humidifier	Notes, x-rays, and consent
Portable suction	Observation chart
Yanker sucker + suction catheters	Mobile phone
Stethoscope	Resuscitation drugs if required
Fluid boluses	Extra sedation and paralysis

ECG, Electrocardiography; *ETT*, endotracheal tube; *ICP*, intracranial pressure; *I/O*, intraosseous; *IV*, intravenous.

incidents should be noted as well as a record of the personnel under-taking the transfer.

Helicopter/fixed-wing air retrieval

From 2018 there will be two children air ambulance helicopters – one based in North of England and the other in the South – providing cover across the mainland of the United Kingdom. It is a resource that is therefore becoming more widely available and will be used for transporting critically ill infants and children where time can be saved due to distances involved. These are run by charities, so the cost to referring hospitals is not increased if the helicopter is used. Fixed-wing transports may also be used. Air retrieval can add another dimension of things to worry about for the transport team, so planning and checklists can help alleviate the worry so you won't be taking off realising that your suction unit is stored in the hold. For further information see http://www.thechildrensairambulance.org.uk.

Paediatric Intensive Care Society UK has developed standards for Air Transfer 2016 – see http://www.picsociety.uk.

CHOICE OF AIRCRAFT

Helicopters offer very rapid response time; good for shorter distances; can often pick up and drop off very close to hospital; can fly at lower altitude (usually 1000 m) so the impact of higher altitudes is minimised; however, the interior is often cramped and noisy; vibration and climate control can be issues; they may need to stop and refuel; may not be able to fly over a sea as extra equipment (e.g., life jackets) would be needed; may not be able to take a parent due to few seats available; the crew will need total weight of all equipment and the weights of all members of the retrieval team.

Fixed-wing air ambulance – may have some medical equipment aboard; may have a power and gas source; has a small cabin but better light and climate control than a helicopter; may need to refuel; often lands at small airfields, requires being met by ambulance for ongoing transport.

Commercial flight – time pressured as cannot delay commercial flight; cruising cabin altitude around 2400 m; all equipment and oxygen cylinders must be stowed securely at all times and this can be more challenging on a commercial flight; however, light, climate control, and space are not so challenging.

PLANNING FOR FLIGHT TRANSFER

The following ABCDE provides guidance for transport teams' undertaking a flight transfer. Box 13.2 highlights potential problems that may

> ## Box 13.2   Effects of gas expansion at altitude
>
> Gas volume at altitude can be increased by up to 30% and can have the following effects:
> - Sinus or ear pain with blocked sinuses or rupture of tympanic membrane (Ruskin et al 2008)
> - Pneumothoraces with ventilatory compromise
> - Spontaneous rupture of bronchogenic cysts and bullae (Closon et al 2004)
> - Abdominal pain and or perforation with increased gas in loops of bowel
> - Surgical wound dehiscence (Skjenna et al 1991)
>   Medical devices may also be affected by:
> Air-filled splints, air-filled balloons, for example, on catheters, ETT, or tracheostomy tubes

Table 13.4   Oxygen cylinder size, capacity, and weight

Cylinder size	Cylinder capacity	Cylinder weight when full
CD	460	3.5 kg
ZD	600	4.0 kg
E	680	6.5 kg
F	1360	17.0 kg

NB Of these cylinders, the CD and ZD sizes have both flow meter and Shrader valve, and the E and F have Pin Index outlet connections.
Data from Medical Gas Cylinder Data BOC, 2016. Medical gas cylinder data chart.
<http://www.bochealthcare.co.uk> (accessed 24/01/16).

be caused by the effects of gas expansion at altitude and Table 13.4 provides information about the capacity and weight of oxygen cylinders. Careful and clear communication with the parents/family/guardians of the infant or child being transferred must occur, and consent gained prior to transfer. The family members may or may not be able to accompany their child depending on space available and the consent of the flight and medical crew. The family must be given telephone numbers of the receiving hospital and must be informed and updated about their child's condition wherever possible throughout the journey. The referring hospital must arrange transport for the parents if required.

Airway

- ETT position must be confirmed radiologically and adequately secured.
- If a cuffed ETT or tracheostomy tube is used, deflate the cuff if possible, but if not, ensure the cuff is filled with saline instead of air. (The air in cuffs will expand and can cause pressure necrosis to tracheal mucosa.)

- Suction the patient prior to take-off and ensure the suction unit (plus backup hand-operated suction for longer flights) is to hand in the aircraft cabin.

Breathing

- Exclude any pneumothorax – any air leak, however small, must be drained prior to flying as trapped air within the pleural space at altitude will expand and could result in a life-threatening tension pneumothorax.
- End-tidal CO_2 monitoring is essential (auscultation is impossible during helicopter flight).
- Oxygenation will be affected by changes in barometric pressure. Anticipate and expect oxygen saturations to fall once airborne, and increase FiO_2 and ventilator as required. At high altitude in a pressurised cabin, inspired PO_2 falls and is equivalent to breathing 15% oxygen at sea level (Currie et al 2007).
- Calculate oxygen requirements – total journey time in minutes × ventilator or flow metre usage (litres/minute) then DOUBLE it and ensure you bring correct cylinders that can be stowed. Check user guides for relevant ventilator (but between 8 and 15 L/min is often used depending on pressures and oxygen requirement). Ensure all chosen oxygen cylinders have both a flow metre AND a Schrader valve outlet if the child is ventilated, or you may need to take a spanner key to change PIN index valves, which is far from ideal midflight.
- Use a Heimlich valve on any chest drain and ensure the end is not occluded (can use a drainage bag if an effusion).
- Never clamp a chest drain for a flight.
- Have emergency equipment to hand in case a needle thoracocentesis is required to treat a tension pneumothorax. This may be a life-saving procedure with a tension pneumothorax and should precede chest drain placement.
  Information taken from Advanced Paediatric Life Support (ALSG 2016): Absolute minimum equipment required: alcohol swabs, large over-the-needle intravenous cannula (16 gauge or commercially available product), 20-mL syringe
  Needle thoracocentesis procedure:
- Identify the second intercostal space in the midclavicular line on the side of the pneumothorax.
- Swab the chest wall with surgical preparation solution or an alcohol swab.
- Attach the syringe with saline to the cannula. Fluid in the cannula will assist in the identification of air bubbles.
- Insert the cannula vertically into the chest wall, just above the rib below, aspirating all the time (Fig. 13.2).
- If air is aspirated, remove the needle leaving the plastic cannula in place.
- Tape the cannula in place and proceed to chest drain the insertion as soon as possible.

Fig. 13.2 Needle thoracocentesis. (From Advanced Life Support Group (ALSG), 2016. Advanced Paediatric Life Support, sixth ed. Wiley Blackwell, Chichester.)

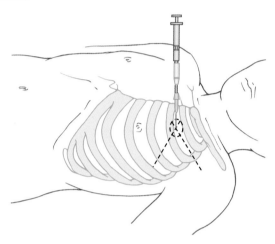

Cardiovascular

- Invasive arterial and central venous pressure monitoring is preferred. Attach the pressure monitoring set to a pump, not an air-filled pressure bag.
- Ensure all intravenous lines are free from even the smallest air bubbles as they will expand, coalesce, and dampen the trace on monitoring lines, or cause irregular/inaccurate delivery of infused drugs on the intravenous line.
- If using a cuff BP, deflate and remove, or open the cuff after each use.
- Relative or absolute volume depletion causing hypotension may be revealed at take-off; therefore anticipate and manage this, have fluid boluses drawn up for use, and give if indicated.

Disability and everything else

- Ensure the child is adequately sedated (and muscle relaxed if required) with additional drugs drawn up.
- Deceleration during landing may expose raised ICP – so anticipate this and have hypertonic saline bolus (3 mL/kg) prepared for use if concerned about acutely raised ICP.
- Decompress the stomach with nasogastric tube and leave on free drainage.
- Vacuum mattress will lose vacuum at altitude and will need to be revacuumed.

- Consider temperature control and ensure infant/child is kept warm.
- Provide ear defenders for all babies and children in a helicopter.
- Ensure all documentation accompanies the child and contemporaneous notes and observations should be documented where possible throughout the journey.
- Any critical incidents should be noted and reported.

EFFECTS OF GAS EXPANSION AT ALTITUDE

Some effects of gas expansion at altitude are summarised in Box 13.2.

It is essential to ensure you will not run out of oxygen in midair, so Table 13.4 provides cylinder capacity to aid the planning of cylinder requirements.

REFERENCES

Advanced Life Support Group (ALSG), 2015. Advanced Paediatric Life Support, fifth ed. Chapter 13 Wiley Blackwell, Chichester. http://www.alsg.org.

Advanced Life Support Group (ALSG), 2016. Advanced Paediatric Life Support, sixth ed. Wiley Blackwell, Chichester.

BOC, 2016. Medical gas cylinder data chart. http://www.bochealthcare.co.uk. Accessed 24 January 2016.

Closon, M., Vivier, E., Breynaert, C., et al., 2004. Air embolism during an aircraft flight in a passenger with a pulmonary cyst: a favourable outcome with hyperbaric therapy. Anesthesiology 101, 539–542.

Currie, G.P., Kennedy, A., Paterson, E., et al., 2007. A chronic pneumothorax and fitness to fly. Thorax 62, 187–189.

Davies, J., Tibby, S.M., Murdoch, I.A., 2005. Should parents accompany critically ill children during inter-hospital transport? Arch. Dis. Child 90, 1270–1273.

Kim, J.S., 2013. Acute abdominal pain in children. Pediatr. Gastroenterol. Hepatol. Nutr 16 (4), 219–224.

NHS Acute Abdominal Pain Pathway, 2016. Clinical assessment management tool for children. http://www.what0-18.nhs.uk/health-professionals/front-line-hospital-staff/clinical-pathways/abdominal-pain/. Accessed 22 September 2016.

NHS England – Paediatric Intensive Care Retrieval, 2015, http://www.england.nhs.uk, Accessed 11 October 2015

NICE, 2014. Head injury: assessment and early management. NICE guidelines (CG176), National Institute for Health and Care Excellence. January 2014, https://www.nice.org.uk/guidance/cg176.

Pearson, G., Shann, F., Barry, P., et al., 1997. Should paedaitric intensive care be centralised? Trent vs Victoria. Lancet 349, 1213–1217.

Ruskin, K.J., Hernandez, K.A., Barash, P.G., 2008. Management of in-flight medical emergencies. Anesthesiology 108, 749–755.

Saito, J.M., 2012. Beyond appendicitis: evaluation and surgical treatment of pediatric acute abdominal pain. Curr. Opin. Pediatr 24, 357–364.

Skjenna, O.W., Evans, J.F., Moore, M.S., et al., 1991. Helping patients travel by air. CMA 144, 287–293.

South Thames Retrieval Service (STRS), 2016, http://www.strs.nhs.uk.

Tasker, R.C., Morris, K.P., Parslow, R.C., 2006. Severe head injury in children: emergency access to neurosurgery in the United Kingdom. Emerg. Med. J 23 (7), 519–522.

USEFUL CONTACT INFORMATION – TRANSPORT

NISTAR (Northern Ireland Specialist Transport and Retrieval service) – covers Northern Ireland and is a combined service for paediatric and neonatal transport

Referral Hotline for Paediatric Intensive Care Transport: 02890 632449

Neonatal Transport Co-ordinator (08:00–20:00) 07825 147266 or 02890 632499 out of hours

ScotSTAR – covers Scotland by ambulance and air

Referral Hotline: 03333 990 222

Website, http://www.snprs.scot.nhs.uk.

Nectar – (North East Children's Transport and Retrieval) covers North East England

Referral Hotline: 0191 282 6699

Website – work in progress as new service

Northwest and North Wales Paediatric Transport Service – a collaborative service between Royal Manchester Children's Hospital and Alder Hey Children's Hospital

Referral Hotline@ 0800 084 8382

Website: http://www.nwts.nhs.uk

Embrace (The Yorkshire and Humber Infant and Children's Transport Service) – provides ambulance, fixed-wing, and helicopter transport for neonates and paediatric patients

Referral Hotline: 0845 147 2472

Website: http://www.embrace.sch.nhs.uk

KIDS Intensive Care and Decision Support – serving the West Midlands

Referral Hotline: 0300 200 1100

Website: http://www.kids.bch.nhs.uk

CATS Children's Acute Transport Service – covers North Thames region and East Anglia. Uses ambulance and flight retrieval

Referral Hotline: 0800 085 0003

Website: http://www.cats.nhs.uk

SORT Southampton Oxford Retrieval Team – a collaborative service between and Southampton and Oxford covering South central region – by ambulance and flight retrieval

Referral Hotline: 02380 775502

Website: http://www.sort.nhs.uk

STRS South Thames Retrieval Service – based at Evelina London Children's Hospital and covering the South Thames Region and South East England by ambulance and flight retrieval

Referral Hotline: 0207 188 5000

Website: http://www.strs.nhs.uk

WATCh Wales and West Acute Transport for Children – covers South
    Wales and Southwest England by ambulance and flight retrieval
Referral Hotline: 0300 0300 789
Website: http://www.watchtransport.uk

SAFEGUARDING CHILDREN AND YOUNG PEOPLE

14

The United Nations Convention on the Rights of the Child includes the requirement that children live in a safe environment and be protected from harm. To protect children and young people from harm, all health care staff must have the competencies to recognise child maltreatment and take effective action as appropriate to their role (Royal College of Paediatrics and Child Health [RCPCH] 2014b). In short, safeguarding children is everybody's responsibility (Department of Health [DH] 2015a).

This is supported in British law: The Children Act (DH 1989) was followed by an updated version, also called the Children Act (DH 2004), as a result of Lord Laming's enquiry into the murder of Victoria Climbie – an 8-year-old girl – and section 11 placed a statutory duty on organisations and individuals to safeguard and promote the welfare of children. It highlighted the need to work openly, endeavouring to achieve partnership with parents to support them in parenting their child. It also stressed that the welfare of the child is paramount.

In order to fulfil this responsibility, effective communication (particularly accurate documentation and information sharing) and teamwork are essential both within and outside of the clinical areas where critically ill children are cared for.

This is emphasised by the DH (2015b) who state that no single professional can have a full picture of a child's needs and circumstances and, if children and families are to receive the right help at the right time, everyone who comes into contact with them has a role to play in identifying concerns, sharing information, and taking prompt action.

Children and young people may be admitted to a children's critical care unit as a direct result of abuse. Examples could include a baby with a severe head injury; a toddler with multiple fractures and visible injuries, such as bite marks or burns; a young person who has tried to commit suicide by hanging following online bullying; a looked-after child who has been found unconscious following allegations of sexual exploitation; and a child who has serious stabbing injuries following an incident involving two rival gangs.

The role of health care staff in relation to safeguarding children may therefore include the following:

- Having concerns about a child and/or the family, which you will need to escalate in accordance with your local policies

- Responding to concerns raised by other agencies, for example, children's social care or the police, about a child in accordance with multi-agency information-sharing protocols
- Participating in your local child death processes in the event that a child passes away; if there are safeguarding concerns, it is likely that you will need to ensure that you meet the requirements of your local policy for managing child death, your local safeguarding policies, and any risk management processes together with multiagency involvement as above

Principles of practice for health care staff in relation to safeguarding children include the following:

- Make sure you are alert to the signs of abuse and neglect
- Question the behaviour of parents/carers and don't necessarily take at face value what you are told
- Know where to turn if you need to ask for help
- Refer to children's social care or the police if you suspect that the child is at risk of harm or is in immediate danger (DH 2015a)

SAFEGUARDING CHILDREN POLICIES AND TRAINING

Each Health Trust should have a safeguarding children policy that provides guidance on what constitutes cause for concern, and the actions to be taken if concerns are raised. This should include what constitutes abuse, how it should be managed, the escalation and referral processes for each organisation, and the contact details for key individuals: the named nurse, the midwife and the doctor, and 24/7 safeguarding advice within the Trust together with other agencies, including duty social workers.

In order to support staff in implementing the policy, safeguarding training is mandatory for all health care staff and should form part of their core training. The minimum training numbers achieved in every organisation are generally set by commissioners and reported at Trust Board level.

Robust training programmes should therefore be in place, and for children's critical care clinical staff this should be at level 3. Further guidance relating to the content and duration of the training for various professionals and their roles is provided by the RCPCH (2014b) intercollegiate document. Specific guidance has also been produced for anaesthetists (Royal College of Anaesthetists 2014).

TYPES OF CHILD ABUSE

There are four main types of child abuse; the following is a summary guide.

Physical abuse

Physical abuse is deliberately physically hurting a child. It might take a variety of forms, including hitting, poisoning, burning or scalding, drowning, or suffocating a child. Physical abuse can happen in any family, but children may be more at risk if their parents have problems with drugs, alcohol, and mental health or if they live in a home where there is domestic abuse. Babies and disabled children also have a higher risk of suffering physical abuse. Physical harm may also be caused when a parent or carer fabricates the symptoms of, or deliberately induces, illness in a child. Physical abuse can also occur outside the family environment.

Signs that may be indicators of physical abuse include children with frequent injuries; children with unexplained or unusual fractures or broken bones; and children with unexplained bruises or cuts, burns or scalds, or bite marks. The Royal College of Paediatrics provides a list of systematic reviews of clinical evidence (child protection evidence), which may help distinguish accidental injuries from deliberate harm (RCPCH 2014a).

Emotional abuse

Emotional abuse is the persistent emotional maltreatment of a child. It is also called psychological abuse and it can have severe and persistent adverse effects on a child's emotional development. Emotional abuse may involve deliberately telling a child that he or she is worthless, unloved, and inadequate. It may involve serious bullying – including online bullying through social networks, online games, or mobile phones – by a child's peers.

Signs that may be indicators of emotional abuse include children who are excessively withdrawn, fearful, or anxious about doing something wrong; parents or carers who withdraw their attention from the child, giving him or her the 'cold shoulder'; parents or carers blaming their problems on the child or humiliating the child, for example, by name calling or making negative comparisons.

Sexual abuse and exploitation

Sexual abuse is any sexual activity with a child. Sexual abuse may involve physical contact, noncontact activities, and may include grooming a child in preparation for abuse (including via the internet). A child may not understand what is happening and may not even understand that it is wrong. Sexual abuse can have a long-term impact on mental health. It is not solely perpetrated by adult males. Women can commit acts of sexual abuse, as can other children.

Signs that may be indicators of sexual abuse include physical sexual health problems including soreness in the genital and anal areas, sexually transmitted infections, or underage pregnancy.

Child sexual exploitation is a form of sexual abuse where children are sexually exploited for money, power, or status. It can involve violent, humiliating and degrading sexual assaults. Child sexual exploitation doesn't always involve physical contact and can happen online. A significant number of children who are victims of sexual exploitation may be missing from home, care or education at some point.

Signs that may be indicators of sexual exploitation include sexually transmitted infections or underage pregnancy, changes in emotional well-being, and children who misuse drugs and alcohol.

Neglect

Neglect is a pattern of failing to provide for a child's basic needs, whether it be adequate food, clothing, hygiene, supervision, or shelter. It is likely to result in the serious impairment of a child's health or development. Children who are neglected are likely to also suffer from other types of abuse.

Signs that may be indicators of neglect include children who are undernourished with poor hygiene; who are late in reaching developmental milestones for no medical reason; who fail to receive basic health care; and those who are angry or aggressive, or who self-harm (Adapted from DH 2015a).

In addition to the four categories of abuse, there are some other key issues related to safeguarding children, which children's critical care staff need to be aware of:

LOOKED-AFTER CHILDREN

In England and Wales, the term 'looked-after children' (LAC) is defined in law under the Children Act 1989. In Scotland, the term is defined under the Children (Scotland) Act 1995. A child is looked after by a local authority if he or she is under their care or is provided with accommodation for more than 24 hours by the authority.

LAC fall into four main groups:

- Children who are accommodated under voluntary agreement with their parents (section 20)
- Children who are the subject of a care order (section 31) or interim care order (section 38)
- Children who are the subject of emergency orders for their protection (sections 44 and 46)
- Children who are compulsorily accommodated, including all children remanded to the local authority or subject to a criminal supervision order with a residence requirement (section 21)

The term 'looked-after children' includes unaccompanied asylum-seeking children, children in friends and family placements, and those children where the agency has the authority to place the child for adoption.

It does not include those children who have been permanently adopted or who are on a special guardianship order (RCPCH 2015).

It is particularly important that children's critical care staff are aware of the status of any of their patients who are LAC, due to the increased vulnerability of this group and also aware of their responsibility in relation to safety and well being of these children. Local policies should guide the procedures to be followed, including those related to consent and discharge planning, in order to protect and support these children.

FEMALE GENITAL MUTILATION

The World Health Organisation (WHO) defines female genital mutilation (FGM) as follows:

> *'All procedures that involve partial or total removal of the external female genitalia, or other injury to the female genital organs for non-medical reasons' (WHO 2014).*

The Royal College of Nursing (RCN) clearly states that FGM is child abuse and is illegal in the United Kingdom. It also states that the practice has no health benefits and can often lead to serious morbidity and mortality in girls and women (RCN 2016). Furthermore, the Serious Crime Act (2015) brought in a range of actions related to FGM including a new statutory duty: mandatory reporting by all health care professionals, social workers and teachers, who must now report to the police cases of FGM, or suspected FGM, on girls under the age of 18 years.

Clearly it is vital that those working in children's critical care have a working knowledge of this practice in order to be able to recognise, manage, and report it appropriately. Trusts should have local policies and procedures in place as part of their approach to safeguarding children, which clarifies for staff their individual roles, the legal requirements and, again, the importance of multiagency working.

The importance of FGM being included in safeguarding children training programmes is emphasised as a core competency for health care staff by the RCPCH (2014b).

Sensitivity around this subject is essential. This practice is culturally embedded as it is viewed as a form of cultural expression among those who support it. FGM may be upheld as a religious obligation by some Muslim populations, even though the practice predates Islam and it is practised by some Muslims, Christians, and followers of African religions (RCN 2016).

HUMAN TRAFFICKING

The National Crime Agency (2015) highlights that in 2013 the term 'modern slavery' was introduced in the United Kingdom to describe all offences previously described as human trafficking, slavery, forced labour, and domestic servitude. Traffickers and exploiters use whatever means they have at their disposal to coerce, deceive, and force individuals into a life of abuse, servitude, and inhumane treatment. Modern slavery is a global problem, and a hidden crime. In order to address this robustly, the Modern Slavery Act came into force in July 2015 and addresses both the pursuit and prosecution of perpetrators and the defence of and support for victims (NCA 2015).

The most widely used definition of human trafficking is referred to as the Palermo Protocol Article Three, and the following is an abridged version.

Trafficking in persons means the recruitment, transportation, transfer, harbouring, or receipt of person. By means of threat or use of power or to a position of vulnerability or the giving or receiving of payments of benefits to achieve the consent of a person having control over another person, for the purposes of exploitation.

Exploitation shall include, at a minimum, the exploitation of prostitution of others or other forms of sexual exploitation, forced labour or services, slavery or practices similar to slavery, servitude, or the removal of organs.

The recruitment, transportation, transfer, harbour, or receipt of a child for the purpose of exploitation shall be considered 'trafficking in persons' and any apparent consent given by the victims will be considered irrelevant.

In relation to children (i.e., <18 years of age), of the 3309 potential victims of trafficking reported in 2014, 732 (22%) were children at the time of exploitation. Of those, the most prevalent country of origin was the United Kingdom (16%). Of the children, 61% were female and were most commonly being used for sexual exploitation; 36% were males, and were most commonly being exploited for criminal purposes. The gender of 3% was not recorded (NCA 2015).

Again, with any concern that a child or young person may be a trafficking, or indeed slavery, victim, the importance of following local safeguarding policies is essential in ensuring immediate multiagency involvement to both protect the victim and to pursue the perpetrator.

CONCLUSION

In summary, if you have any concerns at all about children that relates to safeguarding you must:

Report them – to the nurse in charge, consultant, safeguarding children team

Document them in the child's health records

Follow your local safeguarding children policy to ensure these concerns are effectively addressed

Discuss them with the child's parents or carers if possible; on occasion this initially would not be appropriate as it may put the child at further risk of harm. The safeguarding children team will advise.

Communicate effectively – be persistent, be thorough – Managing safeguarding issues effectively in the children's critical care environment is challenging and can be distressing, even for experienced and expert practitioners. In addition to effective policies and training, it is important that support is provided, which could include debriefing, case review teaching, supervision, and counselling.

REFERENCES

Department of Health, 1989. The Children Act. www.legislation.gov.uk/ukpga/2004/31/contents.

Department of Health, 2004. The Children Act. www.legislation.gov.uk/ukpga/1989/41/contents.

Department of Health, 2015a. What to do if you're worried a child is being abused: advice for practitioners. https://www.gov.uk/government/publications/what-to-do-if-youre-worried-a-child-is-being-abused--2.

Department of Health, 2015b. Working together to safeguard children. https://www.gov.uk/government/publications/working-together-to-safeguard-children--2.

National Crime Agency, 2015. NCA Strategic Assessment: the Nature and Scale of Human Trafficking in 2014. www.nationalcrimeagency.gov.uk/publications/656-nca-strategic-assessment-the-nature-and-scale-of-human-trafficking-in-2014/file.

Royal College of Anaesthetists, 2014. Child protection and the anaesthetist – safeguarding children in the operating theatre. www.rcoa.ac.uk/document-store/child-protection-and-the-anaesthetist.

Royal College of Nursing, 2016. Multi agency practice guidelines: female genital mutilation. www.rcn.org.uk/-/media/royal-college-of-nursing/documents/publications/2016/april/005447.

Royal College of Paediatrics and Child Health, 2014a. Child protection evidence. https://www.rcpch.ac.uk/search?keywords=Child+Protection+evidence.

Royal College of Paediatrics and Child Health, 2014b. Safeguarding children and young people: roles and competencies for health care staff. www.rcpch.ac.uk.

Royal College of Paediatrics and Child Health, 2015. Looked after children: knowledge, skills and competencies of health care staff. www.rcpch.ac.uk.

World Health Organisation, 2014. Female Genital Mutilation. Factsheet. www.who.int/mediacentre/factsheets/fs241/en.

DEATH OF A CHILD

15

Although the overall survival from paediatric intensive care unit (PICU) in the United Kingdom is excellent (>96%), paediatric deaths are 10 times more likely to occur in PICU than in any other hospital wards. It is therefore important that staff working in PICU have the necessary skills to care for dying children and provide support for families and friends. There are many different circumstances surrounding an infant or child dying in PICU, which may include a sudden unexpected event in a previously well child, gradual deterioration in a child with a chronic medical condition, or following a prolonged hospital or ICU admission.

EXPECTED DEATH IN PAEDIATRIC INTENSIVE CARE UNIT

In the circumstance in which it is clear to medical and nursing staff that a patient is unlikely to survive the PICU admission or is diagnosed with a life-limiting condition, it is important for a senior member of the medical team and the nurse caring for the child to sit down with the parents and have frank and honest discussion.

The discussion with the family should include:

- An opportunity for the family to explain their current understanding of their baby/child's illness
- An explanation of the cause of the patient's illness and predicted outcome
- Explanation of treatment administered to date and other potential treatments and their side effects
- Explanation of the limitation of therapy (point at which ceiling of care has been reached)
- A gentle and compassionate choice of words, but if the baby/child is dying, then it is important to say that directly and avoid euphemisms
- Discussion about resuscitation, and document parental wishes, including if a 'Do not resuscitate order' has been agreed
- Involvement of palliative care team, if appropriate, including an advanced care plan
- An opportunity to contact members of the extended family and allow them to visit/spend time with the patient and his or her family
- Ask the family if they would like a religious leader to be present to provide spiritual support and perform any important religious ceremonies

- Depending on the situation and resources available, it may be possible to allow the parents to make some key decisions regarding the place of withdrawal of intensive care support, such as in a private room/cubicle on PICU, at home, or in a children's hospice
- If death is imminent, it is really important to say to the family that you think that their baby/child may only have a few hours left to live, because most families will have no idea of terminal signs and symptoms. The family may then have the opportunity to spend the limited time remaining with their child and should be offered the opportunity to hold the child in their arms in a chair or lie beside the child on a bed, ensuring the comfort of the patient and relative
- Encourage the family to ask any questions and explain that you will be available to them at any time.

Unexpected death in paediatric intensive care unit

Occasionally a baby or child may die suddenly and unexpectedly in PICU and the family may or may not be present.

As soon as the child's condition deteriorates, the parents/carers should be contacted and asked to return to the PICU.

When the parents arrive, they may want to see their child immediately.

The most senior clinician should be available to talk with the parents to break the news about the death of their child.

A private space should be made available for the parents to be with their child for as long as they wish – a place to talk and receive family members and, if desired, religious leaders. They should be given time and space to grieve in privacy.

A nurse should be available to stay with the family if they wish. If safeguarding concerns have been raised, then a nurse or other health care professional must remain with the child at all times.

The parents may want immediate answers to why their child has died, and it is important to give honest answers; if the cause of death is not clear, this should be explained. In this situation, it is very likely that the child will be referred to the coroner to determine the cause of death.

Everybody will have a different reaction to death, and this may be expressed by anger, distress, grief, disbelief – a range of emotions may be expected.

Staff should acknowledge parents' feelings and be respectful and sensitive toward varying cultural norms and rituals surrounding death (ALSG 2016).

PALLIATIVE CARE

The National Institute for Health and Care Excellence (NICE 2016) in the United Kingdom has developed guidelines which cover the planning and management of end-of-life and palliative care for infants and children aged 0–17 years with life-limiting conditions, and these guidelines include:
- Advanced care planning
- Emotional and psychologic support and interventions

- Managing distressing symptoms
- Hydration and nutrition
- Recognising that a child or young person is likely to die within hours or days
- Care and support for parents, carers, and health care professionals after the death of a child
- Care at home

See http://www.nice.org.uk for further details because the constraints of this text limit further details of palliative care.

NURSE'S ROLE

When a child dies suddenly in hospital, nurses play a central role in caring for the parents and providing essential information. Parents should be offered a private place to hold, wash, dress, or just be near their child for as long as they wish, and a nurse should be available to support the parents, if desired. A telephone should be made available for their use to contact close family and friends, if required. It is important to refer to local and national policies when caring for a family following the death of a child. Often, when babies or young children die, parents like to have hand and footprints made to treasure and keep. Many parents like to keep a lock of their child's hair, but permission should be sought before taking either. If the parents wish, a photograph may be taken of the child, where possible, when all invasive lines and medical equipment have been removed and after the child has been washed and dressed, but, again, it is vital that permission is given by the parents. A photograph including the family also may be helpful for the parents to keep. Some parents want the keepsakes at the time, but a few may call after several weeks asking for them, and therefore they must be safely stored. Often a favourite toy, a piece of jewellery, a rosary, or a handmade card from a sibling is left with the child who has died and may be buried with them. It is important to offer the support of a chaplain, priest, or spiritual leader, according to the needs of the particular family.

In the United Kingdom, if a postmortem is not required, it may be possible for parents to take their child's body home soon after death, if they so wish. A death certificate must have been completed and given to the parents. Nurses must follow local policy, paying particular attention to all documentation (e.g., ensuring that the mortuary paperwork is completed even if the child's body is not actually taken to the mortuary). A small child may be wrapped in a blanket and transported home in a family member's car. A letter should be given to the parents to take in the car explaining, in case of an accident, that their child died in hospital and that the body is being transported home. Parents should also be given an information sheet about caring for their child's body. Larger children can be taken home with the assistance of a funeral director, and, in all cases, early contact with the funeral directors is vital. Some children's hospices have cold rooms or specific cots/beds so that families may spend extended periods of time with their baby/child before the funeral.

It should be noted that there are some infections, particularly viral haemorrhagic fevers, which if confirmed or suspected will mandate that the child who has died be placed immediately in a sealed coffin (Advisory Committee on Dangerous Pathogens 2014).

It is very important that relevant people have been informed of the child's death as soon as possible so that appropriate care may be given by all agencies (e.g., general medical practitioner, health visitor, school, social worker, and referring hospital). It is also important that future scheduled appointments for the patient are cancelled so that family members are not distressed by unnecessary contact. The specialist nurses/bereavement worker (e.g., a family support sister), if in post, should be informed of each child's death and given all the relevant details and particular circumstances so that they can maintain contact with the family and provide follow-up care. Many children's hospitals have a charity-run 'home from home' (e.g. 'Ronald MacDonald House') where parents can stay while their child is in hospital, and they should also be informed of a child's death.

DOCTOR'S ROLE

The doctor providing care for the patient may be required to withdraw intensive care support such as ventilation and inotropes once a palliative care pathway has been decided. It is important to ensure that the patient is comfortable during this procedure, without hastening death. The symptom management plan should be carefully discussed and agreed, ideally with palliative care specialists, prior to withdrawal of support. The General Medical Council 'Treatment and care towards the end of life: good practice in decision making (2010)' provides clear guidance regarding some of the challenging decision at this point. The doctor providing bedside care should confirm the time and cause of death in the patient's clinical records. A postmortem may need to be discussed with the family, as outlined in the following section.

If no postmortem is required, a medical cause of death certificate should be completed and signed in accordance with local and national guidance. It is recommended to offer the family a bereavement appointment to discuss the events and any additional information (such as postmortem reports) 6–8 weeks after the child's death.

Postmortem

If cause of death is unknown and the doctor is unable to write a death certificate, the death may be referred to a coroner and a postmortem examination will be carried out to establish the cause of death. In such circumstances, the parents are not able to refuse a coroner's postmortem. An external examination and internal examination of all major organs of the deceased is undertaken, and usually results may be available within a few days; however, often, small samples may be taken from organs or

DNA analysis (genetic testing) may be required, which may also delay the final results. If a coroner's postmortem is required, please check with the coroner before any line or invasive tube is removed because, in some cases, the coroner requires all medical equipment left in situ for postmortem (including endotracheal tube (ETT), central lines, etc.).

Occasionally, a doctor or even parents may request a hospital postmortem even though a coroner's postmortem is not necessary, usually when the patient has died of natural causes. This examination can only be performed with informed consent from the parents or legal guardians. Consent for this process should only be taken by those with specific training and a good understanding of the postmortem examination.

ORGAN DONATION

Approaching the family of potential organ donors

When a child is dying, the team caring for the child should consider whether the child could potentially be an organ donor. Best Practice Guidance suggests that approaching families should be adjusted to suit particular circumstances, but three key stages have been identified: planning, confirming understanding, and acceptance of loss, before discussing donation (NHS Blood and Transplant 2017). The Paediatric Intensive Care Society (PICS) has published standards for organ donation (PICS 2014).

Ethical issues in paediatric organ donation

An ethical framework for making decisions about paediatric organ donation in the United Kingdom has been presented in a position paper and can be found at http://www.aomrc.org.uk. This paper discusses legal issues and consent and provides nine recommendations (UKDEC 2015). The key message reminds clinicians that, in the tragic situation of a dying child, full consideration should be given to the possibility of organ donation, and where appropriate, families should be involved in decision making, including decisions about donation because this may help a feeling of control and can result in positive memories about what their child achieved, even in death (Sque et al 2013).

 Where a family is willing to consent to the removal of organs that are viable for transplantation, then the hospital has a responsibility to make this happen if possible (UKDEC 2015).

Donation after circulatory death (nonheartbeating donation)

Donation after circulatory death (DCD) was previously known as nonheartbeating organ donation and refers to the retrieval of organs for transplantation purposes in patients whose death is confirmed using cardiorespiratory criteria. In the United Kingdom an average of 2.8

Table 15.1	The modified Maastricht classification of donation after circulatory death		
Category	**Description**	**Type of DCD**	**Location**
I	Dead on arrival	Uncontrolled	ED
II	Unsuccessful resuscitation	Uncontrolled	ED in a transplant centre
III	Anticipated cardiac arrest	Controlled	ICU and ED
IV	Cardiac arrest in a brain-dead patient	Controlled	ICU and ED
V	Unexpected arrest in ICU patient	Uncontrolled	ICU in transplant centre

DCD, Donation after circulatory death; *ED,* emergency department; *ICU,* intensive care unit.
From Koostra, G., Daemen, J.H., Oomen, A.P., 1995. Categories of non-heart beating organ donors. Transplant. Proc. 27, 2893–2894.

transplantable organs are retrieved from DCD donors, compared with 3.9 from donation after brainstem death (DBD) donors. The biggest contribution of DCD is to kidney transplantation. The Modified Maastricht classification of Donation after Circulatory Death (Koostra et al 1995) is used to categorise DCD (Table 15.1).

Resolution of apparent legal, ethical, and professional obstacles to DCD in the United Kingdom has led to substantial increases in organ donation. The underpinning principal implies that organ donation can, on many occasions, be legitimately viewed as part of the care that a person might wish to receive at the end of his or her life.

Donation after brainstem death

Organ DBD is possible from patients whose death has been confirmed using neurologic criteria. Neurologic criteria for diagnosis and confirmation of death can be applied in circumstances in which brain injury is suspected to have caused irreversible loss of the capacity for consciousness and irreversible loss of the capacity for respiration before terminal apnoea has resulted in hypoxic cardiac arrest and circulatory standstill. This diagnosis is only possible on ventilated patients. In the United Kingdom the Academy of the Medical Royal Colleges (AoMRC) in 2008 published the UK Code of Practice for the Diagnosis and Confirmation of Death.

BRAINSTEM DEATH DIAGNOSIS

Brainstem death tests are usually carried out by the senior doctor in charge of the child's care and one other clinically independent doctor, competent in the field and not a member of the transplant team, who has been qualified for at least 5 years. The tests are performed twice and, prior to testing, time must have elapsed to ensure that the patient has no circulating or therapeutic levels of any drug that could cause coma. A diagnosis must have been established, and the cause of the coma must be irreversible. Prior to testing, the child should be normothermic, with no endocrine or metabolic disturbances, and have no effects of muscle relaxants in his/her system, with relatively normal cardiovascular and respiratory parameters supported, as required with inotropes, fluid, and adequate ventilation.

The Royal College of Paediatric and Child Health (2015) published guidelines on the determination of death by neurologic criteria in infants from 37 weeks' corrected gestational age to 2 months postterm (RCPCH 2015). These guidelines use clinical examination criteria to establish death in older infants, children, and adults, but, in view of the immaturity of the newborn infant's respiratory system, a stronger hypercarbic stimulus is used to establish respiratory unresponsiveness (a clear rise in arterial blood partial pressure of carbon dioxide [$P_a\text{CO}_2$] levels of >2.7 kPa above a baseline of at least 5.3 kPa to >8.0 kPa with no respiratory response at that level) (RCPCH 2015).

There are forms now available online specifically for the Diagnosis of Death using Neurological Criteria in Children, with full guidance, and are available at NHS Blood and Transplant Paediatric Care Useful Resources (http://www.odt.nhs.uk).

Clinical tests for brainstem death

- Pupils are fixed and dilated and do not react to light
- Absent corneal reflexes – tested by touching exposed cornea with a piece of cotton wool, but take care to avoid damage
- Absent oculovestibular reflexes – ice-cold water is syringed into each ear in turn, having ensured that the passage to the tympanic membrane is clear. Normally this would produce eye movement, where there is deviation to the stimulated side
- No cranial nerve motor response to deep, painful stimulation within the cranial nerve distribution
- Absent cough or gag reflex – this is tested with deep suction via the endotracheal tube and to the back of the throat
- Apnoea test – the $P_a\text{CO}_2$ should be 6.0 kPa prior to the apnoea test and should rise to at least 6.5 kPa during the test if the patient remains apnoeic. The patient should be preoxygenated with 100% oxygen for 10 minutes prior to testing, and arterial blood gases should be taken. The patient is disconnected from the ventilator but given a continuous supply of 100% oxygen via the endotracheal tube. The patient is observed for at least 5 minutes to note any respiratory effort, and then another arterial blood gas is taken to ensure that the $P_a\text{CO}_2$ has risen above 6.5 kPa. The patient is then reconnected to the ventilator. This test must be discontinued if hypotension, cardiac arrhythmias, or hypoxia occurs.

If the first test shows brainstem death, the legal time of death is recorded on completion of this first set of brainstem tests and must be declared in the medical notes. Death is not pronounced until the second set of tests has been completed.

Spinal reflexes: the spinal cord may continue to function after the death of the brainstem, and the resulting limb movement may be distressing to the family and staff caring for the patient. Nurses should be aware of this potential occurrence and be able to give the family an explanation.

If appropriate, the opportunity for organ donation must be offered to families once brainstem death has been established.

The World Health Organisation (WHO) has published critical pathways for DBD and DCD (Domínguez-Gil et al 2011) (see Fig. 15.1). This is intended to describe a process for deceased organ donation and has been developed by a diverse, multicultural and multiregional working group so that this tool is applicable to every country, region, or hospital, regardless of the level of development of its health care system.

Consider making the specialist nurses in organ donation (SNODs) aware of the potential organ donor prior to brainstem testing so that a collaborative approach can be taken when talking to the family about organ donation. When a child is found to be brainstem dead, the family should be offered the opportunity to donate their child's organs. The family will need time and privacy to discuss the matter. The donor transplant coordinator will come to the unit to discuss all aspects with the family. If the family still wish to continue, full explanations should be given at this time about the likelihood of needing to continue treatment to maintain the organs in the best possible condition. It must be consistently reinforced that the child is brainstem dead and that no treatment can change that. Consent will then be obtained if the family wishes to proceed with the donation of their child's organs.

INVESTIGATIONS THAT MAY BE REQUIRED PRIOR TO ORGAN DONATION

This is the responsibility of the transplant coordinator or SNOD, but it requires teamwork and it may be helpful to liaise with the specialist nurse and to begin to obtain the necessary tests so that the process takes as little time as possible.

- Virology screen – 10 mL of blood in plain blood tube (it may be necessary to take a virology screen from the mother if the child is <2 years)
- Blood group and tissue type
- Urea and electrolytes
- Liver function tests
- Arterial blood gases
- Clotting studies
- Sputum Gram stain
- Chest x-ray
- Electrocardiogram (ECG)
- Amylase
- Cardiac troponin (if cardiac arrest has occurred)
- Echocardiogram
- Culture and sensitivity screens – wounds, sputum, urine.

Fig 15.1 The critical pathway for deceased organ donation. (From Domínguez-Gil, B., et al., 2011. The critical pathway for deceased donation: reportable uniformity in the approach to deceased donation. Transpl. Int. 24 (4), 373–378.)

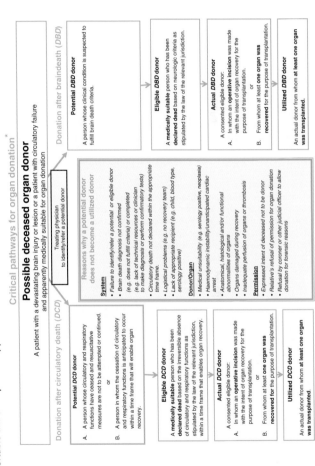

Critical pathways for organ donation*

Possible deceased organ donor

A patient with a devastating brain injury or lesion or a patient with circulatory failure and apparently medically suitable for organ donation

Treating physician to identify/refer a potential donor

Donation after circulatory death (DCD)

Potential DCD donor

A. A person whose circulatory and respiratory functions have ceased and resuscitative measures are not to be attempted or continued.

or

B. A person in whom the cessation of circulatory and respiratory functions is anticipated to occur within a time frame that will enable organ recovery.

Eligible DCD donor

A medically suitable person who has been declared dead based on the irreversible absence of circulatory and respiratory functions as stipulated by the law of the relevant jurisdiction, within a time frame that enables organ recovery.

Actual DCD donor

A consented eligible donor:

A. In whom an operative incision was made with the intent of organ recovery for the purpose of transplantation.

or

B. From whom at least one organ was recovered for the purpose of transplantation.

Utilized DCD donor

An actual donor from whom at least one organ was transplanted.

Reasons why a potential donor does not become a utilized donor

System
- Failure to identify/refer a potential or eligible donor
- Brain death diagnosis not confirmed (e.g. does not fulfill criteria) or completed (e.g. lack of technical resources or clinician to make diagnosis or perform confirmatory tests)
- Circulatory death not declared within the appropriate time frame.
- Logistical problems (e.g. no recovery team)
- Lack of appropriate recipient (e.g. child, blood type, serology positive)

Donor/Organ
- Medical unsuitability (e.g. serology positive, neoplasia)
- Haemodynamic instability/unanticipated cardiac arrest
- Anatomical, histological and/or functional abnormalities of organs
- Organs damaged during recovery
- Inadequate perfusion of organs or thrombosis

Permission
- Expressed intent of deceased not to be donor
- Relative's refusal of permission for organ donation
- Refusal by coroner or other judicial officer to allow donation for forensic reasons

Donation after braindeath (DBD)

Potential DBD donor

A person whose clinical condition is suspected to fulfill brain death criteria.

Eligible DBD donor

A medically suitable person who has been declared dead based on neurologic criteria as stipulated by the law of the relevant jurisdiction.

Actual DBD donor

A consented eligible donor:

A. In whom an operative incision was made with the intent of organ recovery for the purpose of transplantation.

or

B. From whom at least one organ was recovered for the purpose of transplantation.

Utilized DBD donor

An actual donor from whom at least one organ was transplanted.

*The 'dead donor rule' must be respected. That is, patients may only become donors after death, and the recovery of organs must not cause a donor's death

CLINICAL MANAGEMENT GUIDELINES OF THE ORGAN DONOR

(Information adapted from http://www.odt.nhs.uk)

Common clinical problems that may occur in a brainstem dead patient include:

- Hypotension
- Hypothermia
- Diabetes insipidus
- Electrolyte imbalance
- Arrhythmias
- Hypoxia
- Disseminated intravascular coagulation
- Neurogenic pulmonary oedema

Cardiorespiratory instability due to brainstem ischaemia – may be triphasic:

- Cushing reflex of hypertension and bradycardia
- Transient phase of tachycardia and severe hypertension (related to outpouring of catecholamines [sympathetic storm]) that is associated with ECG changes, rises in cardiac troponin, and myocardial impairment
- Hypotension

Hypothalamic failure in brainstem death causes hypothermia as a result of vasodilatation and diabetes insipidus caused by a loss of antidiuretic hormone secretion from the pituitary gland.

Neurogenic pulmonary oedema – a catecholamine surge triggers a surge in the left ventricular end-diastolic and pulmonary capillary pressures, which disrupts the integrity of the alveolar – capillary barrier and results in alveolar flooding.

Physiologic optimisation of the potential donation after brainstem death donor (basic principles)

- Correction of hypovolaemia and maintenance of normal cardiovascular parameters
- Correction of diabetes insipidus, correct electrolyte abnormalities
- Introduction of vasopressin and weaning of adrenaline/noradrenaline
- Recruitment manoeuvres to correct atelectasis post apnoea testing
- Methylprednisolone to attenuate the systemic inflammation of brainstem death
- Maintain blood sugar, temperature, and urine output in normal range

See Paediatric Donor Optimisation Care Bundle at http://www.odt.nhs.uk for further details of physiologic goals and useful paperwork to record hourly parameters achieved.

After recipients have been found for the organs, a team of surgeons will come to retrieve the organs. Major organs will not be removed unless a matched recipient has been identified. The donor's family will usually say their goodbyes at this time, then the child is taken to theatre with cardiopulmonary function being maintained and supported.

Once the organs have been retrieved, they are taken, swiftly, to be transplanted into the recipients. The donor child's body will be carefully sutured and then taken to the mortuary or back to the ward if the parents wish to spend more time saying their goodbyes. The time taken between parents deciding to donate their child's organs and the child being actually taken to theatre is usually less than 12 hours, and parents have the right to change their mind at any time. The process described is concerned with solid organ donation, because some tissues (e.g., heart valves and corneas) may be retrieved the following day.

NB The parents may wish to come back to see their child in the hospital chapel following donation of their child's organs, and they may wish to hold their child, so it may be advisable to gently inform them that:

- their child will feel cold to the touch
- their child will look very pale
- their child will have a suture line where the organs have been removed, but this will be covered with a dressing
- their child may feel lighter in weight if they pick him/her up for a cuddle
- their child's abdomen may appear flatter or concave if large organs have been donated

RELIGION

The major religions in the United Kingdom support the idea of organ or tissue donation; however, it is advisable to be aware of individual requirements for the care of the deceased. It may be important for the next of kin to liaise with their religious leader regarding donation. This is always respected.

REFERENCES

Academy of Medical Royal Colleges, 2008. A code of practice for the diagnosis and confirmation of death. http://www.aomrc.org.uk.

Academy of Medical Royal Colleges, 2015. Ethical issues in paediatric organ donation – a position paper by the UK Donation Ethics Committee (UKDEC). http://www.aomrc.org.uk.

Advanced Life Support Group, 2016. Advanced Paediatric Life Support. A Practical Approach to Emergencies, sixth ed. Wiley Blackwell, Chichester.

Advisory Committee on Dangerous Pathogens, 2014. Management of Hazard Group 4 viral haemorrhagic fevers and similar human infectious diseases of high consequence. http://www.hse.gov.uk.

Domínguez-Gil, B., Delmonico, F.L., Shaheen, F.A., et al., 2011. The critical pathway for deceased donation: reportable uniformity in the approach to deceased donation. Transpl. Int. 24 (4), 373–378.

Koostra, G., Daemen, J.H., Oomen, A.P., 1995. Categories of non-heart beating organ donors. Transplant. Proc. 27, 2893–2894.

National Institute for Health and Care Excellence, 2016. End of life care for infants, children and young people with life-limiting conditions: planning and management. NG61. http://www.nice.org.uk.

NHS Blood and Transplant, 2017. Approaching the families of potential organ donors: an audiovisual guide for Hospital Clinicians. http://www.odt.nhs.uk/toolkit.

Paediatric Intensive Care Society, 2014. Standards for Organ Donation. Paediatric Intensive Care Society, London. http://www.picsociety.uk.

Royal College of Paediatric and Child Health, 2015. The diagnosis of death by neurological criteria in infants less than two months old. http://www.rcpch.ac.uk.

Sque, M., Walker, W., Long-Sutehall, T., et al., 2013. Bereaved families' experiences of organ and tissue donation, and perceived influences on their decision-making. Final report of a study funded by the Department of Health. University of Wolverhampton.

It is useful for professionals who are unfamiliar with Paediatric Intensive Care to have some knowledge of normal child development in order to be able to assess a child thoroughly on admission. Each child is different and the parents/carers may be the best source of information about the developmental milestones achieved. It has been shown that some children regress developmentally when they are admitted to hospital or in other stressful circumstances. This chapter is intended as a brief guide to normal child development, and it includes a summary of common childhood illness and the current immunisation schedule in England.

NORMAL CHILD DEVELOPMENT

Seven major reflexes of the newborn

Rooting – infant turns towards the touch of a cheek searching for something to suck

Sucking – sucking results when something is put into the infant's mouth

Swallowing – initially not well coordinated with breathing

Moro – when startled, infants will arch their back and throw open their arms

Grasp – infants will curl their fingers around any object that can be grasped

Babinski – if the bottom of the foot is stroked, infants will splay toes out then curl them in

Stepping – if infants are held so that their feet just touch the ground, they will initiate walking movements

Source: From Bee, H., 1989. The Developing Child, fifth ed. Harper and Row, New York.

These reflexes are a healthy sign in a newborn but should not persist beyond the first few months of life. Their presence in an older child may indicate brain injury.

Table 16.1 gives examples of normal developmental progress across ages.

CHILDREN'S DEVELOPMENTAL CONCEPTS OF PAIN

It is important that nurses understand children's cognitive development and their perceptions of pain at each developmental stage.

Hurley and Whelan (1988) describe children's concepts of pain according to Piaget's cognitive developmental stages (Piaget & Inhelder 1969). The sensorimotor stage (0–2 years) is omitted as these children are unable to vocalise their perceptions of pain.

Table 16.1   Normal development across ages

Age	Social skill	Verbal	Physical	Psychological	Play
Newborn	Learning to follow movements, can already recognise mother's voice	Range of cries for hunger, pain	Reflexes as described – totally dependent	Healthy emotional and cognitive development is shaped by responsive, dependable interaction with adults (Center on the developing child 2007)	Best able to focus at distance of around 25 cm
6 weeks	Starts to smile	Starts to coo in response to mother's voice	Developing head control	As above	Can fix and follow on your face. Will reach for objects
3–6 months	Will smile a lot and enjoy interaction	Be vocalising	Full head control, roll onto side, play with fingers		Looks for fallen toys, throws toys, develops pincer grip
6–12 months	Laughs out loud, claps hands, waves goodbye, responds to name	Imitates sounds, can babble, for example, goo, ga, then dada, mama	Sits unsupported, pushes up on elbows when prone, pulls to stand, cruises furniture, may walk	Starts becoming shy with strangers	
1–2 years	Understands simple commands, takes off shoes, indicates toilet needs	Can speak a few words and at 2 may put 2 words together and use about 50 words	Anterior fontanelle closes around 18 months, can walk, run	Sometimes clingy, sometimes resistant, temper tantrums	Can jump, build a tower of 3–4 cubes, kick a ball
3–4 years	Starts to play with other children and understands but does not like sharing, starts showing concern for others	Good conversation and lots of questions, can count to 10, name 3–4 colours	Can hop, dress and undress, walk downstairs, can ride a tricycle, balance bike or bike	Wanting to explore the surroundings	Starts using a pencil, plays imaginatively, uses scissors

5–6 years	Actively helps others	Fluent speaker	Can dress alone	Begin to try to exert power and control through play and have influence	Likes to follow rules, prefers to play with same sex
8–10 years	Keen to be involved in clubs, likes company of others, likes to help	Able to classify and count backwards from 20	Increasing manual dexterity, gaining height and weight	Gaining logical thinking	Best friends are important
Adolescent	Friends very important	Use of social media for communication	Bodily changes associated with puberty	Mood swings, conflict with parents, increasing capacity for abstract reasoning	Friends very important

Preoperational stage (2–7 years)

- These children may think that pain is a punishment for something they have done wrong
- They may blame someone else for their pain
- They relate to pain primarily as a physical experience
- They often have feelings of sadness when in pain so may feel comforted if held and given reassurance

Concrete operational stage (7–10 years)

- These children can understand physical pain and can locate the pain to the relevant part of the body
- They fear bodily harm and death
- They like to feel they have some control over the pain so they should be encouraged to ask for help to find the most comfortable position or to ask for pain relief

Formal operational stage (12+ years)

- These children are able to use reasoning, for example, 'my head hurts because I banged it'
- They fear loss of privacy and control when in pain
- They need to be given as much information as they require and choices about how best to control the pain

Table 16.2 shows the routine immunisation schedule in England for 0–16 years from Spring 2016.

In addition to this schedule, there are selective immunisation programmes for target groups, such as babies born to hepatitis-infected mothers, or babies born in areas where there is a high incidence of tuberculosis where additional vaccines may be given. There is also an additional vaccine schedule for individuals with underlying medical conditions and this may be found at www.gov.uk (search complete routine immunisation schedule from Spring 2016).

Table 16.3 is a useful reference and can guide the need to isolate the child if contagious.

Rare but serious complications of these childhood illnesses

- Measles can be complicated by ear infections, diarrhoea and vomiting, conjunctivitis, optic neuritis, pneumonia, meningitis encephalitis, subacute sclerosing panencephalitis, and death (Orenstein et al 2004).
- Mumps can lead to viral meningitis, temporary or rarely permanent hearing loss, oophoritis, orchitis and possibly sterility in men, acute pancreatitis, and encephalitis (Dayan et al 2008).
- Rubella can cause a range of birth defects, which is called congenital rubella syndrome, in unborn babies.
- Chickenpox encephalitis, toxic shock, and necrotising fasciitis post-chickenpox are potentially life-threatening complications (Sultan et al 2012). (May cause foetal varicella syndrome in unborn babies, and the earlier in pregnancy the greater the risk.)

Table 16.2 Routine immunisation schedule

Age due	Diseases protected against	Vaccine given
2 months	Diphtheria, tetanus, pertussis, polio, Haemophilus influenza type b (Hib) Pneumococcal (13 serotypes) Meningococcal group B Rotavirus gastroenteritis	DTaP/IPV Hib Pneumococcal conjugate vaccine PCV Men B Rotavirus
3 months	Diphtheria, tetanus, pertussis, polio, Hib Meningococcal group C Rotavirus	DTaP/IPV/Hib MenC Rotavirus
4 months	Diphtheria, tetanus, pertussis, polio, Hib MenB Pneumococcal (13 serotypes)	DTaP/IPV/Hib MenB PCV
1 year	Hib and MenC Pneumococcal (13 serotypes) Measles, mumps, and rubella (MMR) MenB	Hib/MenC booster PCV booster MMR MenB booster
2–6 years (including children in year 1 and year 2)	Influenza (each year from September)	Live influenza vaccine
3 years and 4 months	Diphtheria, tetanus, pertussis, polio Measles, mumps, and rubella	DTaP/IPV MMR (check first dose given)
Girls aged 12–13 years	Cervical cancer caused by human papilloma virus (HPV) types 16 and 18 (and genital warts caused by types 6 and 11)	HPV (2 doses 6–12 months apart)
14 years (school year 9)	Tetanus, diphtheria, polio Meningococcal groups A, C, W, and Y disease	Td/IPV (check MMR status) MenACWY

Public Health England, 2016. The complete routine immunisation schedule from Spring 2016. <www.gov.uk/collections/immunisation> (accessed 17.09.2016).

Table 16.3 General features of common childhood illnesses

Disease	Type	Spread	Signs/symptoms	Incubation	Contagious
Measles	Viral	Coughs/sneezes	Fever, coryza, cough, watery, sore red eyes, may have grey spots in mouth, small red spots all over body that may join into larger patches after a few days	10–12 days after exposure	4 days before rash to 4 days after *Highly contagious*
Mumps	Viral	Direct contact with saliva or discharge from nose/throat	Fever, swelling, and tenderness of salivary glands (sometimes orchiditis in boys)	Usually 16–18 days after exposure	3 days before and up to 4 days after onset of symptoms
Rubella	Rubella virus	Close contact with coughs/sneezes	Usually a mild disease, slight fever, red/pink spots for 2–3 days	12–23 days after exposure	1 week before rash to 1 week after rash, but most contagious while rash visible
Chickenpox	Varicella zoster	Through air by coughs/ sneezes or by direct contact with fluid from vesicles	Fever, itchy rash all over body, first raised pink bumps, forming fluid-filled vesicles which finally crust and scab. Lesions may form in throat, eyes, and mucous membrane of urethra, anus, and vagina	14–21 days after exposure	1–2 days before rash appears until all blisters have dried up (usually 4–5 days)
Pertussis	Bordetella pertussis bacterial infection	Personal contact/ coughs/sneezes	Coryza, fever, cough which becomes severe and paroxysmal and can last for 3 months (whooping noise)	7–10 days after exposure	1 week from exposure until up to 3 weeks after the severe cough starts

- Pertussis, with high or rapidly rising white cell counts, indicates more severe disease and possible death (may need to consider exchange transfusion) (Murray et al 2013).

 NB Measles, mumps, rubella, whooping cough, diphtheria, and tetanus are all notifiable diseases. There is a long list of notifiable diseases. See https://www.gov.uk/guidance/notifiable-diseases-and-causative-organisms-how-to-report.

REFERENCES

Bee, H., 1989. The Developing Child, fifth ed. Harper and Row, New York.

Center on the developing child, 2007. The impact of Early Adversity on Child Development. Retrieved from: www.developingchild.harvard.edu.

Dayan, G.H., Quinlisk, M.P., Parker, A.A., et al., 2008. Recent resurgence of mumps in the United States. N. Engl. J. Med. 358 (15), 1580–1589.

Hurley, A., Whelan, E.G., 1988. Cognitive development and children's perceptions of pain. Pediatr. Nurs. 14, 21–24.

Murray, E.L., Nieves, D., Bradley, J.S., et al., 2013. Characteristics of severe Bordatella pertussis infection among infants ≤90 days of age admitted to pediatric intensive care units – Souuthern California, September 2009–June 2011. J. Pediatric. Infect. Dis. 2 (1), 1–6. https://doi.org/10.1093/jpids/pis105.

Orenstein, W.A., Perry, R.T., Halsey, N.A., 2004. The clinical significance of measles: a review. J. Infect. Dis. 189 (1), S4–S16.

Piaget, J., Inhelder, B., 1969. The Psychology of the Child. Routledge and Kegan Paul, London.

Public Health England, 2016. The complete routine immunisation schedule from Spring 2016. www.gov.uk/collections/immunisation.

Sultan, H.Y., Boyle, A.A., Sheppard, N., 2012. Necrotising fasciitis. BMJ 345, e4274.

Infants and children may present in accident and emergency department (A&E) or a paediatric intensive care unit (PICU) with an unusual collection of signs that lead to the diagnosis of a syndrome. There are also an increasing number of children with syndromes who are surviving infancy and more likely to require PICU for a variety of reasons. The following chapter provides an alphabetical list and quick reference to the more common syndromes, but it is not exhaustive. These are 'congenital' syndromes which exist at, and before, birth due to genetic mutations, but the symptoms may only cause problems at a later stage.

Many of the patients with the congenital syndromes will require extra special care and consideration at the time of intubation for a multitude of reasons that include:

- craniofacial malformations (e.g., small chin, large tongue)
- laryngotracheo–oesophageal malformations
- cardiac conditions
- instability in atlantoaxial joint
- subglottic stenosis

Check the Airway chapter to plan a safe intubation strategy.

Web links for support groups have been given where possible. Many are voluntary groups and as such no responsibility can be taken for any information provided on these sites.

ALAGILLE SYNDROME

Alagille syndrome is a genetic disorder that can affect the liver, heart, kidney, skeleton, and other organs of the body. Some, but not all, of the genetic mutations that cause this condition have been identified. It affects boys and girls evenly, and there is a wide variation in the severity and presentation of the condition even within the same family.

The most common problem associated with Alagille syndrome is a reduced number (paucity) of bile ducts within the liver. This causes children to present within the first 6 months of life with jaundice, itching, an enlarged liver, and pale stools. In a very small number of cases this may lead to end-stage liver disease due to progressive liver cirrhosis requiring a liver transplant (Kamath et al 2010).

A heart murmur is the second most common feature of Alagille syndrome. This is usually due to a narrowing of the pulmonary arteries. Narrowing of other blood vessels, such as the head and neck vessels, increases the risk of stroke. Some children with Alagille syndrome may also have valvular heart defects and should therefore all be referred to a cardiologist.

The typical facial features of Alagille syndrome include a prominent forehead, deep-set eyes, and a small chin. Their eyes may have an opaque ring in the cornea which looks like a transparent cover on the eyeball (posterior embryotoxon) but it does not affect vision. A skeletal abnormality associated with this syndrome is butterfly vertebrae, which gives some vertebrae the shape of flying butterflies.

Support for families with children with liver disease can be found at: www.childliverdisease.org.

CHARGE ASSOCIATION

CHARGE syndrome is an autosomal dominant genetic disorder often caused by mutation or deletion in the CHD7 gene.

Diagnosis: CHARGE is an acronym of congenital defects that can occur together and it has been suggested that for a diagnosis to be made, at least four major features, or three major features and three minor features, are present (Blake et al 1998):

C   Coloboma – this is a malformation that results in a cleft in one of the structures of the eye, most commonly the iris
H   Heart defects
A   Choanal atresia
R   Retarded growth and development
G   Genital hypoplasia
E   Ear anomalies/deafness

Children with CHARGE association may also have renal anomalies, tracheo-oesophageal fistula, and orofacial problems.

Treatment: A multitude of specialities may be involved in the care of infants and children with CHARGE association and these include ear, nose, and throat (ENT), cardiology, ophthalmology, gastroenterology, audiology, neurology, speech therapy, physiotherapy, orthopaedics, and occupational therapy.

CHARGE Family Support Group is found at: www.chargesyndrome.org.uk.

CRI DU CHAT SYNDROME

Cri du chat syndrome occurs as a result of partial deletion of the short arm of chromosome 5. A characteristic of this syndrome is a high-pitched cry, which resembles a mewling kitten, due to abnormal development of the larynx.

Diagnosis: Often diagnosis is made in hospital at birth with this characteristic cry, then a blood test will be taken for chromosomal analysis.

Appearance: Craniofacial abnormalities, microcephaly, and a moon-shaped face with hypertelorism (increased interpupillary distance).

These children have severe learning difficulties, feeding problems, behavioural problems, hypotonia, communication difficulties, and an increased incidence of congenital heart defects (septal defects, tetralogy of Fallot [TOF], and a patent ductus arteriosus [PDA]).

Treatment: There is no specific treatment available, but supportive therapy is given as required.

Cri du Chat Syndrome Support Group is found at: www.criduchat. org.uk.

DIGEORGE SYNDROME

DiGeorge syndrome is usually a sporadic malformation but most patients show a microdeletion of chromosome 22.

Diagnosis: A blood test called fluorescence in situ hybridisation (FISH) can be used for diagnosis.

The thymus and parathyroid glands are absent because of defective development of the third and fourth embryonic pharyngeal pouches. This is characterised by neonatal tetany, hypocalcaemia, learning disability, seizures, and immune disorders leading to frequent viral infections. These may be recalled by the mnemonic CATCH22 (Burn 1999):

Cardiac anomalies – TOF, interrupted aortic arch (IAA), ventricular septal defect (VSD), or PDA most common

Abnormal facies – long narrow face, wide-set eyes, broad nasal bridge, small mouth, small low-set ears that are folded over at the top, cleft lip and palate

Thymic aplasia

Cleft palate

Hypocalcaemia/hypoparathyroidism

Appearance: Dysmorphic features. NB: Laryngotracheoesophageal anomalies

Treatment: Corrective surgery for heart conditions, cleft lip and palate, calcium supplementation, monitoring of autoimmune conditions and prophylaxis, physiotherapy, speech and language therapy.

DiGeorge Syndrome Support Group is found at: www.22crew.org.

DOWN SYNDROME (TRISOMY 21)

An extra chromosome 21 characterises the best recognised chromosome disorder.

Diagnosis: There are often clear physical signs of typical characteristics found in Down syndrome but a blood test will confirm the diagnosis.

Appearance: Small, slanting eyes, low-set ears, prominent epicanthic (neck) folds, small mouth causing frequent tongue protrusion, and commonly there is a single transverse palmar crease.

These children will have learning difficulties with a reduced IQ. Down syndrome is often associated with a congenital heart lesion (40%), the most common being atrioventricular septal defect (AVSD) and VSD, mitral valve problems, TOF and PDA, hypotonia, umbilical hernia, higher than normal incidence of duodenal atresia, thyroid problems, Hirschsprung disease, and leukaemia.

NB: If intubation required, take extra care due to macroglossia; consider the need for smaller endotracheal tube (ETT) due to possible subglottic stenosis; 20% of children may have ligamentous laxity of the atlantoaxial joint so avoid neck flexion and extension during laryngoscopy, care of child with either cyanotic or acyanotic cardiac defect, increased risk of reflux (Meitzner & Skurnowicz 2005).

Treatment: Some babies and children with Down syndrome will require corrective surgery for congenital heart defects; all will need early input from speech and language therapists, physiotherapists, and occupational therapists.

Down Syndrome Association is found at: www.downs-syndrome. org.uk.

EDWARDS SYNDROME (TRISOMY 18)

Edwards syndrome is a random chromosomal disorder known as trisomy 18, caused by an additional copy of chromosome 18 in some or all the cells in the body. Approximately 95% of babies diagnosed with Edwards syndrome have the extra chromosome 18 in every cell in their body and most of these babies will sadly die before infancy. The other 5% of babies with Edwards syndrome have a less severe form called mosaic trisomy 18 where only some of the cells are affected. These babies could be mildly affected or severely disabled; many may survive for a year and rarely a child could survive into adulthood.

Appearance: The baby will have protruding eyes, low-set malformed ears, a receding chin, flexion deformities of the hands with the index finger overlapping the third digit, and characteristic feet with a prominent heel and convex sole ('rocker-bottom feet'). Infants usually have major cardiac anomalies.

Treatment: Depending on the wishes of the parents, treatment is largely supportive. Hospice care may be offered to the most severely affected babies.

Support Organisation for Trisomy 13 and 18 is found at: www.soft. org.uk.

HUNTER SYNDROME – MUCOPOLYSACCHARIDOSIS TYPE 2

Hunter syndrome is a lysosomal storage disease caused by a deficient or absent enzyme called iduronate-2-sulfatase. It has X-linked recessive inheritance and mostly affects males. The symptoms in Hunter syndrome are generally milder than those in Hurler syndrome.

Signs and symptoms: Changes in facial features, facial abnormalities (broad nose, protruding tongue), delayed development, clawlike hands, respiratory difficulties including sleep apnoea, cardiovascular problems (hypertension, thickening of heart valves), aggressive behaviour, joint stiffness, angular kyphosis, nodular skin lesions but generally no clouding of the corneas.

These children may also have retinitis pigmentosa, optic atrophy, progressive deafness, and pulmonary hypertension. Large quantities of dermatan or heparin sulphate may be present in the urine.

Diagnosis: Blood, urine, and tissue samples are sent to identify excess glycosaminoglycans, and genetic testing can provide a diagnosis.

Treatment: There is no cure for Hunter syndrome and treatment is focused on managing symptoms. Emerging treatments include:

- Enzyme therapy
- Bone marrow transplantation
- Gene therapy

The Society for Mucopolysaccharide Diseases Support is found at: www.mpssociety.co.uk.

HURLER SYNDROME – MUCOPOLYSACCHARIDOSIS TYPE 1

Hurler syndrome is also a lysosomal storage disease and is the most severe of the mucopolysaccharidosis. A deficiency of the enzyme alpha-L–iduronidase results in a buildup of heparin sulphate and dermatan sulphate, which damage organs and can lead to early death. It is an autosomal recessive disorder resulting from a deficiency of the enzyme α-L-iduronidase.

Signs and symptoms: Babies appear normal at birth, but around 9 months of age they begin to develop the following symptoms:

- Coarse facial features, short neck, large head, and short stature
- Developmental delay evident by the end of the first year, progressive intellectual disability, and loss of physical skills
- Hearing loss, limited language
- Enlarged heart, liver, spleen
- Respiratory difficulties: obstructive airways, recurring infections that can lead to early death before the age of 10 years

Diagnosis: Clinical examination, enzyme assays, and urine tests. Large quantities of dermatan sulphate are present in the urine.

Treatment: There is no cure but the following therapies are being used:

- Enzyme replacement therapy (ERT)
- Bone marrow transplantation
- Gene therapy

The Society for Mucopolysaccharide Diseases Support is found at: www.mpssociety.co.uk.

KLINEFELTER SYNDROME

Klinefelter syndrome affects males only and means that their chromosome pattern is Klinefelter syndrome (XXY) and they are infertile. It is often undiagnosed until adolescence.

Appearance: Tall in stature with unusually long legs, hypogonadism, and gynecomastia. There is increased incidence of learning difficulties.

Treatment: May include testosterone replacement therapy, breast tissue removal, speech therapy, physiotherapy, educational support, psychologic support, and fertility treatment.

Klinefelter Association is found at: www.ksa-uk.net.

MORQUIO SYNDROME – MUCOPOLYSACCHARIDOSIS TYPE 4

This is a rare form of mucopolysaccharidosis that again is an autosomal recessive trait. A deficiency of either galactosamine-6-sulfatase or beta-galactosidase enzymes leads to a buildup of keratin sulphate, which causes damage to organs.

Signs and symptoms: Short stature, short neck, large head, prominent sternum, scoliosis, waddling gait, protruding mandible with widely spaced teeth, and short nose.

These children have normal intelligence but may have mild deafness, clouding of the cornea, and perhaps aortic valve disease.

Diagnosis: Genetic testing, urine tests for presence of excess mucopolysaccharides, x-rays of long bones, ribs and spine.

Treatment: There is no cure for Morquio syndrome and, at present, enzyme therapy is not yet available. Treatment is focused on relieving symptoms as they occur.

The Society for Mucopolysaccharide Diseases Support is found at: www.mpssociety.co.uk.

NOONAN SYNDROME

Noonan syndrome is an autosomal dominant trait that affects both sexes, but is sometimes known as male Turner syndrome.

Diagnosis: In most cases, genetic blood tests can confirm various mutations that identify Noonan syndrome, but sometimes a negative blood test cannot rule out this syndrome where other signs and symptoms indicative of it exist.

Appearance: Downward slanting eyes, low-set ears, webbed neck, and short stature.

Learning difficulties and congenital heart defects (most commonly hypertrophic cardiomyopathy or pulmonary stenosis) are often present.

Treatment: Cardiology input and drug therapy for impaired cardiac function (may require surgery); monitoring of growth and vision, with treatment if required; physiotherapy; speech and language therapy; possible need for lymphatic problems; testosterone replacement therapy.

Noonan Syndrome Association is found at: www.noonansyndrome.org.uk.

PATAU SYNDROME (TRISOMY 13)

Patau syndrome is a trisomy syndrome caused by the presence of an extra chromosome 13 in all cells in 70–90% of babies born with it. This is a devastating syndrome where the median survival is days and the babies are born with a range of clinical features including failure of the forebrain to develop into two hemispheres, micro-ophthalmia, cleft lip and palate, disrupted development of the midface, proboscis nose, polydactyly, rocker-bottom feet, cardiac malformation (commonly VSD, PDA, atrial septal defect [ASD], dextrocardia), severe growth and intellectual disability, kidney malformation, and low birthweight. In some babies, only some cells have the extra chromosome 13 (mosaicism) and these babies may have a longer-term survival.

Diagnosis: May be made antenatally due to abnormalities identified on the 20-week scan, or postnatally due to characteristic clinical features; however, genetic testing is required. Patau syndrome is associated with a high rate of spontaneous loss during pregnancy.

Treatment: There is no cure for babies with Patau syndrome and care of these babies is focused on comfort care and feeding.

Patau support from Support Organisation for Trisomy 13 and Trisomy 18 (SOFT UK) is found at: www.soft.org.uk.

PIERRE ROBIN SYNDROME

Pierre Robin syndrome may be caused by genetic anomalies in chromosomes 2, 11, or 17 (Jakobsen et al 2006). In this syndrome there is underdevelopment of the lower jaw, micrognathia, and glossoptosis (downward displacement of the tongue), often associated with cleft palate and absent gag reflex. Breathing and feeding difficulties may pose problems for some babies born with this condition, so specialist help should be provided. Infants should be nursed on their sides or prone as the tongue is at risk of occluding the airway.

Diagnosis: It is usually diagnosed clinically just after birth when the baby develops respiratory difficulties. Genetic testing will then follow.

Treatment: Parents should have access to the Cleft Lip and Palate Team, specialist health visitor, speech and language therapy, and a feeding clinic if required.

There is no support group for Pierre Robin syndrome in the United Kingdom yet, but The Cleft Lip and Palate Association has an area of its website dedicated to this condition: https://www.clapa.com/what-is-cleft-lip-palate/related-conditions-and-syndromes/pierre-robin-sequence/.

POMPE SYNDROME OR GLYCOGEN STORAGE DISEASE TYPE 11

This is an autosomal recessive metabolic disorder caused by mutations in the glucosidase alpha acid (GAA) gene located on chromosome 17. The GAA gene stores information for producing the enzyme acid alpha-glucosidase, which is active in lysosomes and normally breaks down glycogen into the simpler sugar, glucose. Therefore, mutations in this gene reduce the activity of the acid alpha glucosidase, and prevent the enzyme breaking down glycogen effectively. This can lead to a buildup of glycogen to toxic levels; can damage muscles, organs, and tissues throughout the body; and impair their ability to function normally.

Signs and symptoms:

   Classic Infantile-onset Pompe – begins within a few months of birth. Infants may present with:

- Myopathy – legs in froglike position due to weak muscles
- Hypotonia – overall floppy baby

- Heart problems – enlarged heart from excess glycogen building up in heart muscle, rhythm changes due to weak heart muscle with inadequate function, heart failure
- Failure to thrive – difficulty feeding
- Breathing problems – difficulty breathing, tendency to respiratory infections
- Hepatomegaly

If no treatment is given, then death as a result of heart failure is likely to occur before the infant is 1 year old.

Nonclassic Infantile-onset Pompe – usually appears before the first birthday. It is characterised by:

- Progressive muscle weakness
- Delayed motor skills
- Cardiomegaly
- Serious breathing problems

In Pompe disease, the pelvic muscles are more severely affected than the muscles of the shoulder girdle. Facial muscles may also be affected with dysphagia or ptosis.

Late-onset Pompe Disease – may become apparent at any time from later childhood into adulthood. Usually symptoms are milder than in early-onset Pompe as these patients generally have more acid–alpha glucosidase in muscle cells than the severely affected infants with classic infantile Pompe.

- Slowly progressive muscle weakness in legs and trunk, leading to breathing problems and respiratory failure.

Diagnosis: Diagnosis of classic-onset Pompe is usually made easily due to the severity of the symptoms, but late-onset Pompe may take a decade due to the gradual onset of symptoms. The American Association of Neuromuscular and Electro Diagnostic Medicine (2009) has developed an algorithm to aid the diagnosis of Pompe disease.

Treatment: Although there is no cure for Pompe disease, the introduction of ERT may prolong survival and improve respiratory function (Kishnani et al 2007). This is sometimes combined with immune modulation. Diet therapy may be used in some cases; high protein diets may sometimes be used in noninfantile Pompe. In some patients, a liver transplant may correct electrolyte abnormality.

The Association for Glycogen Storage Disease (UK) for information and support is found at: www.agsd.org.uk.

PRADER–WILLI SYNDROME

In approximately 50% of patients with Prader–Willli syndrome there is a small deletion in the long arm on chromosome 15 (Connor & Ferguson-Smith 1987).

Diagnosis: A clinical suspicion of Prader–Willi syndrome may be identified in a newborn if hypotonic, and unable to suck. Genetic testing can confirm the diagnosis.

Appearance: Round face with a prominent forehead and a pronounced nasal bridge, short stature, small hands and feet, obesity, and hypogonadism.

These children are initially hypotonic and have delayed motor development, feeding difficulties, and developmental delays. They have rapid weight gain aged 1–6 years, excessive overeating, small genitalia, scoliosis, sleep disturbances, a high pain threshold, and an inability to vomit.

Treatment: There is no cure for Prader–Willi syndrome and all therapies depend on individual's symptoms. Growth hormone therapy has been shown to increase height, lean body mass, to improve movement, and to decrease fat, and is usually given from infancy to adulthood (Carrel et al 2002). Other therapies include feeding and diet advice, physiotherapy, orthopaedic, ophthalmic, and endocrine consultation, and early intervention from programs for intellectual disability.

The Prader–Willi Syndrome Association is found at: www.pwsa. co.uk.

RETT SYNDROME

Rett syndrome is a rare, progressive neurologic disorder usually caused by a mutation in the MECP2 gene, which is located on the X chromosome. This gene contains instructions to make a particular protein MeCP2 that is essential for brain development. Nerve cells in the brain do not develop properly and this can cause severe physical and intellectual disability. It affects approximately 1:10 000 females (Leonard et al 1997) but is only rarely seen in males (in Klinefelter syndrome where there is an extra X chromosome XXY) (Leonard et al 2001). It is thought to be a sporadic genetic mutation, so it occurs without a family history of the disease.

Signs and symptoms: Four stages of Rett syndrome have been described, but symptoms will overlap between stages.

Stage 1 – Normal early development, but generally from 6 to 18 months the following changes may appear:
- Slow development
- Hypotonia
- Feeding difficulties
- Poor coordination of trunk and limbs
- Abnormal hand movements (e.g., repeated wringing)
- Lack of interest in toys

Stage 2 – This stage usually begins between the ages of 1 and 4 years and may last weeks or months. It is known as the regressive stage where the child will start to develop severe problems with communication, coordination, language, learning, and other brain functions. Other signs include:
- Loss of purposeful hand movement
- Social withdrawal and avoidance of eye contact
- Unsteady gait when walking
- Altered respiratory pattern

- Periods of irritability and distress including screaming
- Sleeping problems
- Difficulty with eating, chewing, and swallowing
- Slowing of head growth

Stage 3 – This usually begins between 2 and 10 years and may last for years; it is considered a plateau stage where regression has ended. Signs include:

- Hypotonia of limbs with associated difficulty in moving around
- Poor weight gain
- Teeth grinding and abnormal tongue movements
- Persistent repetitive hand movements
- Some children may develop seizures
- Some may develop cardiac arrhythmias

Also there may be some improvement during this stage such as:

- Increased alertness and interest in surroundings, people, and communication
- Improvement in behaviour, less crying and irritability
- Improvement in walking ability

It is thought that most girls remain in this stage for most of their life. Stage 4 – This can last for decades and the main symptoms are:

- Scoliosis
- Spasticity – especially in the legs
- Loss of ability to walk

Diagnosis: This is usually made on the presenting symptoms, but a blood test looking for the genetic mutation will be taken. However, the genetic mutation is not found in every child with Rett syndrome. As previously discussed, Rett syndrome is not usually familial as the vast majority of cases occur randomly, but the risk of having a second child with Rett syndrome is estimated at 1%, so genetic counselling is available to parents planning another pregnancy.

Treatment: There is no cure for Rett syndrome and whilst symptoms can be difficult to manage, many health professionals are available to help manage symptoms. Some of the following therapies may be useful:

- Physiotherapy
- Assistance with diet and feeding (often a feeding tube is required and a high calorie diet)
- Occupational therapy
- Communication tools, such as picture board, eye gaze technology
- Splints and braces for hands, back brace, possible spinal surgery for scoliosis
- Antiepileptic medication
- Beta-blockers for arrhythmias

Rett Syndrome Support is found at: www.rettuk.org.uk.

SANFILIPPO SYNDROME – MUCOPOLYSACCHARIDOSIS TYPE 3

Sanfilippo syndrome has autosomal recessive inheritance. There is a deficiency of either heparin sulphate sulphamidase or N-acetyl-α-D-glucosaminidase.

Diagnosis: Symptoms may appear after the first year of life, and there is a decline in learning between the ages of 2 and 6. Urine tests will show large amounts of heparin sulphate.

These children have severe progressive learning difficulties with a low IQ and neurologic symptoms. They may have coarse facial features with thick eyebrows that join together but have no corneal clouding and no cardiac defects.

Treatment: There is no cure and no specific treatments – only those supportive of symptoms.

The Society for Mucopolysaccharide Diseases Support is found at: www.mpssociety.co.uk.

STURGE–WEBER SYNDROME

Sturge–Weber syndrome (SWS) is a congenital syndrome that affects the brain, skin, and eyes.

Diagnosis: A haemangioma on the forehead or scalp is an indication of possible SWS so magnetic resonance imaging with contrast can confirm the diagnosis.

Appearance: Facial haemangioma (port-wine stain) may occur on both sides of head

Intracranial haemangioma is associated with facial haemangioma, epilepsy, learning difficulties, hemiplegia, and glaucoma may also occur.

Treatment: Can include laser treatment for the port-wine stain, medication to control epilepsy, regular monitoring for glaucoma, care by neurologists and physiotherapists.

Sturge Weber UK Support Group is found at: www.sturgeweber.org.uk.

TREACHER COLLINS SYNDROME (MANDIBULOFACIAL DYSOSTOSIS)

Treacher Collins syndrome is an autosomal dominant trait.

Diagnosis: Characteristic features of this condition make it recognisable at birth. Genetic testing will be carried out as well as a craniofacial computed tomography scan.

Appearance: Characteristic facial appearance – sloping downwards eyes, flat cheeks, hypoplastic mandible, receding chin, large mouth, high palate (sometimes cleft), low-set ears and deficient cartilage, sometimes with no auditory meatus.

These children may have difficulty in swallowing and feeding, and have impaired vision due to underdeveloped lateral and extraocular muscles, and conductive hearing loss.

Treatment: The most severe problems may be airway compromise and feeding difficulty. Tracheostomy may be performed and nasogastric or gastrostomy feeding may be required. Hearing aids may be fitted to promote communication and bonding.

Treacher Collins Family Support Group is found at: www.treachercollins.net.

TURNER SYNDROME

Turner syndrome (X0) affects females only. They have only 45 chromosomes and have a chromosome pattern of X0.

Diagnosis: May be suspected due to clinical signs (e.g., webbed neck, lymphedema of hands and feet, widely spaced nipples). A blood test can confirm the diagnosis. Some children may not be diagnosed until teenage years when puberty does not occur due to nonfunctioning ovaries.

Appearance: Short stature, micrognathia (small jaw), webbing of the neck, lymphoedema, widely spaced nipples, failure to develop breasts.

Normal lifespan and intelligence but increased incidence of congenital heart defects, particularly coarctation of the aorta and atrial septal defect. Most females with Turner syndrome are infertile.

Treatment: Care under a paediatric endocrinologist; growth hormone may be given to promote growth, oestrogen may be given at around 12 years of age to promote breast development, and ENT may be involved as some girls experience hearing loss due to repeated ear infections.

Turner Syndrome Support Society is found at: www.tss.org.uk.

VACTERL ASSOCIATION

This is an acronym for a combination of birth defects:

V   Vertebral defects
A   Anal atresia
C   Cardiac defects (ASD, PFO, TOF, VSD)
TE   Tracheo-oEsophageal fistula
R   Renal defects
L   limb defects in up to 70% of babies with VACTERL (absent or displaced thumbs, digits missing, syndactyly, radial aplasia)

Diagnosis: This is a diagnosis of exclusion and the cause of which remains unknown. These children have normal intelligence, but will have at least three or more of the above birth defects.

Treatment: Focuses on specific problems related to the individual children. Surgical treatment is often required in the first few days of life to correct anal atresia, tracheo-oesophageal fistula, some congenital heart defects, or renal obstruction. A multidisciplinary team approach of different specialties is required.

VACTERL Association Support Group is found at: www.vacterl-association.org.uk.

REFERENCES

American Association of Neuromuscular and Electrodiagnosis Medicine, 2009. Diagnostic criteria for late onset (childhood and adult) Pompe disease. Muscle Nerve 40, 149–160.

Blake, K.D., Davenport, S.L., Hall, B.D., et al., 1998. CHARGE Association: an update and review for the primary paediatrician. Clin. Pediatr. (Phila) 37 (3), 159–173.

Burn, J., 1999. Closing time for CATCH22. J. Med. Genet. 36 (10), 737–738.

Carrel, A.L., Myers, S.E., Whitman, B.Y., et al., 2002. Benefits of long-term GH therapy in Prader-Willi syndrome: a 4-year study. J. Clin. Edocrinol. Metab. 87, 1581–1585.

Connor, J.M., Ferguson-Smith, M.A., 1987. Essential Medical Genetics, second ed. Blackwell, Oxford.

Jakobsen, L.P., Knudsen, M.A., Lespinasse, J., et al., 2006. The genetic basis of the Pierre Robin Sequence. Cleft. Palate Craniofac. J. 43 (2), 155–159.

Kamath, B.M., Loomes, K.M., Piccoli, D.A., 2010. Medical management of Alagille syndrome. J. Pediatr. Gastroenterol. Nutr. 50 (6), 580–586.

Kishnani, P.S., Corzo, D., Nicolino, M., et al., 2007. Recombinant human acid alpha-glucosidase: major clinical benefits in infantile-onset Pompe disease. Neurology 68, 99–109.

Leonard, H., Bower, C., English, D., 1997. The prevalence and incidence of Rett syndrome in Australia. Eur. Child Adolesc. Psychiatry 6 (Suppl. 1), 8–10.

Leonard, H., Silberstein, J., Falk, R., et al., 2001. Occurrence of Rett syndrome in boys. J. Child Neurol. 16, 333–338.

Meitzner, M.C., Skurnowicz, J.A., 2005. Anaesthetic considerations for patients with Down syndrome. AANA J. 73 (2), 103–107.

ABBREVIATIONS

AAF	Amino acid formula	BIVAD	Biventricular assist device
ABC	Airway, breathing, circulation	BM	Blood glucose measurement
ABG	Arterial blood gas	BP	Blood pressure
ACE	Angiotensin converting enzyme (inhibitor)	bpm	Beats per minute
ACT	Activated clotting time	BSA	Body surface area
ADEM	Acute disseminated encephalomyelitis	BSE	Bovine spongiform encephalopathy
ADH	Antidiuretic hormone	BT	Blalock–Taussig (shunt)
A&E	Accident and Emergency	cAMP	Cyclic adenosine monophosphate
AED	Automated external defibrillator	CBF	Cerebral blood flow
AKI	Acute kidney injury	CBV	Cerebral blood volume
ALCAPA	Anomalous left coronary artery arising from the pulmonary artery	CPB	Cardiopulmonary bypass
		CEN	European Committee for Standardisation
ALP	Alkaline phosphatase	CFAM	Cerebral function analysing monitor
ALS	Artificial liver support		
ALT	Alanine transaminase	CHB	Congenital heart block
APTT	Activated prothrombin time	CHF	Congestive heart failure
ARDS	Acute respiratory distress syndrome	CK	Creatinine phosphokinase
ARF	Acute renal failure		
AS	Aortic stenosis	CMPA	Cow's milk protein allergy
ASD	Atrial septal defect		
AST	Aspartate aminotransferase	CMV	Controlled mandatory ventilation; cytomegalovirus
AV	Atrioventricular		
AVSD	Atrioventricular septal defect	CNS	Central nervous system
BAL	Bronchoalveolar lavage	CO	Cardiac output
		CO_2	Carbon dioxide
BFR	Blood flow rate	COHb	Carboxyhaemoglobin
BiPAP	Biphasic positive airways pressure	CPAP	Continuous positive airways pressure

CPB	Cardiopulmonary bypass	EEG	Electroencephalogram/ electroencephalography
CPDA	Added citrate, phosphate, dextrose and adenine	EHF	Extensively hydrolysed formula
CPP	Cerebral perfusion pressure	ELSS	Extracorporeal liver support system
CPR	Cardiopulmonary resuscitation	EMD	Electromechanical dissociation
CRO	Carbapenemase resistant organism	EMG	Electromyography
		ENT	Ear, nose and throat
CRP	C-reactive protein	EPAP	Expiratory positive airways pressure
CSF	Cerebrospinal fluid	ERT	Enzyme replacement therapy
CT	Computed tomography	ESR	Erythrocyte sedimentation rate
CVC	Central venous catheter	ET	Endotracheal
CVP	Central venous pressure	$ETCO_2$	End tidal carbon dioxide
CVVH	Continuous veno-venous haemofiltration	ETT	Endotracheal tube
		FFP	Fresh frozen plasma
CVVHD	Continuous veno-venous haemodiafiltration	FGM	Female genital mutilation
DBD	Donation after brainstem death	F_iO_2	Fractional concentration of inspired oxygen
DBS	Deep brain stimulation	FRC	Functional residual capacity
DC	Direct current	GBS	Guillain-Barre syndrome
DCD	Donation after circulatory death	GCS	Glasgow Coma Scale
DCM	Dilated cardiomyopathy	G.E.T.	Gastric emptying time
DDAVP	1-deamino 8-D arginine vasopressin	GFR	Glomerular filtration rate
DIC	Disseminated intravascular coagulation	GGT	Gamma-glutamyl transpeptidase
		GI	Gastro-intestinal
DKA	Diabetic ketoacidosis	GMC	General Medical Council
DNA	Deoxyribonucleic acid	GP	General practitioner (doctor)
DO_2	Oxygen delivery	GTN	Glyceryl trinitrate
DORV	Double outlet right ventricle	GvHD	Graft versus host disease
ECG	Electrocardiogram/ electrocardiography	G6PD	Glucose-6-phosphate dehydrogenase
ECMO	Extracorporeal membrane oxygenation	H^+	Hydrogen ion
		Hb	Haemoglobin
Edi	Electrical activity of the diaphragm	HCM	Hypertrophic cardiomyopathy

HCO₃	Carbonic acid	LMWH	Low-molecular-weight heparin
HCU	Homocystinuria		
HEV	Hepatitis E virus	LRD	Living related donor
HF	Hemi Fontan	LV	Left ventricle/ventricular
HFO	High-frequency oscillation	LVEF	Left ventricular ejection fraction
HFOV	High-frequency oscillation ventilation	MAP	Mean airways pressure; mean systemic arterial pressure
HFNC	High-flow nasal cannula (oxygen)	MARS	Molecular absorbent recirculatory system
Hib	*Haemophilus influenzae* type b	MCAD	Medium chain acyl-CoA dehydrogenase deficiency
HIV	Human immunodeficiency virus	MCH	Mean corpuscular haemoglobin
HLA	Human leucocyte antigen	MCS	Mechanical circulatory support
HLHS	Hypoplastic left heart syndrome	MCV	Mean corpuscular volume
HR	Heart rate	MDT	Multidisciplinary team
HRS	Hepatorenal syndrome	MMR	Measles, mumps and rubella
HUS	Haemolytic–uraemic syndrome	MRI	Magnetic resonance imaging
IAA	Interrupted aortic arch	MRSA	Methicillin resistant *Staphylococcus aureus*
ICP	Intracranial pressure	MSUD	Maple syrup urine disease
ICU	Intensive care unit		
IHSS	Idiopathic hypertrophic subaortic stenosis	NaHCO₃	Sodium bicarbonate
IM	Intramuscular	NAI	Non-accidental injury
INR	International normalised ratio	NAVA	Neurally adjusted ventilatory assist
IO	Intraosseus	NET	Neonatal exchange transfusion
IPAP	Inspiratory positive airways pressure		
IT	Inspired time	NG	Nasogastric
ITP	Immune thrombocytopenia purpura	NICE	National Institute for Health and Care Excellence
IUT	Intrauterine transfusion	NIRS	Near-infrared spectroscopy
IV	Intravenous	NIV	Non-invasive ventilation
IVC	Inferior vena cava	NJ	Naso-jejunal
JET	Junctional ectopic tachycardia	NMC	Nursing and Midwifery Council
LA	Left atrium/atrial	NO	Nitric oxide
LAC	Looked after child	NO₂	Nitrogen dioxide
LAP	Left atrial pressure		
LDH	Lactate dehydrogenase		

NSAID	Non-steroidal anti-inflammatory drugs	PO_2	Partial pressure of oxygen
O_2	Oxygen	PR	Per rectum
OH^-	Hydroxyl ion	PRES	Posterior reversible encephalopathy syndrome
OI	Oxygenation index		
OLT	Orthotopic liver transplantation	PS	Pulmonary stenosis
PA	Pulmonary artery	PS (V)	Pressure support (ventilation)
P_aCO_2	Partial pressure of carbon dioxide in arterial blood	PT	Prothrombin time
		PTFE	Polytetrafluorethylene (Gore-Tex®)
P_aO_2	Partial pressure of oxygen in arterial blood	PTLD	Post-transplant lymphoproliferative disorder
PAP	Pulmonary arterial pressure	PTT	Partial thromboplastin time
PAPVD	Partial anomalous pulmonary venous drainage	PTV	Patient trigger ventilation
		PVC	Polyvinyl chloride
PCO_2	Partial pressure of carbon dioxide	PVR	Pulmonary vascular resistance
PCR	Polymerase chain reaction	RA	Right atrium/atrial
PD	Peritoneal dialysis	RAP	Right atrial pressure
PDA	Patent ductus arteriosus	RBC	Red blood cells
		RDS	Respiratory distress syndrome
PCV	Packed cell volume		
PCV	Pressure controlled ventilation	RhD	Rhesus D
		ROSC	Return of spontaneous circulation
PD	Peritoneal dialysis		
PDA	Patent ductus arteriosus	RR	Respiratory rate
		RSV	Respiratory syncytial virus
PDEIII	Phosphodiesterase III		
PEA	Pulseless electrical activity	RV	Right ventricle/ventricular
PEEP	Positive end-expiratory pressure	RVOTO	Right ventricular outflow tract obstruction
PEG	Percutaneous endoscopic gastrostomy	SA	Sinoatrial
		SAGM	Added sodium chloride, adenine, glucose and mannitol
PFO	Patent foramen ovale		
PIC	Paediatric intensive care	S_aO_2	Arterial saturation of oxygen
PICC	Peripherally inserted central catheter		
		SBE	Subacute bacterial endocarditis
PICU	Paediatric intensive care unit		
		SIADH	Syndrome of inappropriate antidiuretic hormone secretion
PIP	Peak inspiratory pressure		
PKU	Phenylketonuria		
PO	Per oral		

SIMV	Synchronised intermittent mandatory ventilation		TPN	Total parenteral nutrition
SJS	Stevens–Johnson syndrome		TR-GVHD	Transfusion-related graft versus host disease
SMA	Spinal muscular atrophy		TYR	Tyrosinaemia type 1
SNOD	Specialist nurses for organ donation		UFR	Ultrafiltration rate
			UKCC	United Kingdom Central Council
STRS	South Thames Retrieval Service		UN	United Nations
SVC	Superior vena cava		USS	Ultrasound scan
SvO_2	Mixed venous oxygen saturation		UTI	Urinary tract infection
			VAD	Ventricular assist device
SVR	Systemic vascular resistance		VCV	Volume control ventilation
SVT	Supraventricular tachycardia		VF	Ventricular fibrillation
TA	Tricuspid atresia		VLCAD	Very long chain acyl-CoA dehydrogenase deficiency
TAPVD	Total anomalous pulmonary venous drainage		VOD	Veno-occlusive disease
			V/Q	Ventilation/perfusion
TBSA	Total body surface area		VS	Volume support
TEN	Toxic epidermal necrolysis		VSD	Ventricular septal defect
TGA	Transposition of the great arteries		VT	Ventricular tachycardia
TLS	Tumour lysis syndrome		WBC	White blood count
TMP	Transmembrane pressure		WHO	World Health Organization
TOF	Tetralogy of Fallot		WPW	Wolff–Parkinson–White

INDEX

Note: Page numbers followed by "f" indicate figures and "t" indicate tables "b" indicate boxes.

Diabetic ketoacidosis, 354–359, 355b
  cerebral oedema in, 359
  fluid calculation in, 357–359
  fluid management for, 356–357, 357b
  insulin for, 358–359, 358b
  management of, 356f, 358b
Diagnostic tests, 221–222
  cerebral function analysing monitor, 222
  computed tomography scan, 221–222, 221b
  electroencephalography, 221
  magnetic resonance imaging scan, 222
Dialysate, 176–177, 177b
Dialysis, peritoneal, 175–178
  dialysate composition, 176–177, 177b
  exchange volume, 176
  fill time, dwell time and drain time, 176
  heparin, 177
  potassium, 177
Diaphragmatic hernia, congenital, 80
Diastolic murmurs, 88
Diazepam
  for dystonia, 227
  for pain, 334
Dicrotic notch, 95
Diffusion, solute removal by, 176
DiGeorge syndrome, 419
  absence of thymus in, 51b
Digoxin, in therapeutic drug monitoring, 322t
Dilated cardiomyopathy, 136–137, 137b
Dinoprostone, 316
  standard preparation for, 310t
Disability, transport and, 367
  flight transfer and, 384
  guidance for, 376t–377t
Discordance, aortic valve, 89
Disseminated encephalitis, acute, 232–233
Dobutamine, 316
  pharmacological effect and receptor selectivity of, 312t
  standard preparation for, 310t

Doctor, role of, in paediatric death, 400–401
Documentation
  of fitting, 223
  for intra-hospital transfer, 380f
  during transport, 368
    of audit data, 373
    of medical summary, 372–373
    of nursing summary, 373
    of transfer details, 372–373
Donation after brainstem death (DBD), 402
  physiological optimisation of, 406–407
Donation after circulatory death (DCD), 401–402, 402t
Dopamine, 316–317
  pharmacological effect and receptor selectivity of, 312t
  standard preparation for, 310t
Dopamine resistant shock, 350b–351b
DOPE mnemonic, 18
Double switch procedure, 126, 127f
Double-outlet right ventricle, 131–133, 132f
  diagnosis of, 133
  effect of, 131–132
  management of, 133
  signs and symptoms of, 132–133
Down syndrome, 419–420
Drugs, 307–326
  chronotropic, 311, 312t
  inotropic, 311, 312t
  for intubation, 308–309, 308t–309t
  for raised intracranial pressure, 217–218, 218b
  resuscitation, 307–308, 307t
  therapeutic, monitoring, 321
  during transportation, 367, 371–372
Dysarthria, 235
Dystonia, 225–228
  aetiology of, 227
    acquired, 227
    genetic, 227
  oral medications for, 227–228
  status dystonicus or dystonic storm, 225, 228
  treatment for, 227–228

In all cases of cardiac arrest provide chest compression and ventilation until circulation restored or decision to stop resuscitation reached.

Protocol for management of ventricular fibrillation/pulseless ventricular tachycardia. *CPR*, Cardiopulmonary resuscitation; *DC*, Direct cardioversion; *IV*, intravenous; *IO*, intraosseous; *ROSC*, return of spontaneous circulation. (From Advanced Life Support Group, 2016. Advanced Paediatric Life Support. A Practical Approach to Emergencies, sixth ed. BMJ Books, Wiley and Sons, Chichester.)

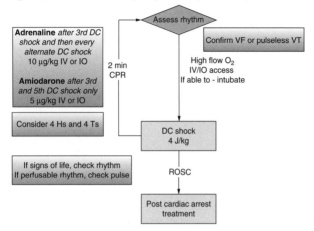

Algorithm for the management of ventricular tachycardia with pulse. *VF*, Ventricular fibrillation. (From Advanced Life Support Group, 2016. Advanced Paediatric Life Support. A Practical Approach to Emergencies, sixth ed. BMJ Books, Wiley and Sons, Chichester.)

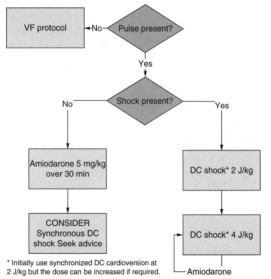